COMPLETE DIABETES GUIDE

SECOND EDITION

Advice for Managing Type 2 Diabetes

KAREN GRAHAM, RD, CDE
Registered Dietitian &
Certified Diabetes Educator

MANSUR SHOMALI, MD, CM
Endocrinologist & Diabetes Expert

Robert
ROSE

Complete Diabetes Guide, Second Edition
Previously entitled The Complete Diabetes Guide for Type 2 Diabetes
Text copyright © 2020 Karen Graham, RD, CDE
Photographs and illustrations copyright © 2020 Durand & Graham, Ltd. *(except as listed below)*
Cover and text design copyright © 2020 Robert Rose Inc.

Some of the content of this book was previously published by Paper Birch Publishing, 2011.

For complete cataloguing information, see page 415.

Disclaimer
The suggestions and information contained in this publication are based on a thorough assessment of the latest research and information. Reasonable steps have been taken to ensure the accuracy of the information presented. However, we cannot ensure the safety or efficacy of any product or service described in this publication. Individuals are advised to consult a physician or other appropriate health care professional before undertaking any diet, exercise, activity or treatment program or taking any herb or medication referred to in this publication. Professionals must use and apply their own professional judgment, experience, and training and should not rely solely on the information contained in this publication before prescribing any diet, exercise, treatment or medication. While we thank the professional expertise of the reviewers of this publication, neither they nor the authors or publisher assumes any responsibility or liability for personal or other injury, loss, or damage that may result from the suggestions or information in this publication.

The recipes in this book have been carefully tested by our kitchen and our tasters. To the best of our knowledge, they are safe and nutritious for ordinary use and users. For those people with food or other allergies, or who have special food requirements or health issues, please read the suggested contents of each recipe carefully and determine whether or not they may create a problem for you. All recipes are used at the risk of the consumer. We cannot be responsible for any hazards, loss or damage that may occur as a result of any recipe use. For those with special needs, allergies, requirements or health problems (such as kidney disease), in the event of any doubt, please contact your medical adviser prior to the use of any recipe.

This book is not intended as a substitute for professional medical care. Only your doctor can diagnose and treat a medical problem.

Use of brand names is for educational purposes only and does not imply endorsement.

Editors: Joanne Seiff and Janice Madill
Robert Rose Proof Editor: Kathleen Fraser
Indexer: Gillian Watts
Food Photographer (except as noted below): Brian Gould, Brian Gould Photography Inc.
Food Stylist: Judy Fowler
Past Design & Page Layout: Rachelle Painchaud-Nash, Fine Line Design
Production & Design Updates: Daniella Zanchetta & Joseph Gisini/PageWave Graphics Inc.
Cover Design: Kevin Cockburn/PageWave Graphics Inc.
Graphic Artwork: Sandi Storen
Nutrient Analysis: Barb Selley and Cathie Martin of Food Intelligence (1st edition); and Karen Graham calculated the net carbs and any recipe and nutrient revisions in this 2nd edition. Canadian Nutrient File and USDA FoodData Central were primary sources of nutrient information.

Additional Image Credits:
Front cover: © Getty Images. Back cover: photo of Karen Graham © David McIlvride; photo of Dr. Shomali © Juliette Bogus.
Photographs on page 43 © Casey Hein; pages 250, 403 and 404 © Rick Durand; page 299 © Grant Mitchell; and page 355 (top) © Roslyn Graham.
Photos on pages: 3, 4, 5, 6, 10, 11, 12, 17, 18, 22, 27, 28, 30, 31, 37, 45, 53, 58, 59, 60, 61, 62, 63, 64, 65, 71, 73, 75, 78, 79, 81, 82, 94 (top), 100, 103, 104, 106 (top), 108, 110, 118, 119, 121, 126, 128, 129 (top), 131, 134 (iced water), 135, 138 (bottom), 139, 145, 147, 148, 150, 177, 180, 181, 196, 201, 204 (bottom), 208, 218, 222, 224, 231, 233, 242, 243, 248, 251, 252, 256 (bottom), 257, 260, 261, 263, 264 (bottom), 266, 267, 268 (left), 269, 272 (top), 273, 281, 288, 289, 290, 295, 297, 300, 304, 308, 313, 314, 315, 316, 318, 319, 320, 321 (top), 322, 331 (middle left), 337, 339, 342 344, 348, 350, 353, 355 (bottom), 356, 359, 362, 364, 365, 366, 368, 370 (left), 371 (bottom), 372, 373 (top), 374, 375, 376, 377, 379, 380 (bottom), 381, 382, 385, 386, 387, 388, 390, 391, 392, 394, 395, 396, 397, 399, 407, 408 © Getty Images. Sidebar illustration (page 321) © Getty Images. Salt icon (pages 196–200) © Getty Images. Any person depicted in Getty Images content is a model.

The publisher gratefully acknowledges the financial support of our publishing program by the Government of Canada through the Canada Book Fund.

Canadä

Published by Robert Rose Inc.
120 Eglinton Avenue East, Suite 800, Toronto, Ontario, Canada M4P 1E2
Tel: (416) 322-6552 Fax: (416) 322-6936
www.robertrose.ca

Printed and bound in China

2 3 4 5 6 7 8 9 LEO 28 27 26 25 24 23 22 21

Special Thanks

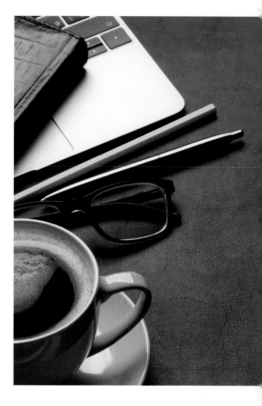

Robert Rose Inc.

Thank you to Bob Dees, president of Robert Rose, who shares our vision to bring you, the reader, practical and exceptional, easy-to-read health books. This book completes our three-book *Health & Wellness Series*. Putting together a book of this size included contributions from the full Robert Rose team. We thank their sales and publicity staff. A special thank you for the dedication and talent of PageWave Graphics, indexer Gillian Watts and editor Kathleen Fraser.

Editors

We are appreciative and grateful for the plain language editing, and expertise and guidance of Joanne Seiff and Janice Madill who edited this edition of the Guide, and have edited earlier editions over the past 12 years. For this edition, Janice provided critical help in the writing of challenging sections and page and chapter organization. Professionals who reviewed the diabetes content of this and earlier editions are listed on pages 4–5.

PageWave Graphics

Under the guidance of Joseph Gisini, designers Daniella Zanchetta and Kevin Cockburn have beautifully designed this edition. The *Complete Diabetes Guide* is created as a stand-alone book, but PageWave also accomplished a harmony in design that flows through all three books in this *Health & Wellness Series*.

Fine Line Design

A special thank-you to Rachelle Painchaud-Nash, who throughout 2019 carefully incorporated our countless text revisions, and who also assisted with design and layout for earlier editions of the book.

Photographer and food stylist

Thank you to Brian Gould, photographer, and Judy Fowler, food stylist, for your humor, skill and creativity at every photo shoot.

Graphic artist

Thank you, Sandy Storen. Your artistic talent gives the book meaningful and beautiful drawings.

Recipe creators and tasters

Karen Graham developed the recipes. She thanks those who contributed recipe ideas and did recipe testing for earlier editions.

Karen Graham includes a special thank-you

To my husband, Rick Durand, for contributing essential inspiration, support and feedback, since the book was first conceived almost 20 years ago.

Thank you to those of you who shared your diabetes stories.

Many of you have overcome challenges, prevented complications and made significant changes in your lives. Others can now learn from your experience and wisdom. This book includes your real stories. To protect contributors' privacy, we did not include your full names or your name was changed.

Most stories were illustrated with models; thank you to each of you.

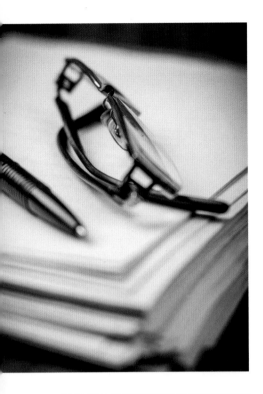

To be sure that this book contained accurate and up-to-date information, health professionals reviewed it on a volunteer basis. These professionals are experts in their particular diabetes or medical specialties. Thank you for taking time out of your busy schedules and providing such essential contributions.

Professional Volunteer Reviewers

Reviewers of this 2020 second edition:

- Nicole Carnochan, Tobacco Wise Lead, Aboriginal Tobacco Program, Cancer Care Ontario, reviewed *Step 3: Becoming a Nonsmoker.*

- Kelly Ciemny, of Thunder Bay, Ontario, provided a consumer review of *Step 7: Sexuality and Diabetes.*

- Dr. Carl Durand, BSc, OD, Optometrist, Selkirk, Manitoba, reviewed sections on eye health.

- Margaret Graham, of Kelowna, British Columbia, a retired nurse and educator, reviewed the whole book.

- Yolande Lawson, Health Promotion Consultant with Baby-Friendly Initiative Implementation for Ontario, reviewed *Step 7: Breastfeeding.*

Reviewers of 2013 and earlier editions:

For this 2020 edition, the authors updated the content from earlier reviews to meet new clinical practice guidelines. We thank past reviewers who reviewed areas of their own particular diabetes or medical specialties. This list includes their work locations at the time of their review; some have now moved, work in a new practice or have retired.

- Teresa Bodin, RN, CDE, diabetes nurse educator, The Pas, Manitoba

- Canadian Association of Wound Care, Toronto: Karen Philp, Chief Executive Officer; Kimberly Stevenson, RN, BN, IIWCC; Heather Orsted, RD, BN, ET, BSc; Marian Botros, DcH (Chiropody)

- Centre for Community Oral Health, University of Manitoba, Winnipeg: Mary Bertone, RDH; and Roxena Trembath, BSc, RDH (dental hygienists)

- Dr. Maureen Clement, MD, CCFP, Vernon, British Columbia

- Dr. J. Robin Conway, MD, Diabetes Clinic, Smith Falls, Ontario

- Diabetes Education Resource for Children team, Winnipeg: Dr. Heather Dean, MD, FRCPC; Dr. E. Sellers, MD, FRCPC; and Dr. B. Wicklow, MD, FRCPC; and Phyllis Mooney, MSW, RSW; Julie Dexter, BN, CDE; Pam Matson, BN, CDE; Nicole Aylward, RD, CDE; and Norma Van Walleghem, RD, CDE

- Dr. Stacy Elliott, MD, Director for the BC Centre for Sexual Medicine, and Clinical Professor, Departments of Psychiatry and Urologic Sciences, University of British Columbia, Vancouver

- Murray Gibson, Executive Director, Manitoba Tobacco Reduction Alliance, Winnipeg

- Roslyn Graham, BA, MSc., Winnipeg

- Casey Hein, BSDH, MBA, Interprofessional Education and Dentistry, University of Manitoba, Winnipeg, and President of Casey Hein & Associates in Evergreen, Colorado

- Wilma J. Koersen, BSc, secondary school teacher, Grand Prairie, Alberta

- Barb Komar, RN, MC, RCC (Masters in Counselling and Registered Clinical Counsellor), St. Paul's Hospital, Vancouver

- Dr. Blair Lonsberry, MS, OD, Med., FAAO, Clinic Director at Portland Vision Clinic and Associate Professor of Optometry at Pacific University College of Optometry, Portland, Oregon

- Dr. Sora Ludwig, MD, FRCPC, Section of Endocrinology and Metabolism, University of Manitoba, Winnipeg

- Pharmacist Scott McGibney, BSc (Pharm), Portage la Prairie, Manitoba

- National Aboriginal Diabetes Association, past Executive Directors, Anita Ducharme and Dina Bruyere, Winnipeg

- Pan Am Clinic, Sports Physiotherapy Centre, Winnipeg: Physiotherapists Sam Steinfeld, Tim Thiessen and Shanna Semler, all BSc BMR (PT)

- Travis Petrisor, BSc (Pharm), BSP, Penticton, British Columbia

- Dr. Jim Price, MD, ChB, CCFP, family physician, Portage la Prairie, Manitoba

- Joan Rew, RD, nutrition educator, Red River College, Winnipeg

- Riverside-San Bernardino County Diabetes Project in California: Dr. Kendall Shumway, DPM (podiatrist and Diabetes Program Director); Marcia Ruhl, RD, CDE (dietitian); Antonia Roots, ACSM, HFS (fitness specialist); and Kristopher Hamlin, BC (fitness assistant).

- Shannon Roode, RD, CDE, Collingwood General and Marine Hospital Diabetes Program

- Stephanie Staples, LPN, Certified Life Coach and Motivational Speaker, Winnipeg

- Gina Sunderland, MSc, RD, dietitian, Winnipeg, Manitoba

- Dr. Sheldon Tobe, MD, FRCPC, FACP, Associate Scientist, Sunnybrook Health Sciences Centre, Toronto

- Holliday Tyson, RM, RN, MHSc (Registered Midwife), Director, International Midwifery Pre-registration Program, Ryerson University, Toronto

- Diane Unruh, RD, CDE, diabetes educator, Carman, Manitoba

- Dr. Richard J. Wassersug, Department of Urologic Sciences, University of British Columbia, Vancouver

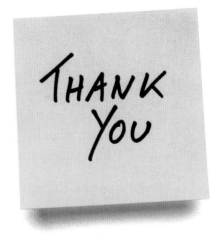

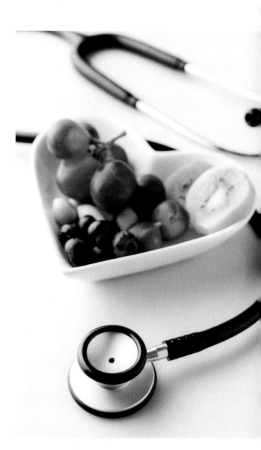

Contents

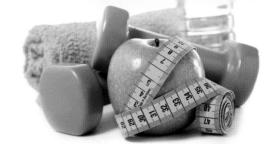

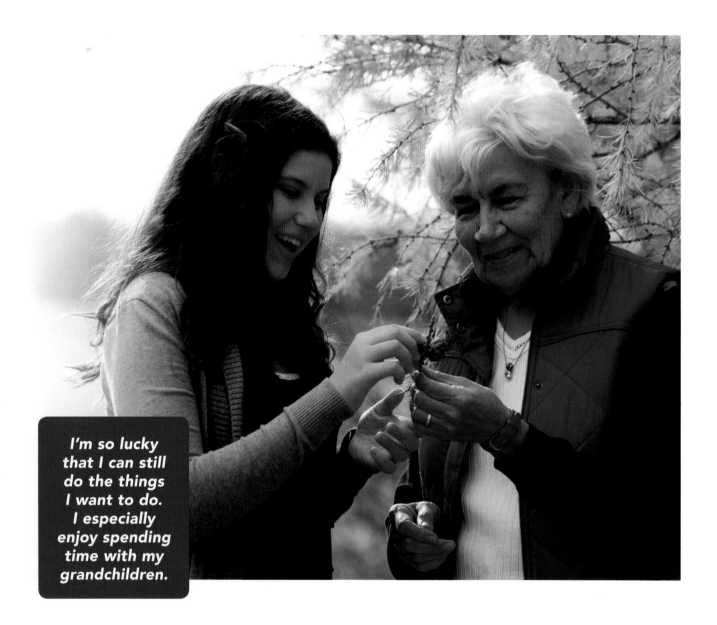

I'm so lucky that I can still do the things I want to do. I especially enjoy spending time with my grandchildren.

 LENA'S STORY: A grandma from Winnipeg shares her diabetes diagnosis story

When I was first diagnosed with diabetes I was in terrible shock. I thought my life would change for the worst. However, what I discovered is that with small changes my life actually got richer in an unexpected way. I think you do appreciate life more and in a different way when you have a crisis in your life or you have to deal with a chronic disease. I don't do things the same way as I did in the past, but I've adjusted to a new way of living. You reflect and enjoy those things and the people you have around you. I still have wonderful foods to eat; I just don't eat as much. I still watch my favorite TV shows, but I turn the TV off in between. I use this time to go for a walk and exercise, and to organize all my pills and medical appointments. I'm so lucky that I can still do the things I want to do. I especially enjoy spending time with my grandchildren.

Introduction

A journey of a thousand miles begins with a single step.

The Chinese philosopher Lao-tzu said these words more than 2,500 years ago. He understood that our difficult journeys in life start with small changes.

From your diabetes diagnosis, you are starting on a new lifetime journey with one small change at a time. As with all journeys, you might need to ask for directions. You may have to give up a favorite food. You may meet new people, learn new skills, try new foods and learn new ways of cooking. You may feel like a stranger in a foreign land at first, but your new experiences will become routine.

Over our combined 50 years as a diabetes educator and doctor, we've learned that people have many similar concerns and questions about diabetes. The next three pages outline some common questions that people have asked when first diagnosed. We've provided some straightforward answers to these questions, and we've suggested pages in this book where you can read more.

This book also includes stories from everyday people with diabetes — stories to inspire you to manage your diabetes.

The book is for you if:
- You are at risk of type 2 diabetes or have prediabetes.
- You are newly diagnosed with type 2 diabetes.
- You have had type 2 diabetes for many years.

In this book, "diabetes" refers to "type 2 diabetes" unless specified otherwise.

Contents, Index and Glossary

The Contents, on pages 6 and 7, list the main subjects covered in this book. This includes *Seven Steps to Prevent or Reduce Diabetes Complications*. Go to the Index at the back of the book for an alphabetical list of topics and recipes and where to find them. If you see a word and you aren't sure what it means, check out the Glossary, also at the back of the book.

What isn't in this book?

This book does not provide individual medical and technical information about diabetes. You need to get that directly from your doctor, pharmacist or diabetes educator. That includes:

- What medications to take
- How to take or adjust insulin
- How to operate a blood sugar machine and other changing technology
- Special needs of people with type 1 diabetes

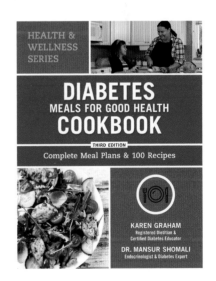

The book you're reading and the one pictured above are part of our diabetes *Health & Wellness Series*. Read more on page 416.

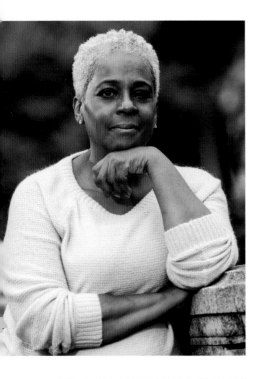

Nowadays, there are many wonderful lighter diabetic desserts that you can enjoy. Save the rich desserts for special occasions.

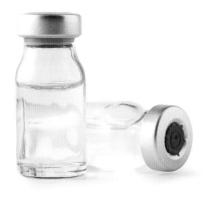

Answers to Common Diabetes Questions

Do I really have diabetes?

You may not feel any different, which makes you wonder whether you really do have diabetes. Many people do not have any symptoms, but blood tests will confirm if you have diabetes. To learn more, read *What Is Type 2 Diabetes?*, pages 16–17; *Symptoms of Type 2 Diabetes*, page 18; *Who Is at Risk for Type 2 Diabetes?*, pages 19–20; and *Lab Tests, Foot Exam and Eye Exam*, pages 301–306.

Do I have to stop eating chocolate bars and desserts?

No, you don't have to stop. You can have all your favorite foods, but in moderation. It's a good idea to limit how often you eat chocolate bars, so if you eat them daily, you'll need to start cutting back. There are many wonderful lighter diabetic desserts that you can enjoy. Save the rich dessert for special times. To learn more, read *Light Desserts and Sweeteners*, pages 100–108; and *A Plan for Special Occasions*, pages 76–77.

What can I eat?

You can mostly eat the same things you have always eaten, but eat less. If you eat a lot of processed foods high in fat, sugar and salt, you'll need to replace some of these with whole foods. Whole foods include whole grains, vegetables and fruit, unprocessed meats, eggs and dairy.

Will I go blind?

Having diabetes does not mean you will go blind. However, if you have chronically high blood sugar levels (high sugar levels over many years) you are more likely to have eye problems. To learn about keeping your eyes healthy, read *Eye Problems*, pages 38–41, 299 and 304.

Will I need to go on dialysis?

Having diabetes does not mean you will need kidney dialysis. You can protect your kidneys with good levels of blood sugar, blood pressure and cholesterol. To learn more, read *Kidney Damage*, pages 33–37.

Will I need to take insulin?

Not everyone who has diabetes needs to take insulin. If your blood sugar levels are high, insulin can be a good way to lower your blood sugar. Some people never need insulin. Some start insulin the day they are diagnosed. Others, take insulin 5, 10 or 20 years after their diagnosis. To learn more, read *Diabetes Medications*, pages 309–320; and *Insulin*, pages 319–328.

Will I lose my leg like my grandpa did?

The good news is that the vast majority of amputations in people with diabetes are preventable. Daily foot care helps prevent infections from happening in the first place. Having good blood sugar is also important to help reduce the risk of infection. With care, you can keep your feet for life. To learn more about keeping your feet healthy, read *Foot and Lower Leg Infections*, pages 29–32; and *Keep Your Feet Healthy*, pages 268–281.

Do I have to stop smoking?

This is a very good question. Please seriously think about quitting. When you have diabetes and you smoke you are more likely to get complications. This would include gum disease, a foot amputation, heart attack, kidney problems or blindness. To learn more, read *Become a Non-Smoker*, pages 247–266.

Can I eat in restaurants?

Yes. Restaurant meals tend to be higher in fat, sugar and salt, so try to order less and choose healthier meal choices. Limiting how often you eat in restaurants and switching to more homemade meals is also a positive step. To learn more, read *Eat Out Less Often*, pages 71–75.

Can I still drink alcohol?

Yes, in moderation. There are good reasons to drink less or not drink at all. You must take precautions if you take insulin or certain diabetes medications. And alcohol has calories, which can cause weight gain. To learn more, read *Alcohol*, pages 134–137; and *Low Blood Sugar*, pages 329–336.

How will diabetes affect the cooking I do for my family?

Diabetes tends to run in families, so you are all at a greater risk for diabetes. It's good if you all eat the same healthy way. If you gradually make small changes to your cooking, your family may not even notice any difference. Experiment with new recipes, new flavors (herbs and spices), and new desserts. To learn more, read *Light Desserts and Sweeteners*, pages 100–108; and *Seven-Day Meal Plan with Recipes*, pages 149–200.

Is diabetes going to make me feel sick?

When your blood sugar is high, you can feel tired and unwell. To learn more, read *Symptoms of Type 2 Diabetes*, page 18. When your blood sugar improves and you begin to exercise and eat better, you may start to feel a lot better. You'll start feeling younger.

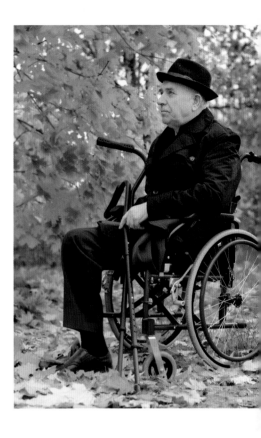

There are tips to prevent and manage diabetes in children (pages 364–376), and during pregnancy (pages 377–389).

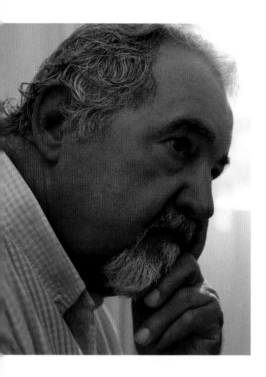

Rx DOCTOR'S ADVICE

Research shows that you are responsible for making changes to improve your health. If a doctor diagnoses your diabetes early, you can learn to manage it. You will have a better chance of living a long and healthy life.

Is diabetes going to shorten my life?

Statistics show that people with diabetes on average have a shorter life. Moderate daily exercise and weight loss will help you live a longer, healthier life. Changing your lifestyle will make a difference.

Will I have to prick my finger for blood every day?

No, not necessarily. Talk to your doctor or diabetes educator. You may do fine with little or no blood sugar checks at home and rely on regular blood tests recommended by your doctor. For others, doing daily blood sugar checks helps to manage their blood sugar, especially if they are on insulin or at risk for low blood sugar. New continuous glucose monitors don't require finger pricks. To learn more about checking your blood sugar, read *Check your Blood Sugar at Home*, pages 337–345.

How am I going to cope with one more thing?

Take one step at a time. Your doctor may diagnose your diabetes at a time when you have other stresses too. This can be difficult, but it's not impossible. Go to see a diabetes education team or your doctor as an important first step. You can tell them how you feel. They will help you work out ways to cope better. To learn more, read *Stay Upbeat*, pages 347–362.

Is this going to stop me from being active?

If you are an active person, that is great. Continue activities, sports and hobbies that you love. Walking and exercise are an essential part of diabetes management. There will be things to do to reduce your risk for injury during exercise, such as wearing supportive shoes. To learn more, read *Step 2: Be Active*, including *Exercise Precautions*, pages 239–246; and *Keep Your Feet Healthy*, pages 268–281.

Will diabetes affect my sex life?

After a number of years of diabetes, some people notice sexual changes. Today there are prevention and treatment options. To learn more, read *Sexuality and Diabetes*, pages 390–409. As you make lifestyle changes and bring your blood sugar down, you will find more energy for everything, including sex. Good health and good sex go together.

How do I get rid of diabetes?

There is no cure for type 2 diabetes. Taking medication and making lifestyle changes help many people bring their blood sugar very close to, or within, the normal range. Your risk for problems will then be low. This book will give you the tools to make gradual, small changes so you manage the diabetes and diabetes doesn't control you.

Learning About Diabetes

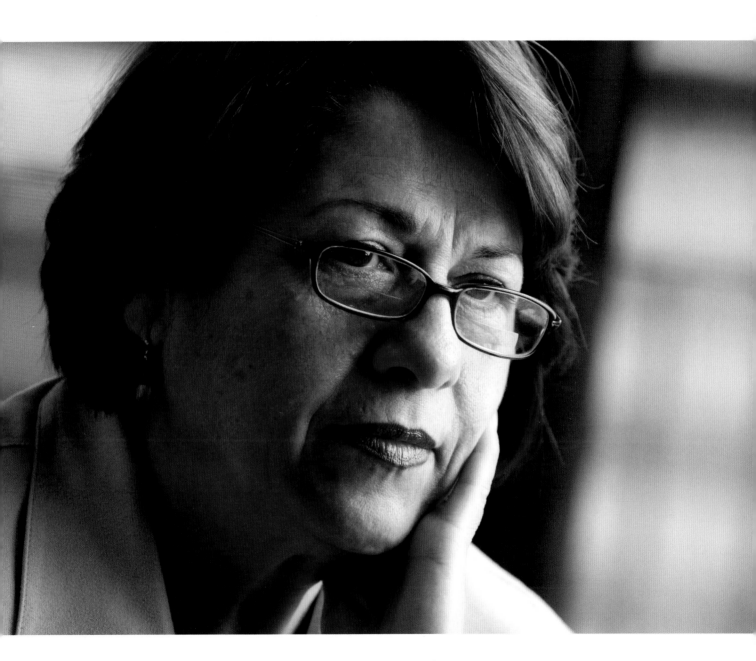

Diagnosis of Diabetes and Prediabetes
Usually, your doctor will order a fasting blood glucose (blood sugar) or an A1C test. See page 16 for information on American and Canadian blood sugar levels, and page 302 to learn about the A1C test.

Fasting blood glucose should be measured in the lab on two different occasions to make certain of the diagnosis.

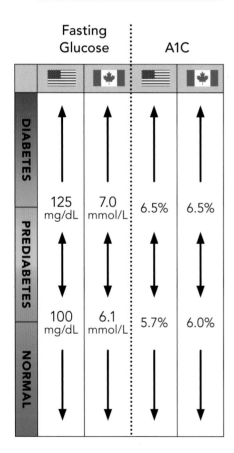

Fasting Glucose		A1C	
🇺🇸	🇨🇦	🇺🇸	🇨🇦
DIABETES			
125 mg/dL	7.0 mmol/L	6.5%	6.5%
PREDIABETES			
100 mg/dL	6.1 mmol/L	5.7%	6.0%
NORMAL			

Types of Diabetes

Diabetes means there is too much sugar in your blood.

Prediabetes

Prediabetes means your blood sugar levels are higher than normal but lower than what is diagnosed as type 2 diabetes. You may hear this condition called:

- borderline diabetes
- impaired fasting glucose, or
- impaired glucose tolerance

If your doctor discovers you have prediabetes, you have the best chance to prevent type 2 diabetes by making healthy changes to your lifestyle. Also, your doctor may recommend that you take a diabetes pill to try to reduce your chance of getting type 2 diabetes.

Type 2 diabetes

Type 2 diabetes is the most common type of diabetes.

Type 2 diabetes is on the rise at all ages

It generally develops after age 40. It now occurs in children, teenagers and young adults — this increase in the young is alarming. People of all ages are gaining too much weight and are less physically active. Only one out of 10 people with type 2 diabetes are lean or underweight when they get diabetes.

It is caused by genetics and how we live

Type 2 diabetes runs in families. If one or both of your parents, or a brother or sister has diabetes, you have a higher risk of getting diabetes. In addition to the genes we inherit, we also learn how to eat and exercise from our families. People in the same household tend to eat similar foods and to be either active or inactive. Children who learn from their parents how to eat healthy foods and to be active will have a decreased risk for diabetes, even if diabetes runs in their family.

Insulin is still made by the pancreas

In type 2 diabetes, the pancreas continues to make some insulin. Therefore, some people will need no medication and can manage their diabetes with their diet and exercise. Others will benefit from taking diabetes medication and/or insulin. Early use can often help improve blood sugar and delay diabetes complications.

Gestational Diabetes

Gestational diabetes develops during pregnancy.

There are two things that happen during pregnancy that can increase a woman's blood sugar:

1. The weight gained during pregnancy means the pancreas needs to make more insulin. The pancreas becomes overworked. It cannot make enough insulin, and blood sugar rises.

2. The hormones produced during pregnancy can result in the insulin not working as well.

After the baby is born, weight loss reduces the workload on the mother's pancreas. Then her blood sugar goes down.

To learn more, read *Type 2 Diabetes Pregnancy and Gestational Diabetes*, pages 377–384.

Type 1 Diabetes

In type 1 diabetes, the pancreas makes less insulin, and eventually makes none. Without insulin, sugar isn't removed from the blood and it builds up quickly. Type 1 diabetes often starts in children over the age of five and in teenagers. The diagnosis of type 1 diabetes is less common in children under age five or adults.

Typical symptoms of type 1 diabetes may look like a severe flu. They include:

- extreme thirst
- frequent urination
- stomach pains
- weight loss
- fruity-smelling breath

See page 18 for a list of other symptoms of diabetes.

Usually within days or several weeks, the pancreas stops making insulin and symptoms rapidly worsen. In order to survive, the person must take insulin every day.

Type 1 diabetes also runs in families. Whites have the highest risk of getting type 1 diabetes. Although the precise cause of type 1 diabetes is not known, having diabetes genes and exposure to certain viruses are risk factors. A virus could have been contracted up to two years before the diabetes onset. These viruses can cause the body's immune system to attack the once-healthy part of the pancreas that makes the insulin. Other possible triggers of the immune response include dietary and environmental factors.

Diagnosis of gestational diabetes
When you are 24 to 28 weeks pregnant, your doctor may order a glucose tolerance test. You will be asked to drink a glassful of sweet liquid, then your blood sugar is tested over one to three hours.

What's the difference between type 1 and type 2 diabetes?
People with type 1 diabetes make no insulin at all.

People with type 2 diabetes still make some of their own insulin.

Rx DOCTOR'S ADVICE

Studies show there is some protection against type 1 diabetes for those who have been breastfed. The protection against type 1 diabetes is greatest when the infant has been exclusively breastfed (no formula, and table foods delayed until four to six months). Another protection may be higher levels of vitamin D through sun exposure or diet.

What Is Type 2 Diabetes?

When you do not have diabetes...

American and Canadian blood sugar levels

- The United States uses mg/dL as the measure for blood sugar.
- Canada and many other countries use mmol/L.
- 18 mg/dL = 1 mmol/L
- To convert from mg/dL to mmol/L, divide by 18.
- To convert from mmol/L to mg/dL, multiply by 18.

Blood sugar levels before you eat

Normal blood sugar is about 70–100 mg/dL (4.0–5.6 mmol/L).

Blood sugar levels after you eat

For a person without diabetes, blood sugar will rise a few points after eating a meal, perhaps up to 150 mg/dL (8 mmol/L), but it quickly returns to normal as insulin removes the extra blood sugar to your tissues and organs.

Your blood sugar goes up because much of the digested food changes into a kind of sugar called glucose. The glucose moves into your bloodstream and is called blood glucose, or blood sugar.

Insulin quickly brings down blood sugar

Insulin is a hormone made by your pancreas. Insulin is extremely important because it enters the bloodstream after you eat and removes extra sugar. Insulin stimulates "receptors" on your body cells (especially in your muscles and liver) to take the extra sugar out of your blood.

When the extra sugar is removed from your blood and stored in your body cells and liver, it can be used later for fast energy.

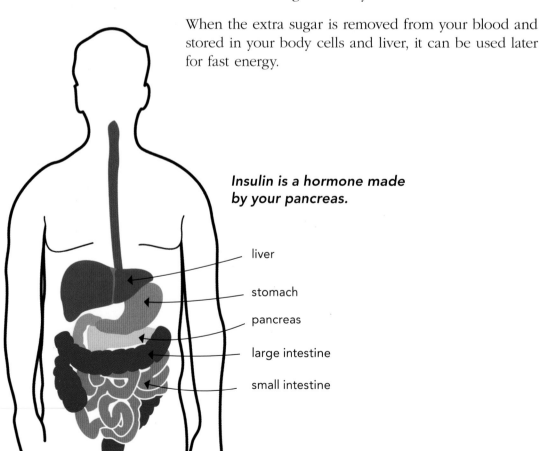

Insulin is a hormone made by your pancreas.

liver

stomach

pancreas

large intestine

small intestine

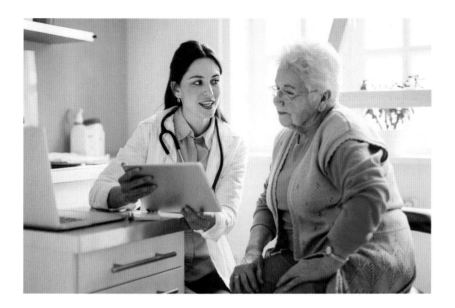

When you do have diabetes...

Blood sugar levels before you eat

Blood sugar is often high in the morning before eating, above 7 mmol/L (130 mg/dL).

Blood sugar levels after you eat

After eating a meal the blood sugar can go up quickly, for example, up to 10 mmol/L (180 mg/dL) or more. Blood sugar levels take longer to come back down.

Extra body fat causes insulin resistance

Insulin resistance means that the "receptors" on your body cells are blocked, most often because of extra body fat, and extra sugar is not being removed from your bloodstream. Your pancreas then makes more insulin to try to remove the extra sugar. Unfortunately, now the extra insulin in your bloodstream can make you feel hungry and overeat.

Extra sugar builds in your bloodstream

This can worsen over time because of changes in how your organs work:

- **Your pancreas** works overtime to make extra insulin and this organ gets worn down. Then it cannot make enough insulin. Too much sugar remains in your bloodstream. Therefore, your muscles do not have an adequate source of energy and you feel tired.

- **Your liver** releases extra stored sugar, even when you don't need it.

- **Your stomach and intestines** make less of certain hormones that would help insulin work better.

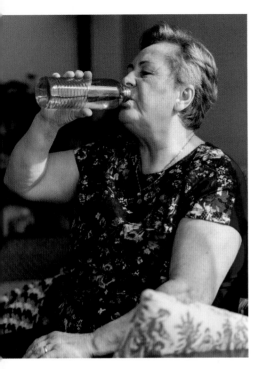

You or your doctor will recognize one or two of the symptoms of diabetes, such as being very thirsty. Blood tests will confirm the diagnosis.

Symptoms of Type 2 Diabetes

Symptoms are what you feel. Some people go to their doctor because they have a symptom of diabetes such as extreme thirst. However, because blood sugar can build up gradually in your bloodstream, you may have no recognizable symptoms of diabetes.

1. Symptoms of high blood sugar

- extreme thirst or hunger
- frequent urination
- unexplained weight loss
- extreme fatigue
- blurred vision
- a urinary tract infection
- a cut that is slow to heal

You or your doctor will recognize one or two of these symptoms. Blood tests will confirm the diagnosis.

2. No symptoms

Diabetes diagnosed at annual checkup at doctor's office

If you go to your doctor once a year for a complete checkup, routine blood tests include a blood sugar test. If your blood sugar test is high, your doctor will assess further for diabetes, even if you have no symptoms of diabetes.

Diabetes diagnosed after diabetes complications

If you don't go to a doctor for checkups, you may have diabetes for many years before a doctor diagnoses it. Your body adapts to high blood sugar so perhaps you were unaware of the symptoms. However, during this time your pancreas has been working too hard, making more insulin to try and remove the extra blood sugar. The extra sugar builds up in your blood vessels, nerves, eyes and kidneys. Eventually, you go to the doctor because you notice symptoms of diabetes complications:

- Nerve tingling or pain in your hands, feet or legs
- An infection or ulcer on your foot or leg
- Men may experience erectile dysfunction
- A change or loss of some vision
- Shortness of breath, swelling in your legs, or pain in your calf (the back of your lower leg) — these could mean circulation or heart problems.

In some cases, it is after a heart attack or stroke that diabetes is diagnosed.

Who Is at Risk for Type 2 Diabetes?

It's important to know who is most at risk of getting type 2 diabetes because the symptoms may not show up for many years. If you have one or more of the risks below, see your doctor once a year for a complete checkup.

- You are 40 or older. Your risk increases with age.
- You already have high blood pressure and/or high blood cholesterol.
- You are overweight, especially if you carry the extra weight around your waist or upper body.
- You don't exercise regularly.
- You are a woman who had gestational diabetes, or gave birth to a large baby that weighed 9 lbs (4 kg) or more.
- You have a parent, sister or brother with type 2 diabetes.
- You are an adult who experienced trauma in your childhood.
- You are Indigenous, Hispanic, African or Asian.

Adverse Childhood Experiences

Genetics, family history and current unhealthy lifestyles all increase the risk of getting diabetes. We now have a better understanding of how mental health stressors that start in our childhood experiences can also increase our risk of getting diabetes.

Children born into families who live with poverty, racism, unemployment, low education, homelessness and violence experience a kind of trauma known as adverse childhood experiences (ACEs). Current research explains how childhood trauma can lead to mental health issues such as addictions, depression and social anxieties in adults. Many adults learn to cope with the stresses and complications of childhood trauma in unhealthy ways. These include overeating, eating unhealthy food and living with little physical activity. These are all high-risk indicators for getting diabetes.

Resources needed to help lower the risk of diabetes

Parents, neighborhoods, schools and communities need resources and funding from government public health programs. These programs must assess for adverse childhood experiences (ACEs) and seek the best outcomes for children's physical, mental and emotional health and well-being.

This means, for example, reducing children's access to unhealthy foods and building activity back into their daily lives as ways to prevent childhood diabetes. This also means understanding childhood trauma and how it affects learning. Public health programs must include counselling and therapy for children identified with a higher risk of developing diabetes.

19

Other Risks for Type 2 Diabetes

- A major life stress, such as death of a spouse, or emotional or physical trauma
- A physical stress, such as a heart attack, stroke or infection
- Tuberculosis (TB) — a bacterial infection
- Pancreas surgery or infection of the pancreas
- Hemochromatosis — a genetic condition where excess iron damages the pancreas
- Medications that increase blood sugar or interfere with how your insulin works, for example, some blood pressure pills and steroids, such as prednisone
- Medications with a side effect of unwanted weight gain, such as drugs given for depression or schizophrenia
- Medical conditions that cause an unwanted weight gain, such as hypothyroidism

- Other conditions related to insulin resistance, such as polycystic ovary syndrome (a hormonal disorder in women), or acanthosis nigricans (darkening of the skin at the back of the neck and armpits), or irregular periods and extra body hair growth (in young women)
- Being a smoker
- If your parent(s) fed you formula rather than breast milk as a baby. Exclusive and extended breastfeeding reduces the risk of type 2 diabetes.
- If you were or are overweight as an infant, child or teenager
- If you have trouble with sleep, such as not enough sleep, sleeping too much or sleep apnea (a condition where you briefly stop breathing while sleeping)

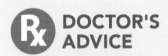

DOCTOR'S ADVICE

If you are at risk for diabetes, have an annual checkup with your doctor.

Your doctor will do routine blood tests that include a blood sugar test.

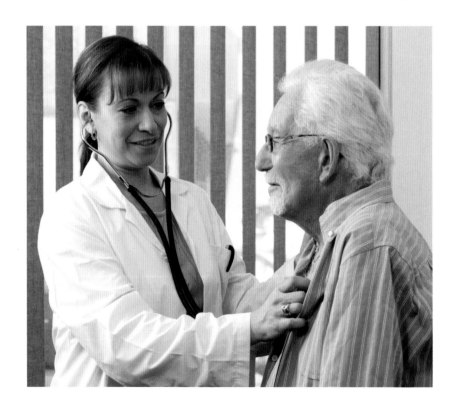

Diabetes Complications

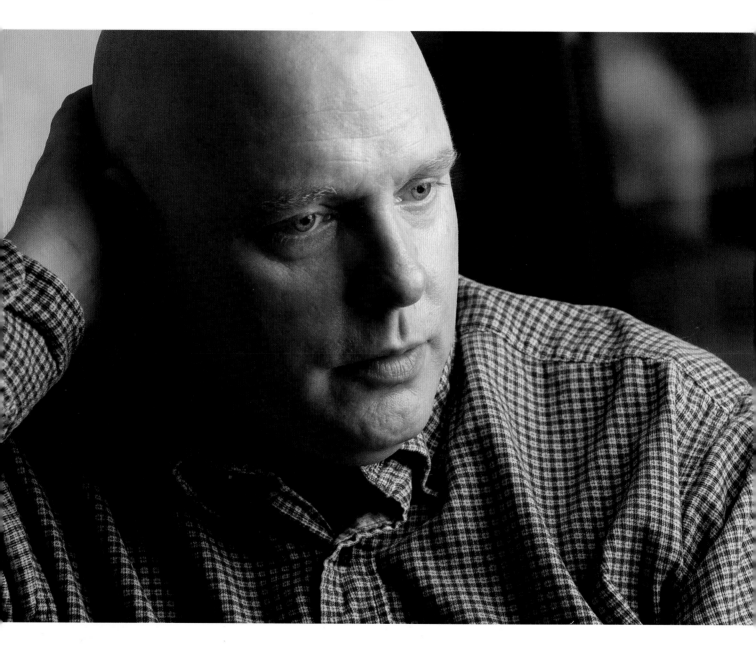

This chapter on the possible complications of diabetes will help you understand why diabetes affects all parts of your body. Taking steps early to prevent these complications is so important.

High blood sugar for many years will harm your blood vessels and nerves. Blood vessels and nerves work together and are everywhere throughout your body. This is why diabetes complications happen to almost all parts of the body.

Diabetes can lead to kidney disease and blindness. Controlling your blood sugar and blood pressure can reduce these problems. Some people say, after having a heart attack, that if they had known that diabetes was a leading cause of heart attacks, they might have made some changes earlier. Knowledge is power. If you know why problems occur, that is the first step in preventing or solving them.

As an example, foot infections and amputations are a serious, yet preventable, diabetes complication. Take time to understand how diabetes affects your feet and why it can cause foot infections. We hope you'll be motivated to check your feet every day. This small change could mean you will have your feet for life, and never have an amputation.

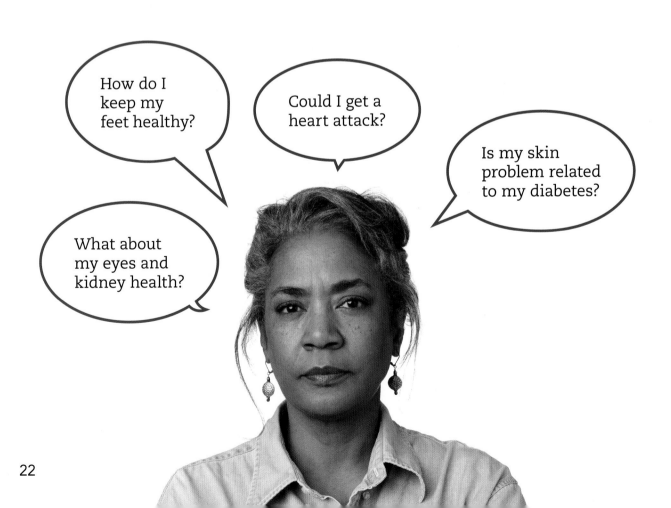

MARY'S STORY: Small changes count!

When I first found out I had diabetes, my doctor sent me to classes at a diabetes education center. In the first class the nurse talked about all the things that could go wrong when you have diabetes. She told us I could lose my vision or I could have my foot amputated. This really scared me. I have an uncle who lost his foot to diabetes. Then she said diabetes is the main cause of stroke and heart attack. I didn't know that. I definitely do not want to have a stroke.

After I got home from this class, I so felt alone that I just sat down and cried. I was upset and worried and didn't understand why this happened to me. What scared me the most was that I didn't want to lose my vision. If I lost my vision I wouldn't be able to drive. And if I couldn't drive I'd be helpless and have to depend on other people to get me around. Back then I had so many family issues to worry about, and looking after my grandkids was like a full-time job, so I didn't have time to think about me. I just kept doing what I was doing and pretended to myself that I didn't have diabetes that bad, that I was okay. After all, I could see and drive fine.

And I didn't go back to any more of those classes.

Three months later I had to go back to my doctor for an appointment, and she told me my blood sugar was still high. She asked me if I had gone to the diabetes classes, and I told her what happened and how scared I was really feeling.

She told me that it was important to know the diabetes complications that the nurse talked about. But she told me not to focus on those complications and instead to think about one change I could make right now. I decided I could start that day with a 15-minute walk, and try every day. My doctor said this small change could make a big difference in my day-to-day blood sugars, and that would reduce my chance of getting diabetes complications later. She asked me to write down my plan and reward myself with a coin in a jar every day that I walked. She gave me an appointment to see her in one month and I had to bring in my record of when I went for a walk.

This is how I began my diabetes plan to better health. I added in more changes over time, like drinking more water, especially after I had gone for a walk. My blood sugars slowly got better. I eventually went back to the diabetes education center and met with the nurse and dietitian; this time I didn't feel so upset and overwhelmed and was able to listen to their other suggestions.

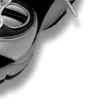

How High Blood Sugar Harms Blood Vessels

As we get older, the walls of our blood vessels thicken, harden and become less elastic. Fatty deposits, cholesterol and cells build up under the inner lining of the blood vessel wall. The medical term for these areas of thickening is plaques. We call this "hardening of the arteries" atherosclerosis.

What do years of high blood sugar cause?

- The inside lining of your blood vessels will absorb more blood sugar than normal.
- More cholesterol and triglycerides (blood fat) will build up in your blood.
- Your blood will be even thicker and more likely to clot.

1. Healthy young blood vessels

When we are young, our blood vessels are clean inside. The blood flows freely. Our blood vessels are elastic. The vessels can easily stretch to pump more blood quickly when we exercise.

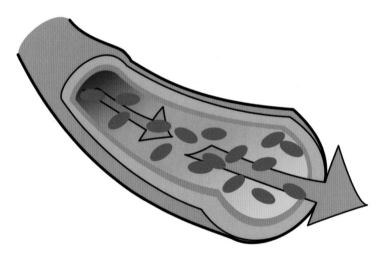

Looking inside a healthy blood vessel.

Factors that contribute to narrowing of blood vessels

- Genetics; some people are more likely to have narrow blood vessels
- Smoking
- Stress
- Eating a high-fat diet
- Lack of vegetables and fruits
- Drinking too much alcohol
- Being overweight
- Being inactive

2. Blood vessels narrow

High blood sugar narrows the blood vessel channel, which causes decreased circulation. With less blood flow, every part of your body will suffer.

The heart must overwork to pump the blood through the narrowed blood vessels. Blood pressure goes up. This high blood pressure places extra stress on the inner blood vessel walls.

The inner blood vessel wall becomes inflamed, rough and weakened from many years of high blood sugar and high blood pressure. Sometimes a plaque can rupture, and the contents will spill out. When this happens, a blood clot can form.

With decreased circulation, you will now have:
- Less oxygen, nutrients and hormones such as insulin circulating to your muscles, tissues and organs
- More waste materials building up

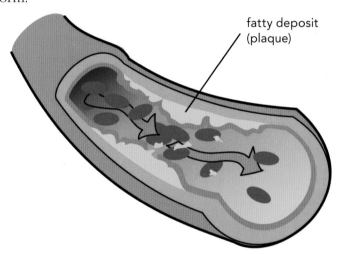

fatty deposit
(plaque)

3. A blood vessel is blocked

This is now very serious. A blood clot or blob of fat can totally block a blood vessel. If the blocked blood vessel is in your leg, you could lose blood flow to your lower leg and foot. Then an infection can't heal, which could lead to an amputation. If the blocked blood vessel goes to your heart, you could have a heart attack. If a blocked blood vessel goes to your brain, you could have a stroke.

Blood clots
Another serious problem is when a blood clot breaks away, and travels in the blood. It can block a blood vessel somewhere else. For example, it could move from a blood vessel in the leg to the lung or brain. When a blood clot moves and lodges somewhere else, it is called an embolism.

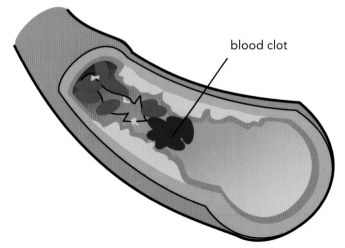

blood clot

How High Blood Sugar Harms Nerves

Healthy nerve

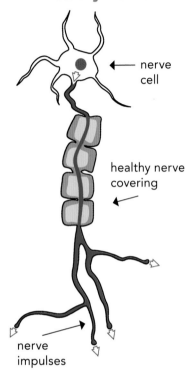

nerve
cell

healthy nerve
covering

nerve
impulses

As the years pass, high blood sugar harms nerves in two main ways:

1. Nerves get less blood flow. The nerve and blood systems are closely connected. To work properly, blood vessels need healthy nerves, and nerves need healthy blood vessels to have a supply of oxygen and nutrients. Damage to blood vessels also means damage to the nerves. As blood vessels narrow, there is nerve damage, especially in the small blood vessels of your hands, feet and eyes.

2. Nerves get direct damage. Extra blood sugar moves into your nerve cells. The sugar changes into unhealthy proteins and other types of sugars, which then damage the nerves. The most damaged part of the nerve is the outside cover. Compare this nerve cover to when the plastic around a covered cord or wire becomes frayed. The longest nerves, which travel from the spine to the hands and feet, are often affected first.

Some nerve damage effects

- Pain in your legs or feet
- Numbness or loss of feeling in your hands or feet
- A sore on your foot that you can't feel, which then becomes infected
- Vision loss
- Poor digestion, constipation or diarrhea
- Bladder control problems
- Sexual changes such as erectile dysfunction in men and decreased lubrication and sensation in women
- Changes in the brain that may lead to dementia, including Alzheimers

**Nerve with
diabetes damage**

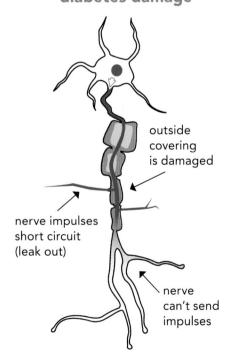

outside
covering
is damaged

nerve impulses
short circuit
(leak out)

nerve
can't send
impulses

Other things that increase your nerve damage

- Smoking
- Drinking alcohol
- High blood pressure
- High blood triglycerides (a type of blood fat that increases when blood sugars are high)
- Weighing too much
- Malnutrition

Symptoms of Narrowed Blood Vessels

It's important to visit your doctor for blood sugar, blood cholesterol and blood pressure tests so the doctor can find any hardening and narrowing of your blood vessels.

Tell your doctor if you have any unusual symptoms that may indicate a blocked large blood vessel, such as:

- **Swelling to your fingers or feet**
  With a weaker heart and narrowed blood vessels, your kidneys get reduced fluid circulation. Your kidneys then hold extra sodium and water. After a long day on your feet, this sodium and water becomes trapped in the tissues of your feet, causing swelling.

- **Shortness of breath**
  You may be out of breath even with small amounts of exercise. This could mean the heart muscle is not able to pump enough oxygen throughout your body. There also may be a more serious problem such as a blood clot in the lungs.

- **Chest pain**
  You could have chest pain, especially when exercising, because of decreased blood flow to your heart. Nerve damage to the heart can result in irregular heartbeats.

- **Difficulty concentrating or headaches**
  Your brain may have lower blood flow, with less oxygen and nutrients. This causes your thinking to be less clear.

- **Calf pain or cramps**
  If you have pain in your calves (the back of your lower legs) when walking and even resting, this may be because of decreased blood flow to your legs.

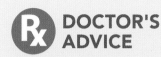

DOCTOR'S ADVICE

Out of shape?
Many people with diabetes get better with medically supervised exercise.

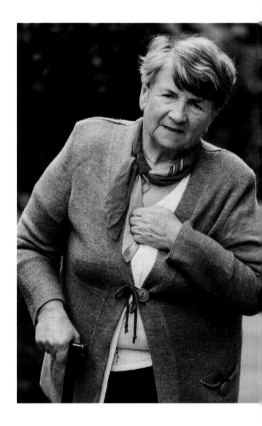

Rx DOCTOR'S ADVICE

You may have nerve damage if you've had diabetes for many years. That means if you have a heart attack, you may not feel all the usual pain.

Many people with diabetes, especially women, do not experience typical heart attack symptoms. Instead, their first symptoms that they are having a heart attack may be fatigue and dizziness.

Have regular checkups with your doctor!

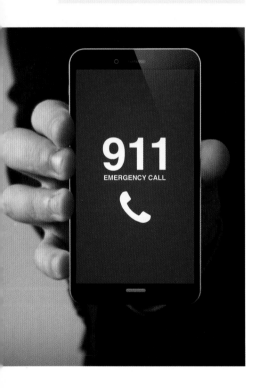

Minutes can make a difference. Call 911 if you think you are having a heart attack or stroke.

Heart Attack and Stroke

If you have think you are having a heart attack:

- First, call 911 right away.
- Then, chew one regular-strength aspirin (325 mg) and swallow it with a drink of water. (A regular-strength aspirin is equal to four low-dose aspirin).

 WARNING SIGNS: Heart Attack

Immediately seek medical help if you have:

- Sudden pain, heaviness or discomfort in your chest, neck, jaw, shoulder, arms or back, lasting more than a few minutes
- Chest pain when exerting yourself
- Shortness of breath
- Nausea, indigestion or vomiting
- Sudden sweating
- Unusual fear or anxiety

⚠ **WARNING SIGNS: Stroke Act Very FAST!**

Immediately seek medical help if you have:

V **Vision** loss, sudden

F **Face** is drooping

A **Arms,** you can't raise both

S **Speech** is slurred

T **Time** to call 911

Foot and Lower Leg Infections

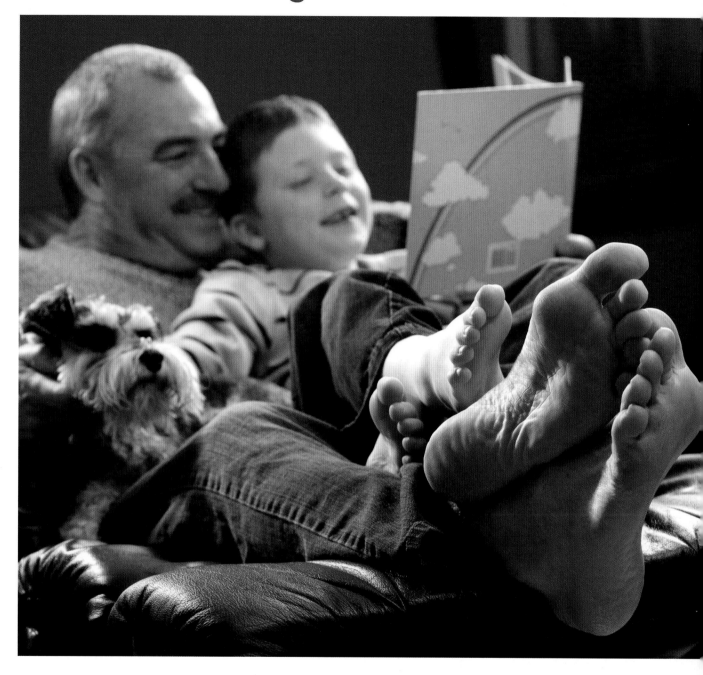

Fight against amputation — keep your feet for life.

With proper foot care, up to 85% of amputations in people with diabetes could be prevented.

You have a 50% chance of developing some nerve damage if you've had diabetes for 10 years.

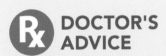 **DOCTOR'S ADVICE**

You may not feel an open sore on the bottom or side of your foot. Check your feet every day.

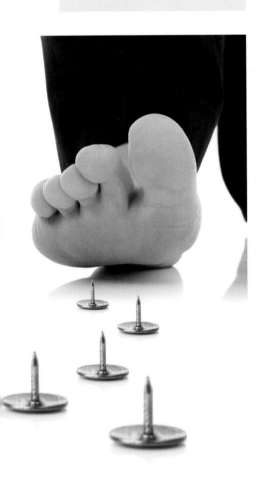

High blood sugar causes a variety of changes to your feet. This puts you at risk for foot and lower leg infections. You'll have a higher risk, depending on how long you've had diabetes and how high your blood sugar has been. It's hard to know your exact risks, or when your risk increases. So look after your feet every day.

Six reasons why you may get a foot or lower leg infection

1. Nerve damage to the feet

- Feeling of pins and needles, or burning and aching (this may also occur in your legs, fingers or arms)
- Extreme sensitivity to touch (for example, when sleeping, the blanket on your feet might be bothersome)
- Loss of feeling on the bottoms of your feet
- Loss of hair growth on your lower leg and on the tops of your feet and toes (hair needs nerve stimulation to grow)
- Dry feet (nerves stimulate oil glands that keep your skin soft)
- Loss of balance and feeling unstable when standing or walking

These symptoms can be mild or severe. When blood sugar improves, nerve damage can be reduced.

Feelings of pins and needles and aching will be uncomfortable or painful, but the greatest risk is when there is a loss of feeling. With loss of feeling, you may not feel pain or dangerously hot water. Pain is your body's way of telling you something is wrong. You may not know that your shoes are too tight. You won't feel the shoe rubbing on your skin, causing a corn or an injury to a bunion. You may not feel an infected hangnail or a stone in your shoe. You will not know that you need to treat the injury right away.

2. Poor blood flow (circulation)

This is when the large blood vessels in your legs and smaller blood vessels in your feet and toes become narrow and less elastic. This causes reduced blood flow. Nutrients, oxygen and white blood cells that fight infection cannot as easily get to your toes. Your nails may become yellowed, brittle or hard. Your feet are often cold or discolored. Cuts don't heal as well.

Smoking decreases circulation. It is a major contributor to the need for amputations. Don't smoke! Read *Become a Nonsmoker*, pages 247–266.

3. High blood sugar feeds germs

Germs (bacteria and fungus) feed on sugar. When you have extra sugar in your blood, germs grow and reproduce fast. Bacterial infections can spread quickly. A serious infection can develop in a short time. Fungus can grow on the foot (athlete's foot), particularly between the toes and under toenails.

4. Dry, cracked skin

Nerves help stimulate oil and sweat glands that moisturize your feet. So, when nerves don't work well, your ability to sweat can be lost and your skin gets dry. Also, if your blood sugar is high, your body pulls fluid out of your tissues (to make extra urine in an attempt to get rid of extra sugar), and this can make dry skin worse. When the skin is dry, you are more likely to get cracks that break open. Once the skin is broken, germs get in and start growing and cause an infection. An infection can cause gangrene and possibly even mean you need an amputation.

Do you have pain, weakness and cramping in your calf muscles?
You may have peripheral arterial disease (PAD). This means a blood vessel to your lower leg is blocked. Talk to your doctor.

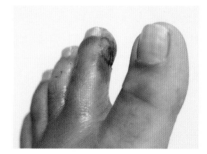

High blood sugar can also decrease your body's ability to fight infection (immunity).

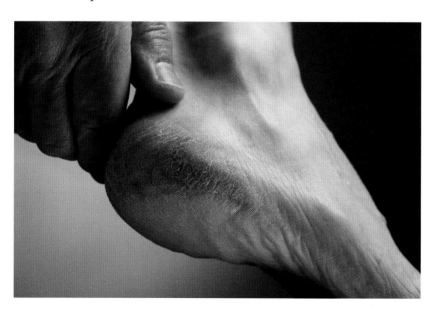

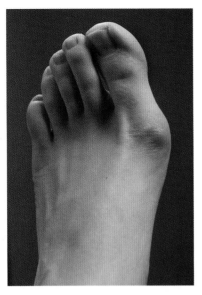

A shoe that is too tight creates a pressure point. This can cause a bunion.

Check your feet daily
Prevent injuries and treat simple injuries immediately.
Read pages 268–281.

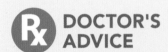
DOCTOR'S ADVICE

Prompt medical care can prevent a minor injury from becoming serious.

5. Distorted foot shape

Nerves control the muscles which hold your foot in place and give you balance. The muscles may get weak because diabetes can damage the nerves in your feet. The bones in your feet (and the joints between your bones) may also weaken in some cases.

For example, most people have a natural arch in the soles of their feet. If your muscles weaken, this arch can fall and you will develop a flat foot. Certain bones and parts of your foot that used to be raised will now touch the ground when you walk. This creates pressure and wear on these parts of your foot.

Here are some other problems that can occur when your foot shape changes:

- Poor balance — you are more likely to fall
- Toes that angle in or out
- Corns or calluses
- Thinning of the pads on the ball of your foot

6. Extra body weight

The more you weigh, the more weight and pressure is on the bottom of your feet as you stand and move around. Doing high-impact exercise (such as running) further increases the weight and pressure on the bottom of your feet.

How infections can lead to gangrene

You lose some feeling in your foot, due to nerve damage.

▼

You get a cut on your toe but you don't feel it.

▼

Germs get into the cut and grow quickly because of the extra sugar in your blood.

▼

The cut becomes infected.

▼

You notice blood on your sock and see that you have a red and infected sore.

▼

Just a few days later, the sore looks worse. It is smelly. You make an appointment with your doctor, but you don't seek help immediately.

▼

Ten days later, when you see your doctor, you may have gangrene.

Kidney Damage

Your kidneys have tiny filtering units. These are surrounded by many tiny blood vessels and nerves. If you have years of high blood sugar and high blood pressure, it harms these vessels and nerves. This harm causes you to lose some of the filtering units. The kidneys won't work as well. With advanced kidney failure, you will feel sick. Some people may need dialysis.

What do healthy kidneys do?

Your two kidneys are like a filter on your furnace or car that removes unwanted compounds and keeps the motor clean. Each kidney has an elaborate network of about a million tiny filters to filter your blood. This keeps fluids and compounds at the right level in your blood and helps control blood pressure.

Your kidneys work to:

- Maintain a healthy balance of water and salts (such as sodium, potassium, calcium and phosphorus) in your body. Extra amounts are filtered out into your urine.
- Maintain normal blood pressure. Damaged kidneys result in extra sodium in your blood and higher blood pressure.
- Filter out waste products from your blood and dispose of them in your urine. This includes compounds that are the result of your body's digestion and metabolism such as urea and creatinine. It also includes excess medications.
- Help make red blood cells. This is why you may be anemic if you have kidney problems.
- Keep these important red blood cells, as well as white blood cells and proteins in the blood. The kidneys don't filter these out.

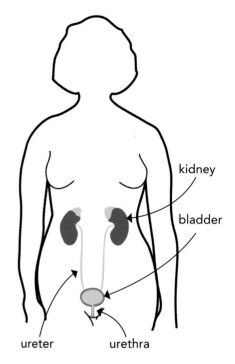

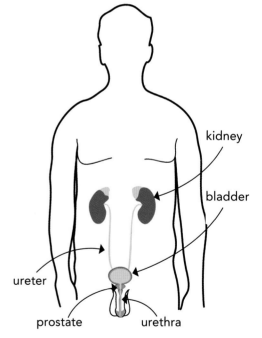

The role of the kidney in regulating blood sugar

Medical researchers are beginning to understand some of the ways that the kidney can significantly affect blood sugar.

- The cells of the kidney can make, store and release sugar. In people with diabetes, the process can be overactive and contributes to high blood sugar.

- As blood flows into the glomerulus, the kidney normally transports any sugar out of the urine and back into the blood stream.

- In people with diabetes, the transport of increased amounts of sugar back into the blood further raises the blood sugar level.

A new group of diabetes medications that block the transport of sugar have been found to be effective in treating diabetes (see page 314). These medications also reduce the risk of heart disease, stroke and kidney damage.

A healthy kidney

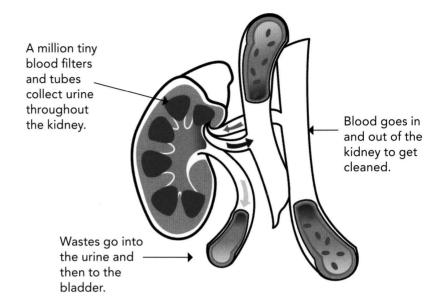

A million tiny blood filters and tubes collect urine throughout the kidney.

Blood goes in and out of the kidney to get cleaned.

Wastes go into the urine and then to the bladder.

What does a kidney filter look like and how does it work?

There are about one million filters in each of your two kidneys. Each of these million filters includes two connected parts: the glomerulus (the main filter) and the nephron (the second filter).

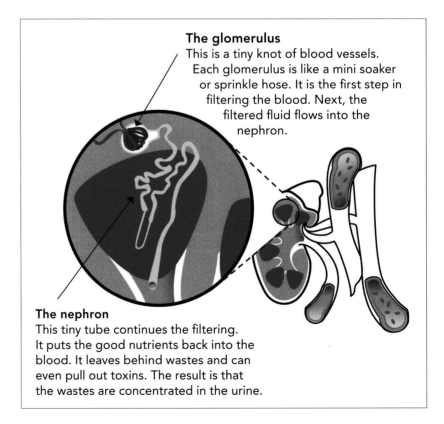

The glomerulus
This is a tiny knot of blood vessels. Each glomerulus is like a mini soaker or sprinkle hose. It is the first step in filtering the blood. Next, the filtered fluid flows into the nephron.

The nephron
This tiny tube continues the filtering. It puts the good nutrients back into the blood. It leaves behind wastes and can even pull out toxins. The result is that the wastes are concentrated in the urine.

Early kidney damage (microalbuminuria)

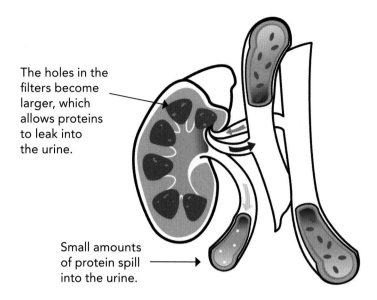

The holes in the filters become larger, which allows proteins to leak into the urine.

Small amounts of protein spill into the urine.

The glomeruli (the main filters) become damaged by the excess blood sugar and high blood pressure. They plug up and no longer work. The nephron that is attached to each of them also stops working and becomes useless. This results in fewer filtering units. The rest try to make up the extra work by filtering more, and the pressure inside the glomeruli increases. This causes holes to grow in the remaining glomeruli, and now they wear out faster. Protein now leaks out into the urine.

If your doctor consistently finds small amounts of protein in your urine, this is an early sign of kidney damage. It can also mean you may be at greater risk of a heart attack or stroke. One type of protein that is measured at the lab is called albumin. "Microalbuminuria" means the loss of small amounts of albumin in the urine.

Page 303 has more information on kidney lab tests.

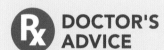 **DOCTOR'S ADVICE**

If you recently have had a kidney or bladder infection, you may have extra protein in your urine. This returns to normal after the infection is cured.

Advanced kidney damage (macroalbuminuria)

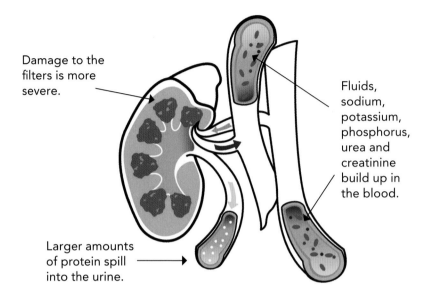

Damage to the filters is more severe.

Fluids, sodium, potassium, phosphorus, urea and creatinine build up in the blood.

Larger amounts of protein spill into the urine.

More glomeruli and nephrons are damaged. More protein leaks into the urine. This is called "macroalbuminuria."

As the kidney function worsens, the remaining filters can't balance the fluids, salts and wastes. Sodium, potassium, phosphorus, urea and creatinine are normal parts of blood, except when their levels are too high. These now build up to dangerous levels in the blood.

As fluids and compounds build up in blood, there will be symptoms of kidney disease:

- swollen ankles or legs
- fatigue
- shortness of breath
- nausea and sometimes vomiting
- dry, itchy skin

Damaged kidneys can no longer remove enough of the toxins building up in your blood. Your symptoms of kidney damage will get worse. You may require dialysis. In some cases you may be a candidate for a kidney transplant.

What is hemodialysis?

You need dialysis when your kidney damage is bad enough that your kidneys are no longer doing their job. You won't feel well. A hemodialysis machine works like a kidney. When you are attached to a dialysis machine, it removes the blood from your body. Your blood is filtered through the dialysis machine, where it's cleaned and returned to your body. Typically, this takes four hours and needs to be done three times a week, either during the day or at night. Hemodialysis is usually done at a hospital or dialysis centre. In some cases, people can dialysis themselves at home. In this case, you would use a special hemodialysis home machine.

Peritoneal dialysis

Peritoneal dialysis is a common form of home dialysis. If this is an option for you, peritoneal dialysis is easier than home hemodialysis. Using a tiny silicone tube in your belly, clean water with added electrolytes, called dialysis fluid, trickles into the tissues. It stays there and the wastes leave your blood and enter the dialysis fluid. The fluid can be exchanged four times a day or at night using a small machine. This gives you more freedom, as you aren't attached to a machine for so many hours. You can do this kind of dialysis at home.

Are you wondering whether you might need dialysis?
This depends on your lab results and how you are feeling. Talk to your doctor, nephrologist (kidney specialist) or kidney nurse.

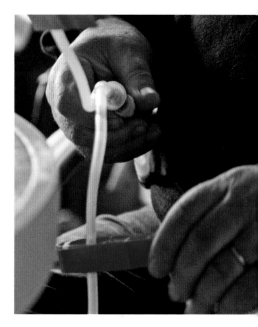

Peritoneal dialysis can be done at home.

Early prevention may protect the kidneys from damage and reduces the need for dialysis

Many doctors now treat blood sugar and blood pressure with medication right away to try to protect the kidneys. You may start taking medication right after your diagnosis with diabetes. Medicines, diet and lifestyle changes are critical to controlling both blood sugar and blood pressure. You and your doctor must work together to prevent or slow down kidney damage.

Eye Problems

Like the kidneys, the eyes have many tiny blood vessels and nerves that can be damaged by high blood sugar and high blood pressure.

Three ways diabetes can affect your eyes

1. **Blurring** of vision

2. **Cataracts** or glaucoma

3. **Retinopathy** (damage to the retina, the back of the eye)

Retinopathy is the most serious diabetes-related eye problem. If not treated, retinopathy can lead to blindness.

1. Blurring of vision

This happens when your blood sugar is high or is swinging from high to low. At the front of your eye is the lens (see diagram on next page). As the level of sugar goes up in your blood, water goes into your lens causing it to swell. This change in shape is what usually causes blurring. This makes it difficult to see long distances (or in some cases, to read), but it doesn't mean you are going blind. Once you get your blood sugar lowered, the lens goes back to its normal shape and your usual vision returns.

2. Cataracts or glaucoma

These eye problems are more likely to develop at an earlier age in people who have diabetes.

- **Cataracts** are when the lens of your eye becomes cloudy. Signs may include blurred vision or a feeling of having a film over your eyes that doesn't clear up when you blink. Cataracts develop slowly. With surgery, doctors remove the cloudy lens and replace it with a new lens.

- **Glaucoma** is damage to the optic nerve that causes a loss of vision. At first, you lose peripheral vision, that is, the edges of what you see. However, you may not notice this damage at this stage. Eventually, you also lose the middle part of your vision. There may not be early warning signs, so a regular eye exam is important. Your optometrist will measure your eye pressure but will also look at the optic nerve for changes. If you have glaucoma, you may need treatment or surgery.

Macular degeneration can affect central vision. It is an eye condition of older adults, but diabetes has not been found to increase it.

When blood sugar improves, there is less blurring of vision.

Factors that affect the development of eye problems:

- age
- diabetes
- smoking
- drinking too much alcohol
- eating an unhealthy diet
- high blood pressure
- excess bright sun exposure
- pregnancy

Side view of the eye (enlarged)

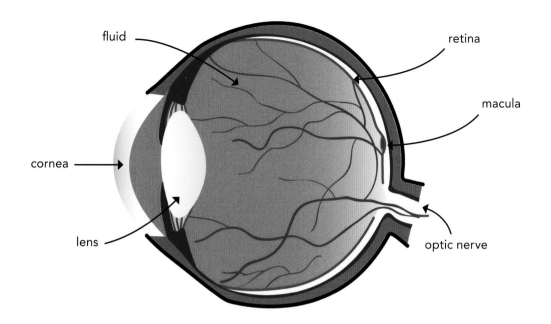

fluid

retina

macula

cornea

lens

optic nerve

What you see with different eye problems

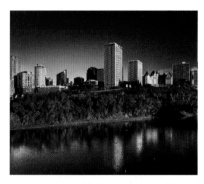

Normal vision

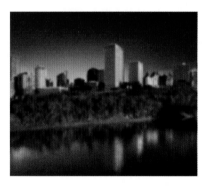

Blurring of vision

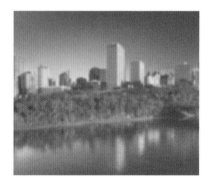

Cataracts

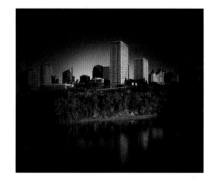

Glaucoma

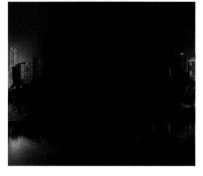

Macular degeneration

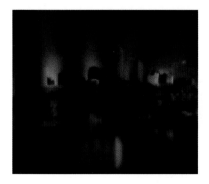

Advanced retinopathy

There are no warning signs of early retinopathy. See your eye doctor once a year. Only the eye doctor will be able to see changes by looking at the back of your eye. *See pages 299 and 304 to learn more about your eye appointment.*

 WARNING SIGNS

Advanced Retinopathy

Immediately seek medical help if:

- You have persistent blurring not associated with blood sugar changes.
- You notice a sudden decrease, or loss of vision, in one or both eyes.
- You see flashing lights, black spots or spider webs.
- Shapes or objects look distorted.
- You see red color (meaning bleeding in the eye).
- You feel unusual fear or anxiety.

3. Retinopathy (damage to the back of the eye)

Retinopathy is when, over a long time, high blood sugar causes damage and abnormal growth of the tiny blood vessels at the back of the eye (the retina).

Changes your eye doctor can see

Early retinopathy (non-proliferative retinopathy)

- *Small bulges in blood vessels.* This can be a sign of reduced blood flow to the retina. Blood vessels can break (hemorrhage) and leak fluid and blood (blood spots). This can cause swelling in the retina. This swelling may affect your macula that gives you detailed vision.
- *Small blobs of hard yellow fat.* This comes from leaking blood vessels.
- *Whitish patches or "cotton wool" spots.* These are caused by reduced blood flow to nerves in your retina.

Advanced retinopathy (proliferative retinopathy)

- *Many new thin and fragile blood vessels* on the surface of the retina. These grow because the retina needs more oxygen and nutrients.
- *Blood spots.* These new tiny blood vessels are weak and tend to break and leak fluid and blood. Broken blood vessels can leave scar tissue behind. These two things, broken blood vessels and scarring, can threaten your vision.
- *Blood in the eye socket.* This is due to bursting of the new fragile blood vessels.

If you do not seek treatment for advanced retinopathy, several things can lead to loss of vision:

- **Retinal detachment.** The retina pulls away from the back wall of the eye (usually as a result of scar tissue).
- **Vitreous hemorrhage.** Blood leaks into the eye socket.
- **Macular edema.** Blood vessels around the macula leak.

Treatment

If an eye doctor catches your retinopathy early, you can get treatment, if needed. The usual treatment uses a laser (high-powered tiny light beams) pointed to the outside of the retina. This helps increase blood flow and reduce leakage to the remaining tissues in the inner part of the retina. Also, there are new medications available to reduce macular edema if you have it.

View of the back of the eye

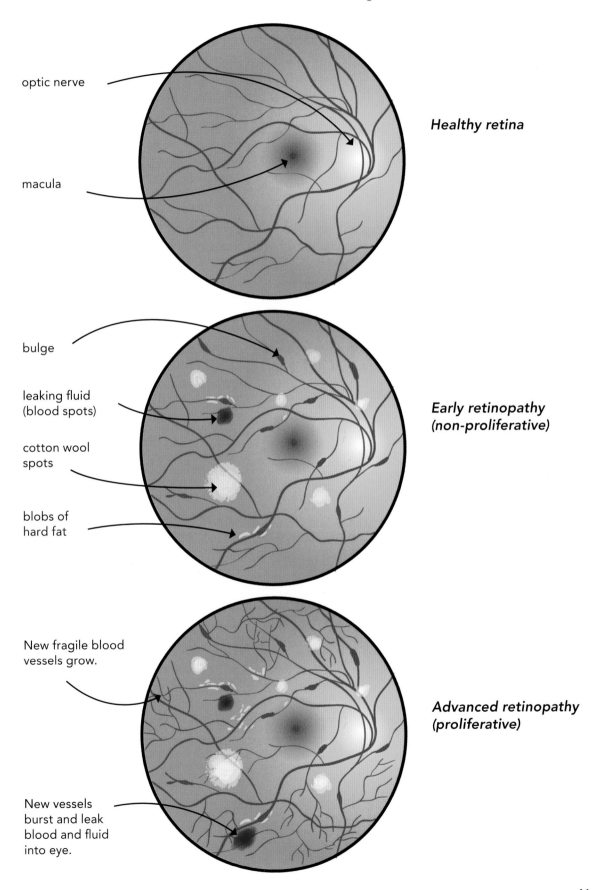

optic nerve

macula

Healthy retina

bulge

leaking fluid
(blood spots)

cotton wool
spots

blobs of
hard fat

*Early retinopathy
(non-proliferative)*

New fragile blood
vessels grow.

New vessels
burst and leak
blood and fluid
into eye.

*Advanced retinopathy
(proliferative)*

Rx DOCTOR'S ADVICE

To prevent and manage skin issues related to diabetes, improve your blood sugar and care for your skin.

Learn more about skin care on page 282.

If you're in pain, you don't have to suffer. If your doctor doesn't offer you support, check with another doctor, your pharmacist or a diabetes nurse for additional advice and a second opinion.

Other Complications

Skin Concerns

High blood sugar and decreased nerve function affect your skin. It particularly affects the skin on your legs and feet. Here are some examples of skin concerns in people with diabetes:

- Small sores on your shins or front lower legs
- Dry, itchy or scaly skin
- Bacterial infections that can develop into sores
- Fungus infections that develop under the breasts or folds of skin, in armpits, in the groin area, or on hands.
- Blisters or boils (most often on feet, lower legs or hands)
- Darkened skin on the neck, armpits, hands, elbows or groin
- For those who take insulin, bumps or pits can occur on your skin if you inject in the same spot over and over. It is important to rotate your injection sites (see page 321).

Report to your doctor any skin condition that doesn't go away. A skin concern can look different on you than someone else. Some skin conditions are uncommon or rare.

Painful skin

If you have painful skin, it can be caused by damaged nerves in your skin because of high blood sugar over a long time. This nerve pain is also called neuropathic pain. You may have numbness or tingling, or you may have a burning or deep pain. You are most likely to have pain in your feet or legs. Some people have pain in their hands. The pain can be mild or severe.

Things that may reduce painful skin
- Keep active to improve circulation.
- Quit smoking to improve your circulation.
- If your blood sugar is high, bring it down.
- Try gentle massage.
- Place warm or cold compresses on your skin.

If your pain becomes severe, talk to your doctor. Ask about the cause of your pain and what to do about it. Your doctor may recommend an ointment to put on your skin, to dull the pain, or prescribe a pill. Medications include pain killers, antidepressant pills or other pills. If your pain makes it difficult to cope, your doctor may refer you to another doctor who is a pain specialist.

Gum Disease

- Gum disease is a serious bacterial infection of your gums and jawbone, which support your teeth.
- You are more likely to get gum disease when your blood sugar is high.
- Gum disease is one of the most common infections in people with diabetes. Yet we often miss diagnosing it.
- If your gum disease is not treated, you may lose teeth.

How do I know if I have gum disease?

At first, you may not know you have gum disease. This is because it doesn't usually hurt in the beginning.

Early warning signs
- Red, puffy gums
- Gums that bleed when you brush, floss, or eat hard food

Later signs
- Gums that pull away from your teeth and make your teeth look longer
- Bad breath
- Raised blood sugar levels
- Sores or pain in your mouth
- Pus between your gums and teeth
- Loose teeth or toothaches
- Poor bite: your teeth or dentures may not fit together properly
- Trouble chewing raw fruits and vegetables.

Early gum disease

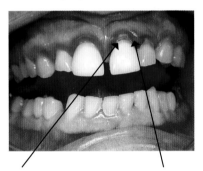

plaque   red, puffy gums that bleed easily

Are you having a hard time bringing down high blood sugar? Gum disease might be part of the cause.

There are two reasons for this:

1. If you have a gum infection with inflammation or redness, your insulin may not work as well.
2. A gum infection, like all infections, may cause your body to make stress hormones; these may increase your blood sugar.

It's important to see your dentist or dental hygienist at least two times a year.

Healthy gums and teeth begin in infancy.

We can't change how we were fed as infants. However, here are important things to know to protect your children and grandchildren's teeth.

- Breastfeeding is best for an infant's healthy gums and teeth (learn more about infant health on pages 384–388).

If a baby is bottlefed, take steps to protect baby's gums and teeth:

- Don't feed babies or toddlers bottles with juice, soft drink or sweetened beverages.
- Don't give a baby a bottle when putting them to bed.
- Don't put sugar, honey or other sweet liquids on a soother (pacifier).
- Also, don't give a child a soother after age two.
- Gently clean a baby's gums daily with a clean, soft moist cloth. Once baby's teeth appear, gently brush every day. Use an infant toothbrush. Ask your dentist when to start using toothpaste with fluoride.

Three main causes of gum disease

Plaque

Bacteria (germs) are normal in your mouth and attach to your gums and teeth every day. Gum infections begin when the buildup of bacteria turns into a sticky, clear film, called plaque. When you don't brush and floss your teeth, plaque builds up around the gum line. Often the plaque attaches to tartar, a hard deposit that builds up under your gums, around the roots of your teeth. When this happens, your gums and the bone that supports your teeth are covered all the time by the plaque bacteria. This causes gum infection. That's why it's so important to clean your teeth every day. You also need to have your teeth cleaned by a dental hygienist every six months. This removes the plaque.

Smoking and vaping

The nicotine from smoking, vaping, JUULing or chewing tobacco constricts blood vessels, reducing blood circulation. This decreases your ability to fight infection and makes you more likely to get gum disease.

High blood sugar

Years of high blood sugar can damage blood vessels and nerves. Even over a short period of time, high blood sugar causes more sugar in your saliva.

Damaged blood vessels: You are less able to fight infections.
As with other parts of your body, your mouth's blood vessels can be damaged by high blood sugar. When blood vessels become narrow, less blood reaches the gums. This makes it difficult to fight infection and heal the gums.

Damaged nerves: Your glands make less saliva.
Nerves stimulate your glands to make saliva, especially when you eat. Saliva helps wash away bits of food. This reduces the bacteria and plaque that start gum disease. Saliva also keeps your mouth clean and moist. With high blood sugar, nerves in your glands may be damaged. As a result, your body may make less saliva in your mouth.

More sugar in your blood and saliva: More germs grow.
Extra sugar in your blood feeds the growth of bacteria in infected areas. Also, when your blood sugar is high, some of this extra sugar goes into your saliva. This sweeter saliva around the infected area offers even more sugar for growing bacteria. Your infection can get worse or be difficult to heal.

Thrush

Thrush is a yeast infection. It can be in the mouth, gums, lips or tongue.

It's normal to have some bacteria and yeast in your mouth. However, too much yeast can grow when you take antibiotics, have a poor immune system, or have high blood sugar. You're more likely to get thrush than someone who doesn't have diabetes.

Common signs of a yeast infection
- You have white or yellow patches on your mouth and tongue, or sides of your lips.
- The corners of your mouth may be dry and cracked.
- It itches or hurts.

Tooth Decay

Tooth decay is when the enamel (white surface) of your teeth breaks down, leaving cavities (holes) in your teeth.

Acid causes tooth decay
When the bacteria in plaque mixes with sugar from the foods that you eat, it makes acid. This acid attacks the enamel. Eating acidic foods, such as lemons or soft drinks, can also break down enamel. These acid attacks last for 20 minutes or more after eating. Over time, this can break down tooth enamel, causing cavities. As a person with diabetes, you have more sugar in your saliva and are more likely to get tooth decay.

The good news!
Studies show that if you keep your blood sugar at a good level, you are less likely to get gum disease, thrush and tooth decay. See targets for blood sugar on page 17. Having good blood sugar is very important. When you treat your gum disease, this may reduce how much insulin you need.

Read pages 283–286 for specific things that you can do to keep your teeth and gums healthy.

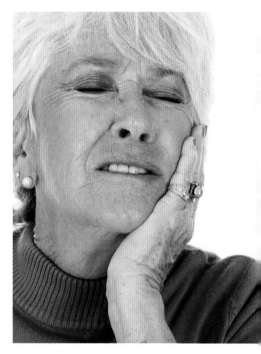

Tooth decay can cause pain.

Urinary Tract Infections

Urinary tract infections (UTIs) are infections that affect the kidneys, ureters, bladder or urethra (the tube that carries the urine from your bladder out of your body). In women, UTIs are often associated with vaginal infections. In men, UTIs can be associated with an enlarged prostate gland or kidney stones. UTIs can occur if your blood sugar is high for even a few days or a week.

When your blood has extra sugar in it, for example, 270 mg/dL (15 mmol/L) or more, your body feels overwhelmed by the extra sugar. Your kidneys filter it into your urine, which goes to your bladder and you pee it out.

Bacteria and yeast can feed and multiply rapidly when there is extra sugar in your kidneys, bladder and urine. An infection can develop. When your blood sugar is high, your body has reduced immunity due to slow-moving white blood cells. This means your body is less able to fight infection.

Two things happen. First, high blood sugars contribute to a UTI. Second, once you have a UTI, the infection increases stress hormones in your body. These make blood sugar go even higher. If left untreated, you can become very sick.

If UTIs occur frequently, they may damage the kidneys. Prompt treatment is important.

UTI Symptoms
- Increased need or urgency to urinate
- Pain during urination or sex
- Blood or pus in the urine
- Abdominal cramps or pain (back pain if kidneys or prostate are infected)
- Smelly urine
- Signs of a vaginal yeast infection: vaginal itching or burning, or a yeasty smell or thick white discharge

---

When you have nerve damage to the bladder, it's more difficult to feel when your bladder is full. Because of that, you may not empty your bladder as often as you should, or as fully. Urine sits in the bladder for a longer time. This gives bacteria more time to grow, so the chance of a UTI increases.

Sometimes, bladder nerve damage can mean you may experience opposite symptoms. For example, you may have to urinate frequently or you may have incontinence.

UTIs in women

Compared to women without diabetes, women with high blood sugar have more sugar in their urine and in their vaginal secretions.

The biggest source of germs is your stool (bowel movements). A woman's vagina is located close enough to the anus that bacteria can easily spread to the vagina. Then germs go up the urethra (the tube between the bladder and opening) and into the bladder and kidneys. A woman's urethra is only about $1\frac{1}{2}$ inches (4 cm) long, so germs can easily travel that distance. The extra sugar in the genital area can also cause a yeast infection.

Sexual activity can increase the infection risk because germs get pushed into the vagina and urethra.

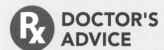

DOCTOR'S ADVICE

Some diabetes medications increase the amount of sugar in the urine (see page 314). Sometimes the extra sugar can cause urinary tract infections and vaginal yeast infections. These infections can be treated in the usual way with medicines, such as antibiotics for a UTI, and anti-fungals for a yeast infection. If infections continue, talk with your health care provider about changing to a different type of medication.

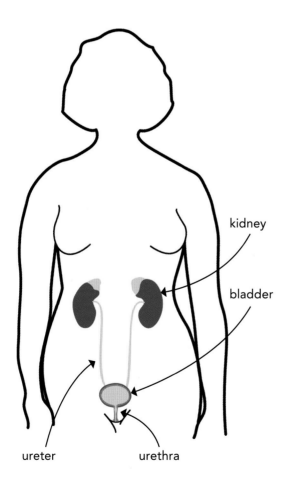

kidney

bladder

ureter   urethra

Read pages 287–291 for prevention and treatment of UTIs.

UTIs in men

Compared to women, men have a significantly lower risk of UTIs, but infections can happen. Men have a longer urethra (about 8 inches/20 cm) compared to women (1.5 inches/4 cm). A man's urethra extends from the bladder down the length of the penis. Usually, bacteria from the outside cannot travel this distance, so infections happen less often. Also, the urethra opening at the end of the penis is separated from the anus. So waste is less likely to contaminate the urethra.

However, the risk for a UTI increases with an enlarged prostate. An enlarged prostate pushes against the urethra or bladder. This makes it hard to fully empty the bladder. Germs then can grow in the urine that is left in the bladder. Using a catheter to drain the bladder increases risks for a UTI.

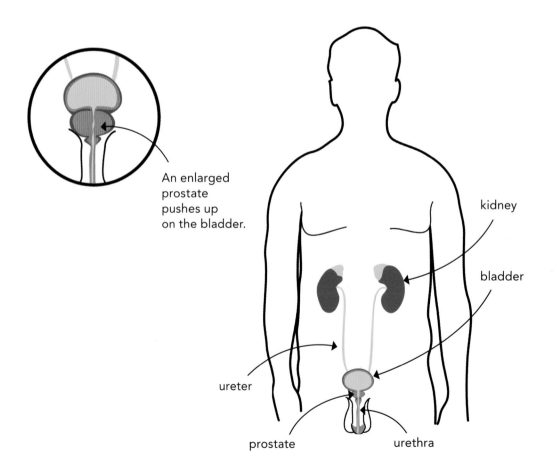

An enlarged prostate pushes up on the bladder.

kidney

bladder

ureter

prostate

urethra

Genital Issues and Sexuality

Our sexual organs are highly sensitive because they have many nerves and blood vessels. However, since diabetes can damage nerves and blood vessels, over time you may lose some sensation or sexual functioning. In some cases, the changes are temporary. Improving your blood sugar and blood pressure can help halt or slow down this damage.

Some people with diabetes experience no changes when it comes to sex.

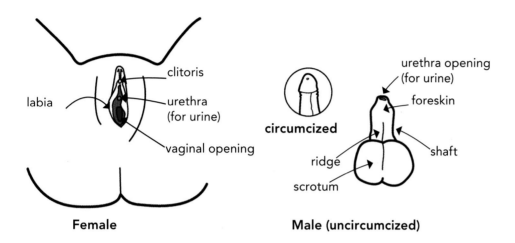

Female   **circumcized**   **Male (uncircumcized)**

Labels: clitoris, labia, urethra (for urine), vaginal opening, urethra opening (for urine), foreskin, ridge, scrotum, shaft

Changes that might affect your sex life

- Feeling tired, depressed and overwhelmed can make it difficult to do things you used to enjoy. You may feel less interested in all things in life, including sex.
- For men, as you age, it's natural to have less of the hormone testosterone, but it's more likely if you have diabetes. A lower level of testosterone can lessen your desire for sex.
- For women, estrogen (and the smaller amount of testosterone) decreases naturally after menopause. This can affect your desire for sex, just as lowered testosterone does with men.
- Some medications, such as pills for treating depression, have been known to lessen the feelings of sexuality.
- Aches and pains, especially in the knees or back, can make your usual sexual activity uncomfortable or painful.

Read pages 390–409 for solutions and approaches to sexual changes to enhance your sex life.

For women, some of these changes might happen

- For a woman with diabetes, nerve damage may reduce sensitivity during sex and decrease lubrication. For those women who have reached menopause, there is less estrogen, also contributing to less lubrication during sex. Intercourse may become less enjoyable and sometimes even painful.
- Diabetes can cause vaginal tract or urinary tract infections. During the time of the infection, the itching, pain or odor can affect a woman's interest in sex.

For men, some of these changes might happen

- A man with diabetes is more likely to have a low testosterone level, which means it can take longer to reach orgasm.
- Diabetes causes nerve and blood vessel damage, so it becomes more difficult to get and maintain an erection. This is called erectile dysfunction, and it can be mild or severe. Over time this may get worse if your high blood sugar and high blood pressure continues or worsens.

Causes of erectile dysfunction
- Psychological stress
- Physical stress, such as fatigue, pain, illness or surgery
- Side effects of medications, such as those taken to treat pressure and depression
- Smoking and heavy drinking
- Diabetes

Stomach and Bowel Problems

Our stomach, small intestine and large intestine (bowel) are muscles that digest food. To work well, they need:

- A network of nerves
- A healthy flow of blood, and
- Digestive enzymes and acids

As a result, diabetes nerve and blood vessel damage also affects the stomach and intestines.

A decrease in nerve function may mean that the muscles in your stomach and intestines don't contract as well or, in some cases, they over-contract. If there are damaged bowel nerves, you may have either constipation (a slowing down of the bowel) or diarrhea (a speeding up of the bowel). You may feel nausea and bloating because food sits in your stomach too long. Carbohydrates and nutrients may be absorbed at a fluctuating rate because of uneven nerve or blood function. This results in fluctuating blood sugar levels.

For constipation prevention, try a high-fiber diet along with lots of water and exercise. For information on high-fiber foods, see pages 56 and 91–93. For severe gastroparesis with diarrhea, a low-fiber, low-fat diet that is mostly liquids is often helpful. You should consider a visit to a dietitian. You may also need medications for constipation or diarrhea.

℞ DOCTOR'S ADVICE

You may have a bowel or stomach problem not related to diabetes, such as irritable bowl syndrome. Diabetes may worsen symptoms.

Consider that symptoms can be worsened by side effects of medications such as:

- Diabetes medications, including metformin or the non-insulin injectable medications
- Pain medications taken for diabetes pain, including cannabis

Gastroparesis is the term for stomach and intestine changes caused by diabetes. It can cause an uneven absorption of carbohydrate. This can sometimes explain strange blood sugar fluctuations. Serious gastroparesis is more often seen in people with type 1 diabetes.

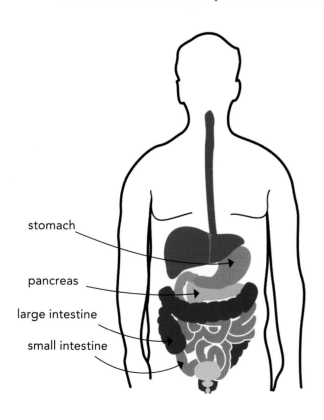

stomach

pancreas

large intestine

small intestine

Read pages 347–360 for information on managing stress.

Stress, Depression, Sleep Problems and Dementia

Stress

Having diabetes can make you feel overwhelmed with feelings of frustration, sadness and anger. This stress can make other diabetes complications worse because it increases both blood pressure and blood sugar.

Depression

We don't know why, but depression is more common in people with diabetes. This doesn't mean you will get depressed, but it does mean you should be aware of signs of depression.

Read pages 361–362 for information on depression.

What are some early signs of depression? You may feel overly tired and less motivated, causing weight gain and rise in blood sugar. Doctors prescribe many pills for depression, and some will cause weight gain. To avoid taking pills, talk to your doctor if you feel you have early signs of depression. This is the time to talk about other ways to manage depression.

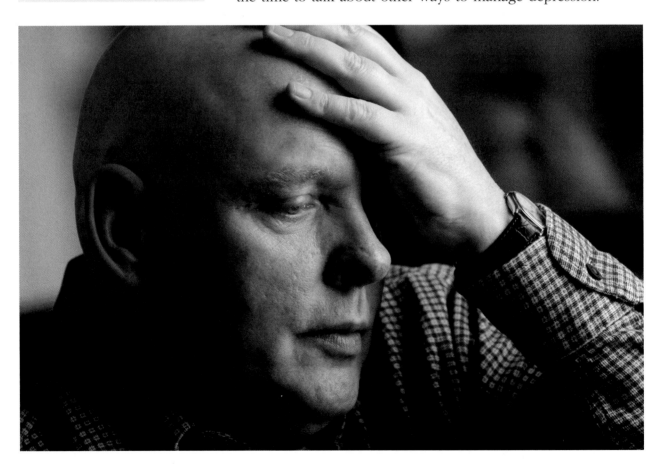

Sleep problems

Lack of sleep, sleep apnea or too much sleep may contribute to diabetes. High blood sugar can make these problems worse.

Lack of sleep

Worry and stress can cause poor sleep. Diabetes nerve damage can cause your legs to be restless or sore. This can keep you awake. High blood sugar can make you thirsty, so you drink more and wake up more during the night needing to pee.

If you don't get enough sleep, it disrupts your appetite hormones, so when you are awake you eat more. It also increases your stress hormones, which increases your blood sugar.

Sleep apnea

If you have sleep apnea, you may be a heavier person who falls asleep quickly and snores a lot. While you are sleeping, you briefly stop breathing many times during the night. This can wake you up, or you can sleep through it, but the result is poor sleep. You don't feel rested when you wake up. Sleep apnea can contribute to high blood pressure, insulin resistance, lack of energy to exercise, weight gain and, for men, erectile dysfunction.

Too much sleep

High blood sugar can cause you to feel very tired and sleep too much. This fatigue will likely mean you will be less active. Your metabolism will go down, and your weight and blood sugar go up.

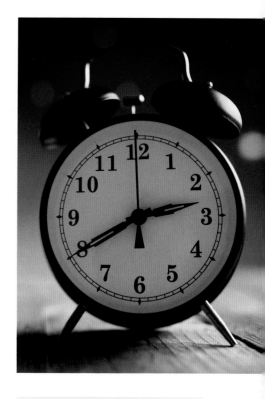

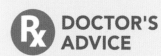 **DOCTOR'S ADVICE**

Do you sleep poorly?
Talk to your doctor. Seek early diagnosis and treatment. It is essential for managing your diabetes.

Read pages 358–359 for tips on sleeping better.

Dementia

Diabetes affects the nerves and the flow of oxygen and nutrients through blood vessels everywhere in the body, including in the brain. People with type 2 diabetes are more likely to have difficulty with attention, concentration and remembering words. They are also more at risk for the two main types of dementia: Alzheimer's type and vascular dementia. Getting the best blood sugar and blood pressure levels will help reduce these risks.

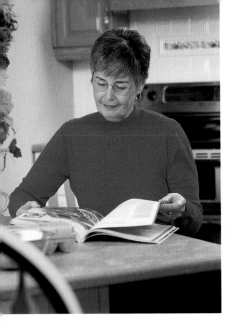

Seven Steps to Prevent or Reduce Diabetes Complications

Step 1: Eat Well

This *Eat Well* section of the book builds on the meal planning information and meal plans found in the *Diabetes Meals for Good Health Cookbook* and *Diabetes Essentials* (see page 416). In this section, you will find a "hands-on" food guide, answers to frequently asked nutrition questions and a seven-day meal plan with recipes. You will also read about challenges to making diet changes, and practical advice for overcoming these.

Hands-On Food Guide

Enjoy a variety of foods. Choose the right portions for a healthy weight.
Eat three balanced meals a day. Include snacks if needed.
Choose high-fiber foods. Drink lots of water. Keep active everyday.

Use your hands as a guide for your portions

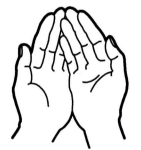

Vegetables: Eat plenty of these, and fruits too.

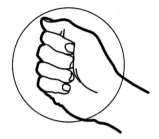

Grains and starches: Include whole grains.

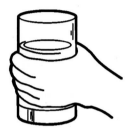

Milk or yogurt: Unsweetened is best.

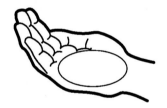

Protein: Include vegetarian sources too.

Added oils and fats: This includes olive and vegetable oils, butter and margarine.

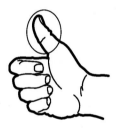

For Infants

If able, offer breast milk exclusively for the first six months. Continue with breastfeeding for one year or more.
At six months, add soft table foods rich in iron and vitamins.

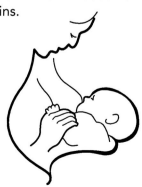

For Children and Teenagers

As children grow, so do their hands — so use their hands as a guide for portions. Offer larger portions during growth spurts.

For Adults

Very active adults may need larger portions than shown in this food guide. Women during pregnancy and breastfeeding may also need more.

For Older Adults

Eat a variety of colorful and nutrient-rich foods, but have smaller portions.

Eat a variety of foods

Vegetables and fruits
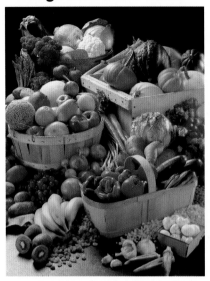

Grains and starches
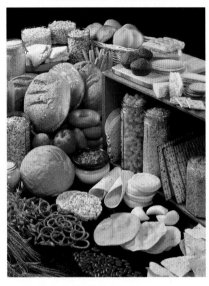

High-fiber foods
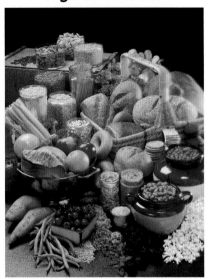

Calcium-rich foods
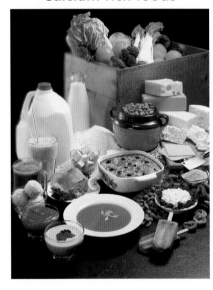

Proteins
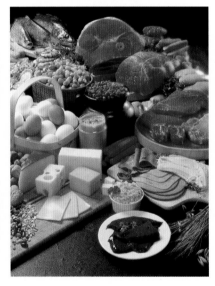

Healthy fats
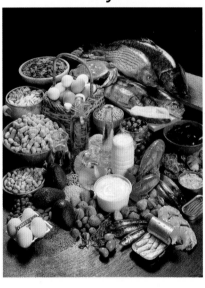

Drink lots of water
Drink six or more glasses of water a day. Drink more if the day is hot or you are active. Tap water with fluoride is good for your teeth and bones. Aim for 6 cups (1.5 L.)

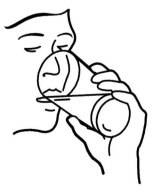

Keep active every day
Walk, bike or play to keep fit.

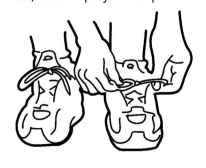

Foods and drinks to limit

Foods high in saturated fats or palm oils

Butter, lard, palm oil, coconut oil, some margarines, fatty meats, fried foods, potato chips and french fries, donuts, chocolates and sweet desserts

Sugar-packed drinks

Cappuccinos, milkshakes, iced drinks, sports drinks, energy drinks, flavored milks, beer, sweet wines, sweetened teas and coffees, juices and sweet drinks

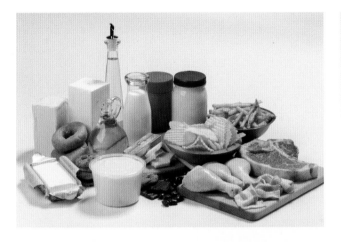

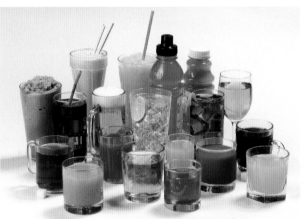

> **These high-fat, sweet foods and drinks taste good — so they are easy to overeat and overdrink. Enjoy them for special treats rather than daily.**

Restaurant meals

These often serve large portions which are high in fat, salt and sugar. Eat out less often. Enjoy healthy and fast homemade meals.

Salty foods

Processed foods and restaurant meals have a lot of salt. Cut back on these as well as table salt.

Alcohol

Talk to your doctor about whether small amounts of alcohol are healthy for you. There is no safe limit for infants, children and pregnant women.

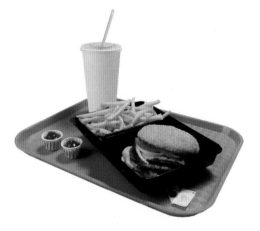

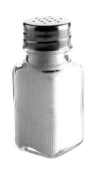

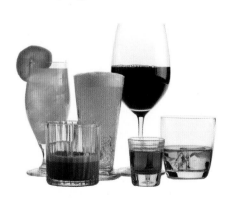

Choosing the right food portions is in your own hands.

Top 10 Nutrition Topics

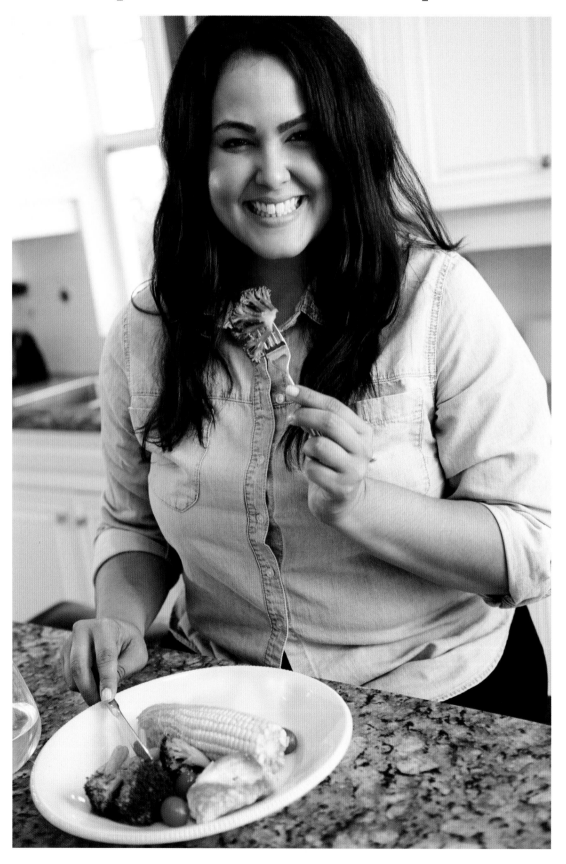

1. A Healthy Weight for You

Begin your journey

You are reading this book, so you are on your way to making gradual healthy changes, and avoiding restrictive and short-term diets.

Stop the weight gain

Have you been gaining a few pounds every year? If so, then halting this continual weight gain will be a tremendous achievement for the first month or two, or even long-term. You will have to reduce your calories or increase your exercise, or do both. You may also have to make other changes like getting a good night's sleep. This balances hormones that affect your appetite. You may need to change your medication.

Make more small changes when you are ready

First your body needs to adjust to not gaining weight, and you need to get used to eating slightly less food and doing more exercise. Then you are ready to work toward losing a few pounds.

Lose weight slowly for a long-lasting benefit

A loss of a pound (0.5 kg) a month will lead to a terrific weight loss of 12 lbs (5.5 kg) over the year. Studies show that a weight loss of 5 to 10 lbs (2 to 5 kg), especially in the prediabetes stage or soon after diagnosis of diabetes, can significantly improve blood sugar.

Keep unhealthy food choices out of sight and out of mind

When we see highly processed, sugary and fried foods on a frequent basis, it sets off triggers and hormones in our brains and stomachs. This makes us think we are hungry. Constant advertising and ready access to fast foods and processed foods are difficult to resist. Step by step, put more healthy foods and less junk food in your shopping cart, make meals at home, and avoid fast food and restaurant meals as much as possible.

Include some favorite foods

Diabetes is for life and so is healthy eating and exercise. Any and all foods can fit in a healthy eating pattern, but smaller portions are critical. Plan for a small indulgence occasionally. Enjoy it. Don't feel guilty about it. Studies show that including some favorite foods is important for a lifelong commitment to healthy eating. We all need a treat once in a while.

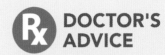

DOCTOR'S ADVICE

Success is losing a few pounds and keeping it off for life, not losing a lot of weight and regaining it within the year. Take it slowly, one step at a time.

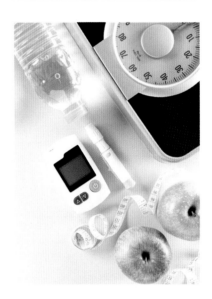

No such thing as a quick fix

Long-term changes need to be made to lose weight and keep it off. Anticipate ups and downs and even standstills. Slowly, you will see benefits. Small easy changes means you are more likely to keep pounds off for life.

TONY'S STORY: Break the yo-yo dieting cycle

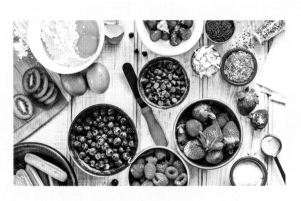

I've lost more than 30 pounds (14 kg) over the past three years, and my blood sugar is now well controlled!

For years, I yo-yo dieted. I would lose and gain, lose and gain, then gain more. When you're dieting, you feel so deprived. When you say "Oh, I'll have something extra, just this one time," it's so easy to fall off your strict pattern. Now that I have diabetes, I know that it's my health at stake. That's why I knew I had to stop my dieting cycle. I didn't just need to lose weight; I needed to change my lifestyle. I knew I could do it. Once I started, it wasn't so hard. I love to bake, so all I had to do was change the recipes a little. These were changes I knew that I could make forever.

I've told family and friends, this probably is the best thing that could have happened to me. Diabetes is a bad thing and I don't wish it on anybody, but it got me under control...and it wasn't that difficult.

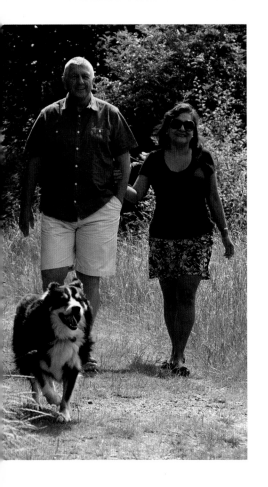

Boost metabolism

Metabolism is how you burn, or use up, your calories. With a higher metabolism, you burn more calories, have more energy and feel better. As we get older, our metabolism generally goes down. This is one reason people gain weight after about age 30. Here are ways to boost your metabolism.

Do aerobic and strengthening exercises

When you exercise regularly, you reduce fat tissue and build muscle, and this results in more energy burning. As you get in shape and can do more, you will benefit more. (See pages 201–246.)

Manage stress

Stress causes the hormone cortisol to rise. This increases blood sugar and insulin resistance (your insulin doesn't work as well). More insulin circulates in your blood. This causes your body to convert sugar into fat. More fat in your body lowers metabolism.

When people are stressed, it's common to overeat. In part this happens because the level of leptin, an appetite-controlling hormone, becomes suppressed during stress. With less stress, leptin goes back up, and your appetite is more controlled. Therefore, it's important to take steps to manage stress. (See pages 201–246.)

Don't miss meals!

Each time you miss a meal, your body's metabolism will temporarily slow down to conserve energy.

Less dieting, more healthy eating

Dieting reduces metabolism as the body slows down to conserve, just as when you miss meals. Strict diets reduce the hormone leptin. This is not good, as leptin helps you to avoid overeating. With less leptin in your system, there is an increase in ghrelin. This is the hormone that makes you want to keep eating. Your weight rebounds and often goes higher after you stop dieting.

Have your thyroid levels checked

The thyroid acts as a thermostat to keep your metabolism at the right level. This controls weight. Many things can cause your thyroid levels to be low. Iodine is essential for maintaining the right, healthy thyroid level. You can get all the iodine you need in a balanced diet that includes milk and milk products, fish and seafood, and a small amount of iodized salt. Do not take an iodine supplement unless recommended by your doctor. Other things that can reduce thyroid function are stress, poor sleep or weight gain. Also, your thyroid can be affected by certain medications, radiation or surgery to the neck area, or because of an autoimmune disease.

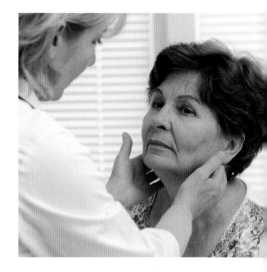

Get a good night's sleep

Adults should get 7 to 8 hours of sleep (8 to 10 hours for youth). During a sound sleep, your body repairs itself and corrects hormone levels, including thyroid and leptin levels. Sleep helps with the release of a healthy amount of melatonin, which can improve insulin production. After a good night's sleep, you wake up with the energy to make healthy meals, go for a walk, and do things you want to do.

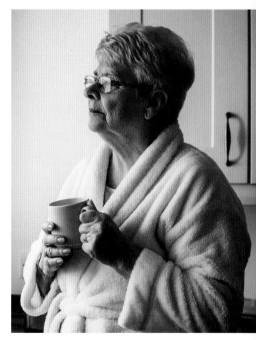

Manage estrogen loss as you age

Estrogen helps a woman's metabolism and weight, but during menopause, estrogen is gradually lost. This is one reason most women gain weight as they get older. To counteract this, become more active.

A full hysterectomy (removal of ovaries and uterus) causes sudden and immediate loss of the hormones estrogen, testosterone and progesterone. If your doctor suggests a full or partial hysterectomy, ask about hormone replacement. Depending on your symptoms, there may be other surgery options, such as endometrial ablation.

Ask about options, such an endometrial ablation. This means the lining of the uterus is destroyed, but your body keeps making more hormones, so you don't have a sudden lowering of your estrogen.

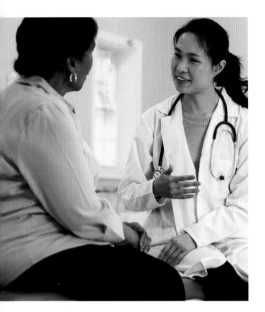
Getting medications reviewed

Manage testosterone loss as you age

Testosterone helps build muscle. Having more muscle increases metabolism. Men have more testosterone than women, so the effect of losing it is greater. The effects of this change can be offset somewhat by keeping physically active. See page 402.

Replace smoking or vaping with exercise

Nicotine speeds up your metabolism. However, it harms your body in more ways than it helps. Replace nicotine with exercise to maintain your metabolism after you quit.

Have your medications reviewed

Medications that can slow metabolism include some antidepressants, steroids like prednisone, and high blood pressure pills that slow your heart rate. Insulin use affects fat storage, which then affects metabolism. The reason medications cause weight gain is not always related to your metabolism. Ask for a review of your medications if you've been gaining weight.

LOSE

W **Weigh** yourself: 75% weigh themselves at least once a week.

E **Eat** breakfast: 78% eat breakfast every day.

I **Increase** exercise: 90% walk or do other exercise each day.

G **Go** for less calories: Some eat less fat and others less carbs, but they all cut calories.

H **Have** a support network: Half of the participants get help from a clinic or program.

T **Turn** off the TV: 62% watch less than 10 hours of TV a week.

Knowing what has helped others can help you lose weight too.

National Weight Control Registry

This ongoing American study began in 1994 and is the largest study of its kind. It tracks over 10,000 people who have successfully lost 30 or more pounds and kept the weight off for at least a year. The registry has shown that these are the key things that have helped the participants lose WEIGHT and keep it off.

Prescription medications for weight loss

People with diabetes, especially those who are heavier, may benefit from medications to help lose weight.

It is important to remember that if you take these medications, you still need to eat well and exercise.

Weight loss drugs should be considered long-term medications that you'll take for the rest of your life. Results from these drugs vary and side effects are common.

Some drugs work by blocking fat from being absorbed into your body. One example is orlistat (Xenical).

Other drugs work by reducing appetite or making you feel satisfied with less food. These include liraglutide (Saxenda), an injectable medication, phenterimine-topiramate (Qsymia), naloxone-bupropion (Contrave) and phentermine.

Weight loss surgery

Weight loss surgery is also known as bariatric surgery. As with all major surgeries, it has benefits and risks. Weight loss medications will usually be tried before surgery. Doctors may consider surgery if you are a very heavy person (diagnosed with obesity) and you have been unsuccessful in losing weight. After bariatric surgery, a large amount of weight is usually lost, resulting in a notable improvement in blood sugar levels. There are three different types of operations.

With laparoscopic adjustable gastric banding, a band containing an inflatable balloon restricts the upper part of the stomach. After the surgery, the balloon can be inflated and deflated to adjust the size of the band. This helps people to feel full with very little food.

In Roux-en-Y gastric bypass, the surgeon creates a small pouch at the top of the stomach that greatly limits the amount that you can comfortably eat and drink at one time. The small intestine is cut and connected to the new pouch. You absorb fewer nutrients and calories because food bypasses a portion of the small intestine.

If you have bariatric surgery, you will need lifelong follow-up after the surgery.

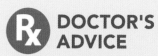

DOCTOR'S ADVICE

Developing new weight loss medications is an area of important research. Doctors are already prescribing these for people who are overweight and have diabetes. The research goal is to find drugs that are more effective with fewer side effects.

Vertical sleeve gastrectomy

In a sleeve gastrectomy, a surgeon separates and removes part of the stomach. The remaining section of the stomach is formed into a small tube-like structure that cannot hold much food. It also produces less of the appetite-regulating hormone ghrelin, which may lessen your desire to eat.

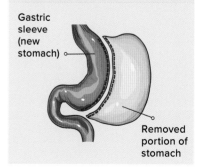

Gastric sleeve (new stomach)

Removed portion of stomach

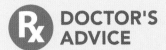

DOCTOR'S ADVICE

Food habits become so normal, we often don't think about what we eat, how much we eat, or the reasons we eat. Once you begin to understand your patterns of eating, you can begin to change them.

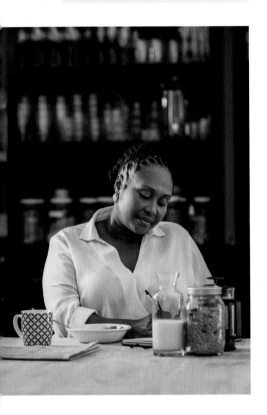

Keep a food record

No matter how much time it will take, write down what you eat and drink each day, for a whole week. Do this once a month, for several months. Our patients tell us that one of the best things about keeping a food record is that it shocks them into realizing their eating habits.

When keeping your food record, count calories of everything you eat and drink for one week, once a month.

- All the meals and portions in this book have the calories counted for you (see page 151).
- Use the Quick Calorie Counter on the next pages for our most common foods.
- To understand how much you're eating, begin by using measuring spoons and cups, a ruler, and a food weigh scale if you have one.
- Count all calories for all added fats and spreads, for example, margarine, peanut butter, gravy and salad dressing.
- Check food labels of packaged foods you eat: they list calories per portions.
- For meals you eat out, check calories per meal on online restaurant menus.

Write down more information:

- What are your emotions when you eat? Bored, happy, upset?
- Where do you eat? On the couch in front of the TV? In bed, in the car?
- What time do you eat? When do you miss meals? When do you overeat?
- When do you exercise?
- How much water do you drink?
- Record your blood sugar before and after your meals
- Weigh yourself at the beginning and end of the week.

After collecting all this information over several months, you will see some patterns in your eating habits. This is the time to consult with your dietitian or diabetes educator. Together you can talk about a few changes that will make a big difference in your calorie intake. Once you feel ready to make more changes, you begin to take real control of your life and your future health. That is the greatest reward.

Quick calorie counter

- Portions are rounded off to 25, 50, 75, 100 and so on to make it easier to add.

- Unless marked, the calories are for the commercial or usual available product, rather than a light, or lighter homemade version. Commercial products vary depending on brand.

- Short forms used: tablespoon = tbsp; teaspoon = tsp; ounce = oz; grams = g.

- Most meat portions are shown in 5-ounce portions, which equals 150 grams.

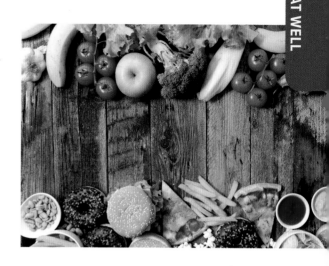

Almonds, 2 tbsp (30 mL)	100
almonds, ½ cup (125 mL)	425
apple, 1 medium	75
applesauce, unsweetened, ½ cup (125 mL)	50
apple juice, unsweetened, 1 cup (250 mL)	125
avocado, ½ medium	100
Bacon, crisp, 2 strips	75
bagel, 6-inch (15 cm)	325
banana, 1 medium	100
bannock, one 3-inch (7.5 cm) piece	200
barley, cooked, ½ cup (125 mL)	100
beans or lentils, cooked, 1 cup (250 mL)	125
beans, canned, baked with tomato sauce, 1 cup (250 mL)	125
beans, kidney, canned, 1 cup (250 mL)	125
beer, regular, Canadian, one 12-oz (355 mL) bottle	175
beer, regular, American, one 12-oz (355 mL) bottle	150
biscuit, tea, 1 medium	250
blueberries, 1 cup (250 mL)	75
bologna, 1 slice (21 g)	50
bread, whole wheat, 1 slice (28 g)	75

bread, white, 1 slice (25 g)	75
bread, 1 thick slice (48 g)	125
bun, hamburger or hotdog bun, 1	125
butter, 1½ tsp (7 mL)	50
Cake, angel food, 1/12 of cake	75
cake, chocolate with icing, 1/12 of cake	200
cake, cheesecake, cherry, 1/12 of cake	325
cappuccino, with whole milk, medium (12 oz/355 mL)	100
carrot, raw, 1 medium	25
cereal, dry, unsweetened, 1 cup (250 mL)	100
cereal, dry, sweetened, 1 cup (250 mL)	150
cereal, granola, commercial, 1 cup (250 mL)	500
cereal, hot, cooked, 1 cup (250 mL)	150
Cheez Whiz, 1 tbsp (15 mL)	50
cheese, Cheddar, 1 oz (30 g)	125
cheese, Cheddar, low fat, 1 oz (30 g)	75
cheese, cottage, 2%, ½ cup (125 mL)	100
cheese, processed, 1 slice (thick)	75
chicken wings, roasted, with skin, 4 wings	400
chicken, baked, breast, no skin, 5 oz (150 g)	225
chicken, deep-fried, drumstick and thigh	500

chili con carne, restaurant, 1¼ cups (300 mL)	300
chocolate bar, standard size, 1 bar (65 g)	275
cinnamon bun, 1 large	500
coffee or tea, black, large	0
coffee, double cream and sugar, large	75
cola, regular, 12-oz (355 mL) can	150
coleslaw, commercial, ½ cup (125 mL)	150
cookies, 2 digestive or 3 graham wafers	75
cookies, chocolate chip, 2 (2½-inch/6 cm)	100
corn on the cob, 1 medium	125
corn, kernel, ½ cup (125 mL)	75
crackers, 4 soda, 2 Breton or 2 melba toast	50
cranberry juice cocktail, regular, 1 cup (250 mL)	125
cranberry juice cocktail, light, 1 cup (250 mL)	50
cream, half and half (cereal cream), 1½ tbsp (22 mL)	25
cream, whipping, whipped, ½ cup (125 mL)	200
croissant, 1 medium	225
Crystal Light beverage, 1 cup (250 mL)	0
Danish pastry, 1	275
donut, cake, 1	200
donut, cream or jelly filled, 1	300
Egg, 1 large	75
English muffin, 1	125
Fish, canned salmon or tuna, ½ can (3½ oz/105 g)	175
fish, fresh, cooked, salmon, 5 oz (150 g)	250
fish, fresh, cooked, white, 5 oz (150 g)	175
french fries, small, with 1 package ketchup	225
french fries, supersize, with 2 packages ketchup	650
fruit, 1 fist-sized	75
fruit, canned in juice, ½ cup (125 mL)	75
Granola bar, single bar	150
grapefruit, half	50

grapes or cherries, 10	50
Ham, cooked, 5 oz (150 g)	250
hamburger with bun, fast food, plain	300
hamburger, equal to a Big Mac size with cheese	700
hash browns, frozen, fried, ½ cup (125 mL)	175
honey, 1 tsp (5 mL)	25
hot chocolate light, 1 cup (250 mL)	50
Ice cream, 1 scoop	125
iced tea, regular, 12-oz (355 mL) bottle	150
Jam, 1½ tsp (7 mL) regular or 1–2 tbsp (15–30 mL) light	25
Jell-O, diet, 1 cup (250 mL)	0
jelly beans, 10	100
Ketchup, 1½ tbsp (22 mL)	25
Lasagna, 4- x 3-inch (10 x 7.5 cm) piece	300
liquor, hard (rye, gin, rum, vodka), 1½ oz (45 mL)	75
Macaroni, plain, cooked, 1 cup (250 mL)	200
macaroni, Kraft Dinner, made per directions, 1 cup (250 mL)	400
macaroni and cheese, homemade, 1 cup (250 mL)	250
milk, skim, 1 cup (250 mL)	100
milk, whole (3.3%), 1 cup (250 mL)	150
milk, chocolate, 2%, 1 cup (250 mL)	200
muffin, commercial, 1 large	400
muffin, homemade, low-fat, 1 small	150
Oil, olive, canola or corn, 1 tbsp (15 mL)	125
olives, small green or black, 4	25
orange, 1 medium	50
orange juice, 1 cup (250 mL)	125
Pancake, 1 small, 4-inch (10 cm)	75
peanut butter, 1 tbsp (15 mL)	100
peanuts (shells removed), ½ cup (125 mL)	450
pie, apple, 2 crusts, ⅛ of a pie (1 piece)	300

pie, apple, 1 piece with 1 scoop ice cream	425
pineapple, 2 rings or ½ cup (125 mL), in juice	75
pizza, thin crust, 2 toppings, 1 piece	300
pizza, thick crust, 2 toppings, 1 piece	400
popcorn, air-popped, 3 cups (750 mL)	100
popcorn, movie-type with butter, large (20 cups/5 L)	1,500
pork chop, cooked, 5 oz (150 g)	300
potato chips, 1 small bag (45 g)	250
potato chips, 1 large bag (300 g)	1,625
potato salad, commercial, ½ cup (125 mL)	200
potato, 1 medium or 1 cup (250 mL) mashed (no butter)	150
potatoes, scalloped, from mix, 1 cup (250 mL)	250
prunes, 2 or ¼ cup (60 mL) prune juice	50
pudding, 2%, regular, ½ cup (125 mL)	150
pudding, skim, no-sugar added, ½ cup (125 mL)	50
Raisins, 2 tbsp (30 mL)	50
ribs, 4 ribs, roasted with sauce	500
rice cake, 1 flavored	50
rice, brown, long-grain, cooked, 1 cup (250 mL)	225
rice, fried, 1 cup (250 mL)	325
rice, white, long-grain, cooked, 1 cup (250 mL)	225
rice, long-grain, instant, cooked, 1 cup (250 mL)	175
Salad dressing, light, 1 tbsp (15 mL)	25
salad dressing, regular, 1 tbsp (15 mL)	75
salad, chef, large, homemade, 2 cups (500 mL)	250
salad, Caesar, restaurant-type, 2 cups (500 mL)	400
salad greens, tossed, 2 cups (500 mL)	25
sandwich, 1 slice of cheese/meat and 2 tsp (10 mL) margarine or butter	350
sausages, breakfast, cooked, 2 links	100
Slushee/Slurpee, small, 12 oz (355 mL)	175
Slushee/Slurpee, jumbo, 40 oz (1.1 L)	550

smoothie, specialty, large, 20 oz (580 mL)	500
smoothie, homemade, low-sugar, skim milk, 1 cup (250 mL)	100
soft drink/soda, 12-oz (355 mL) can	150
soft drink, diet, 12-oz (355 mL) can	0
soup, chicken noodle, ½ 10-oz (284 mL) can with water	100
soup, mushroom, ½ 10-oz (284 mL) can made with milk	150
soup, tomato, ½ 10-oz (284 mL) can made with milk	125
spaghetti sauce, jarred, ½ cup (125 mL)	100
spaghetti, cooked, 1 cup (250 mL)	100
steak, cooked, 5 oz (150 g)	275
strawberries, fresh, 1 cup (250 mL)	50
submarine sandwich, with sauce and toppings, 12-inch (30 cm) sub	1000+
sugar, white or brown, 1½ tsp (7 mL)	25
sweetener, low-calorie, 1 tsp (5 mL)	0
Taco shell or 1 small corn tortilla	50
toast, 1 slice dry (28 g)	75
toast, restaurant, 1 slice buttered	175
tomato juice or vegetable juice, 1 cup (250 mL)	50
tomatoes, canned, 1 cup (250 mL)	75
tortilla, large, 8-inch (20 cm)	175
turkey, light and dark, cooked, 5 oz (150 g)	225
Vegetables such as broccoli, cauliflower, zucchini, cabbage, celery, turnip, tomato, 1 cup (250 mL)	25
vegetables (peas, carrots, beets, or parsnips), ½ cup (125 mL)	50
Waffle, frozen, 1 small (4-inch/10 cm)	100
wine, dry, 4 oz (120 mL)	75
Yogurt, 2%, sweetened, ¾ cup (175 g)	175
yogurt, low-fat, no-sugar added, ¾ cup (175 g)	100
yogurt, Greek, plain, ¾ cup (175 g)	125

Small amounts of extra beverages or foods can cause weight gain when eaten regularly. For example, you could gain 10 pounds (4.5 kg) a year by consuming each week an extra:

- 5 cans of soft drinks, or
- 5 bottles of beer, or
- 2 Big Macs, or
- 2 large servings of fries, or
- 5 scoops of ice cream

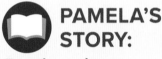 **PAMELA'S STORY:**

Portion sizes matter!

Pamela cooks for her husband and has helped him stick to the small meal plans in *Diabetes Meals for Good Health*:

I had to do it. I put what portions were recommended right on our plates. I dished everything out and went by the measuring spoons and measuring cups. I made up my mind to do it. That's how we cook now. I cooked all the little desserts and stuff. I found that offset not having the seconds. Then there were times when the meals filled us up so nicely that we didn't even need the dessert.

Regular meals and portion control

Enjoy smaller portions

Use smaller plates, smaller glasses and smaller bowls and even smaller spoons. Rather than eating potato chips right out of the bag, portion out your serving into a small bowl and put the rest away. This helps you eat less. The only exception is your water glass and salad bowl — they can be large! Portion out your food servings in the kitchen rather than taking platters of food to the table. If buffets at home or in restaurants lead you to overeat, try to avoid them.

Eat at regular times to control hunger

Develop a routine of eating three meals a day, at regular times, to reduce hunger. You may want to have your dinner at noon and your lunch in the evening. If you get a little hungry, this is your body telling you that you are short of calories and that it will start using up some of your stored fat. Good for you! You want to burn fat.

Eat slowly

Your brain needs time to know that you are full. Chew your food well, especially your first few bites. This sets the pace. Put down your fork between bites. Drink water during your meal.

Put down your phone and turn off the TV when eating

Research shows that we eat more while watching TV. We don't pay attention to how much we eat or that we are full.

Meal plans show you the way

See pages 149–200 and the 70 additional meal plans in *Diabetes Meals for Good Health Cookbook* (see page 416). Choose from the wide variety of favorite meals and snacks. Depending on your calorie needs, choose either the large or small meals. These meal plans include protein and lots of fiber, which keeps you going until the next meal or snack. When you eat more fruit and vegetables and drink more water, you feel more satisfied. You'll start to lose weight, and feel proud of your efforts. Now you'll be able to focus on healthy living, not dieting.

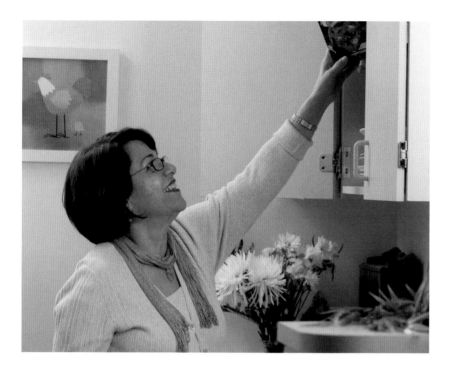

Consider giving yourself a "treat budget"
Keep track of how many treats you eat each week. This might include chips, chocolates, candy, donuts, ice cream, french fries, pie and so on. Then, allow yourself one or two portions a week. It doesn't mean you have to eat them! Sometimes just knowing it's allowed in your budget makes it easier to make it through the week.

Out of sight, out of mind

Put away tempting foods — or better yet, don't buy them. Instead, put low-calorie foods, such as fruits and vegetables, in easy to find places.

What is your weakness? White bread, sweet beverages, beer, potato chips, peanuts, cookies, ice cream or chocolates? Even apparently healthy choices, such as "100-calorie snack packs" become danger foods if you eat all the snack packages in the box. Avoid buying your "danger" foods.

Grocery shop with a list
- Don't shop when you're hungry.
- Only buy what you need.
- Stay away from the most tempting aisles.
- Don't linger near the bakery.
- Say no to buying chocolate bars at the checkout line.

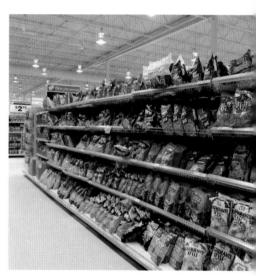

When shopping, stay away from chips and soft drinks. The more you buy, the more you eat.

Pages 260–261 shows you many other practical ways to deal with cravings.

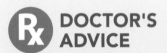

DOCTOR'S ADVICE

Mistakes happen

Don't beat yourself up. These aren't easy changes. Sometimes you'll get fed up, feel anxious or even angry. Get back to your healthy pattern as soon as you can. Try to understand what led to the slip. See if you can prevent it or manage it better next time. Imagine the situation happening again, and plan ahead. How will you react and deal with it differently? If needed, talk to a friend or professional for support.

Conquer your cravings

Most people have experienced cravings and compulsive eating at one time or another. "I meant to eat one piece of chocolate. Before I knew it, I'd eaten the whole box."

What causes cravings?

Sometimes you're hungry. Sometimes you see or smell things which will make your mouth water and make you feel hungry, even if you just ate. For example, ads of luscious looking food, seeing food in the store or on the counter can trigger cravings. How we feel can set off cravings. Are you happy, sad, angry, tired, lonely or bored?

The Four Ds of dealing with cravings

1. **Delay.** Count to ten.

2. **Deeply breathe.** Take a few breaths!

3. **Drink water.** Have a large glass.

4. **Distract yourself.** Go do something else. Eating isn't the only thing in the world to do.

Establish a stop-eating routine

- Eat meals and snacks at about the same time.
- Consider a "no eating" rule in the evening after you're finished eating dinner.
- Try to eat at the same place for each meal, whether you are home or at work. The kitchen table or dining room is the old-fashioned place to eat, and it works! Slowly you will stop associating the couch, the computer, the bedroom, or the car as places to eat.
- After a meal or snack, rinse out your mouth well. A good way to end the eating after your supper or an evening snack is to brush your teeth or dentures and floss your teeth.
- Take a shower or bath to relax yourself for a good night's sleep. Adequate sleep is important for weight loss.

Of course, sometimes you'll overeat. That's okay, but start the next day with a healthy breakfast. Get right back to your healthy pattern, including practicing the Four Ds.

Home cooking can pay off

Homemade meals, as shown in our books, are easy, save money and can be made with healthy ingredients. You can cook a homemade meal in less time than it takes to go to a restaurant. You can freeze leftovers to eat another time. This is "fast food" at home!

Studies show that families that eat together at home are both physically and emotionally healthier. Fast food restaurants and meals-on-the-run are rushed. These kinds of meals don't give families enough chances to learn to cook or talk together.

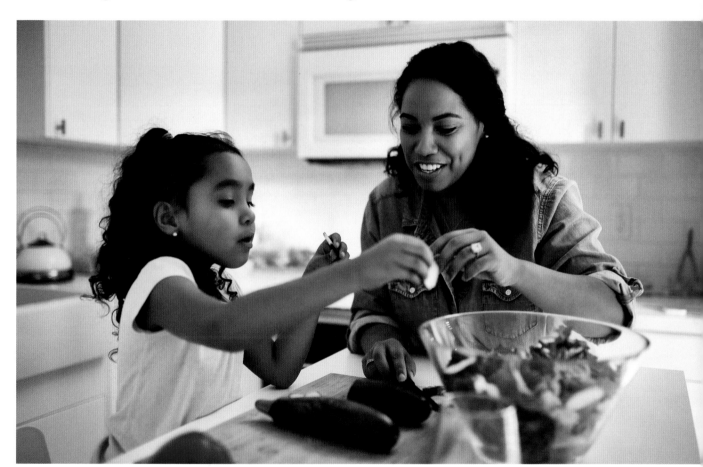

Eat out less often

The most important thing to change about eating in restaurants is to not eat in restaurants, or at least, not very often. North Americans consume almost a third of their food budget outside of home. If you eat in a restaurant daily, consider cutting back to one or two times a week. If you eat out once a week, try to cut it back to once or twice a month. Studies show that taste influences us more than health. In other words, in a restaurant with many good things to choose from the menu, we quickly lose our willpower.

Adult baby food

Fast food restaurants serve addictive soft, processed hamburgers, with fries and large glasses of soft drinks. These are low-fiber foods that require little chewing, so they can be gulped down quickly in large amounts.

Layers of food

Restaurants layer fatty or sugary foods on top of each other. This means that the height of the food, whether it is a burger, sub, dessert or cappuccino, grows and gets more mouth-watering.

Giving you more

Some restaurants constantly refill your basket of buns or bread, or refill your sweet beverages. Even before your meal comes, you will have overeaten on carbs and calories. This way of eating excessive calories in a short time is a cause of weight gain and poor health.

When you do eat out, eat sensibly

Plan ahead where and when you are going to eat. Look at a restaurant's menu online. Choose a restaurant that has some healthier food choices that you like. Restaurants with salad options or meal choices that aren't fried are good. Try to eat within an hour or two of your regular meal time so you're not too hungry. Try to choose a meal that fits into your approximate calorie range. For example, if you normally choose large dinner meals as shown in this book, then look for meals of 700 to 750 calories. Knowing what you want to order when you arrive at the restaurant means you won't have to look at the menu, where browsing can tempt you to order more.

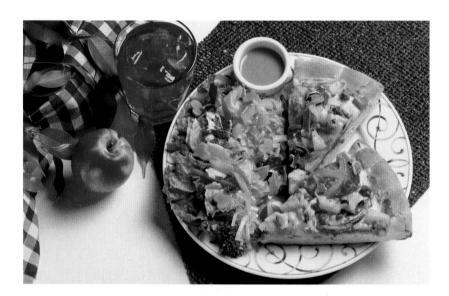

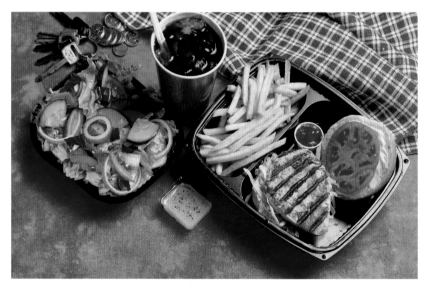

In the *Diabetes Meals for Good Health Cookbook* (see page 416), there are restaurant meal examples for breakfast, lunch and dinner.

Don't go to the restaurant hungry. If you have a chance, before you go to a restaurant have a small snack. Have a fruit, some carrot sticks, 5 to 10 pecans or almonds, or a few crackers with cheese. Then, you won't be so tempted to over order and overeat when you arrive at the restaurant.

Order less. You will eat less! Order smaller meals and avoid supersizing and extras. Instead of calorie-packed "meal deals," order single items, senior meals, junior portions or half-size meals. Or share an order of fries or a dessert; you'll save calories as well as cash. If the meal entrée choices look large, order a salad or soup with a small appetizer instead. Order a smaller steak than you would have in the past. We'd all love to eat more, but we just don't need to.

Take extra care at buffets. Very few people can resist the temptation to overload their plate at buffets. Even salad buffets include "unhealthy choices" that might mysteriously end up on your plate and in your stomach. Try to stick to this buffet rule: go through the line only once. Choose smaller amounts all along the way.

Ask the restaurant to bag it. One large restaurant meal may be enough for two dinners. Solve your problem of what to have for dinner the next day!

Avoid these high-calorie choices, in large or supersized portions:

- french fries
- onion rings
- milkshakes
- burgers
- donuts or muffins
- sweet and creamy coffee beverages

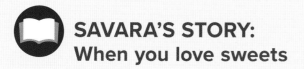

SAVARA'S STORY: When you love sweets

Savara talks about the challenges for her husband and herself when they eat out at buffets:

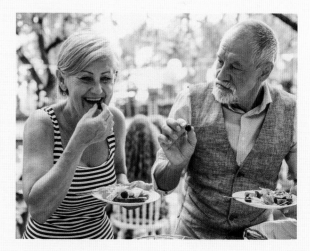

When my husband was diagnosed with diabetes, for the first six months he was not a happy camper. He loved his desserts and, especially at buffets, he'd try them all. But once he cut back on sugary foods, he didn't crave them as much. He was a chocolate cake man, but now he can go by a piece of chocolate cake, and he says nay. When we go to a buffet, we try and eat healthy salads and stuff. He'll look for the reduced-sugar desserts, and he'll have one once in awhile. He eats a lot of fruit. At salad bars, we just hold the dressings, hold everything. I find we're not overeating the way we used to, and we can feel it. If we overeat we don't feel so good, and the next day we go back to our regular habits and we feel a lot better.

Misleading size of bagels and muffins

A 6-inch (15 cm) restaurant bagel is equal to four slices of bread. Low-fat muffins are often so large that they have significant amounts of calories, fat and sugar.

High-fat salads

A Caesar salad with dressing on it can have as many calories as a hamburger and fries. Mayonnaise-laden salads like potato salads and coleslaw are also high in fat and calories. Ask for your low-fat dressing on the side.

Ask for substitutions.

- For breakfast, choose fruit salad or a small glass of tomato or fruit juice instead of hash browns. Ask for a poached or boiled egg instead of fried egg; ham instead of bacon or sausages, and toast (hold the butter) instead of a Danish or large bagel.
- With sandwiches, request bread or toast without butter. Mayonnaise is often added to the fillings so you don't need to double up on the spreads — "one spread per bread."
- Eat a submarine sandwich with no mayonnaise. Have a little mustard instead.
- Drink diet instead of regular soft drinks.
- Try a small serving of low-fat milk instead of a regular soft drink, milkshake or smoothie.
- Order a single hamburger instead of the "meal deal" larger burger.
- Consider getting small fries instead of large fries. Often a baked potato with butter and sour cream on the side, or mashed potatoes or rice are a lighter choice than fries, even though they usually have some fat added.

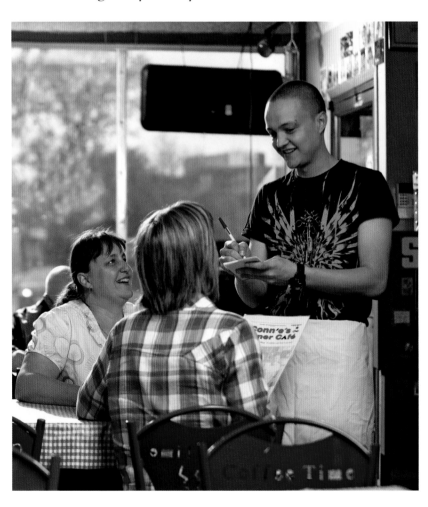

- Get a double order of steamed vegetables without butter. Choose broth-based vegetable soup. Ask for a plain bun, instead of fries or garlic bread.
- Order a green or tossed salad. Ask for some grilled chicken on top and a bun on the side. Try squeezed lemon on the salad instead of dressing.
- Ask for salad dressings, sauces, gravies and butter, "on the side."
- Try plain rice instead of fried rice, a burrito instead of a deep-fried taco shell, or a vegetable stir fry instead of deep-fried foods.
- Choose baked or grilled meat, chicken or fish instead of fried, deep-fried or crispy.
- A thin crust pizza is healthier than a thick crust pizza as long as you don't eat an extra piece because it is "thin." Try it topped with more vegetables. Skip fatty meats and extra cheese.
- Instead of a donut, muffin or Danish with a fancy coffee drink, have two or three donut bites ("holes") and hot or iced coffee or frothy cappuccino made with low-fat milk.

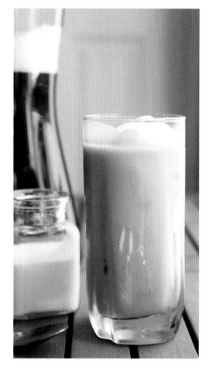

Try a low-fat milk iced coffee with low-calorie sweetener.

Ask for water with your meal, and drink it. Limit alcohol. Alcohol has lots of calories and, when you drink it, you are less likely to care about how much you overeat. Just a few cocktails can add 300 to 600 calories before you even start your meal. If you want to order a drink, consider a glass of dry wine or a light beer. If ordering a mixed drink, choose a diet beverage with it. If you choose to have a nonalcoholic drink, order a diet soft drink, carbonated water or mineral water with lemon.

Consider skipping dessert — except on your own birthday! At other times, if you're craving dessert, a lighter option is one scoop of ice cream, sorbet or ice milk, or to share a dessert. Drinking a coffee or tea after a meal can be an alternative to dessert.

After your restaurant meal, go for a walk. This is especially important if you ate too much.

Birthday parties

Do you have a large family with many birthday meal celebrations? This can be a challenge when you have diabetes as the calories and sugar add up. Could you or your family provide some healthier treats? See pages 77 and 78 for some options to cake.

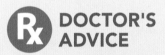

DOCTOR'S ADVICE

Are you taking rapid-acting insulin?

If you are on a flexible insulin regime, you can take extra insulin for extra food. This works for a special day. But if you overeat many times over days or weeks, the extra insulin and food will result in a weight gain.

A Plan for Special Occasions

Celebrate holidays while limiting your eating

We celebrate as many holidays across North America as our diverse ethnic origins. No matter which holidays you and your family celebrate, here are some tips for containing the excess around food.

Holiday food: Is it too much of a good thing?

Most holidays now include homemade "traditional" foods supplemented with store-bought "celebration" foods, often candies and chocolates. Have you noticed how Christmas goodies begin to line the shelves in October and early November? February shelves burst with chocolates for Valentines and even Easter, still two months away. An Easter bunny in the 1970s was the size of your hand, and now it stands a foot tall. If you buy Halloween candy in September, it's all gone by the time October 31 rolls around — so you buy more! Any leftover "celebration" foods from Halloween, Thanksgiving, Ramadan, Nowruz, Hanukkah, Christmas, Super Bowl, Diwali, Chinese New Year, Mardi Gras, Easter or other celebrations can tempt us for many days or weeks until we have eaten them all.

Holiday weight gain can become a diabetes emergency.

An occasional indulgence or large meal causes a temporary blood sugar peak, but is manageable. However, weeks of overindulgence and inactivity can lead to serious blood sugar and weight gain. On average, North American men gain 3 to 5 pounds (1.5 to 2.5 kg) over December, and women gain 2 to 3 pounds (1 to 1.5 kg). That's a lot more than one turkey dinner. Gaining 3 pounds (1.5 kg) equals an extra 10,500 calories. Many doctors consider a sudden 5-pound weight gain a diabetes and health emergency. You need to lose these extra holiday pounds over the next month. Otherwise, the pounds build up, year after year, worsening diabetes.

Fight the holiday food frenzy

1. **Delay.** Wait one or two days before the holiday begins to bring out the holiday food, or offer special foods just on that day. Shop and bake less, so you eat fewer holiday goodies.

2. **Start a new tradition.** Adapt your traditional holiday dessert recipes to make them healthier. See pages 104–105.

3. **Have regular meals.** You may be tempted to skip breakfast and lunch the day of a big family meal and gathering. Unfortunately, this often backfires. You end up too hungry, and eat too much. Eat regular meals, and have a piece of fruit to take the edge off your appetite before the big meal.

4. **Plan for your favorites.** Unless you have super-human willpower, don't plan on going without your favorites. Going without might make you feel deprived, and lead to overindulgence later. Go for one or two of your favorites, in a moderate portion.

5. **Limit the alcohol.** Drinking alcohol piles on calories and makes you more likely to say yes to the extra foods. Have a lighter drink or drinks totalling less than 100 to 150 calories chosen from the list on page 137. Try soda with lemon or a touch of cranberry juice and lime.

6. **Smaller plates work.** We eat more when people serve food on large dishes. For example, if the turkey is on a big platter we take more. If the gravy is in a large gravy boat we pour more on our potatoes. If the host serves us from a small plate, we politely take less. If you are at a buffet, take a lunch plate rather than a larger dinner plate. This will automatically decrease your portion sizes.

7. **Festive fitness.** Exercise is a healthy way to help cope with holiday stress. Plan ahead with your family to go for a walk after a holiday meal to burn off some extra calories you have eaten. Family members of all ages will have a hand to hold on your family walk.

Instead of offering a tray of cakes and sweets, offer:
- A vegetable or fruit plate with low-fat dip
- Shrimp with sauce
- Smoked salmon or oysters on crackers
- Sushi or vegetable-filled rice paper rolls
- Bowl of lightly salted popcorn popped in just a teaspoon of oil
- Crackers and cheese
- Olives and pickles
- Baked tortilla chips with salsa
- Sugar-free drinks

Do you feel pressure from family?
Rehearse how to politely say "no thanks." It's not easy to say no, but with practice it gets easier.

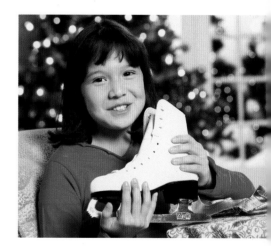

Give the gift of good health!

Manage workplace temptations

At your workplace, do you have junk food tucked in your desk drawer? Are there food and goodies sitting out in common areas, or at coffee breaks or during meetings?

Once you've removed your junk food, talk to your coworkers. How many really want food constantly tempting them? If it's only a few people in the office, perhaps they might consider keeping extra food out of sight.

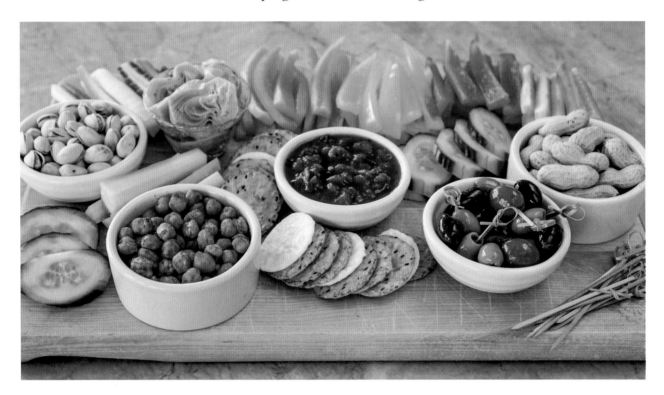

Choose healthier snacks or meals at meetings
- Fresh fruit trays with yogurt dip
- Raw vegetable trays
- Small muffins ($2\frac{1}{2}$-inch/6 cm or smaller)
- Sandwiches on plain whole-grain breads and made with less butter and filling
- Assortment of whole-grain crackers, rice crackers and small chunks of low-fat cheese
- Vegetable-based soups
- Sushi or spring rolls that aren't fried
- Smaller serving sizes of desserts
- Water jug and glasses with ice
- Coffee and tea with low-fat milk

Walk during coffee or lunch breaks

"Coffee breaks" were introduced in the 1940s for North American production line workers. These workers stood on their feet all day, so they were given a break to sit down. Yet today, many of us have an office job where we already sit down most of the day! Now we need to get up, stand, stretch and go for a 15-minute walk. Ask a coworker to join you for a walk-and-talk. You may find you can even give up a coffee on these breaks, and replace it with water.

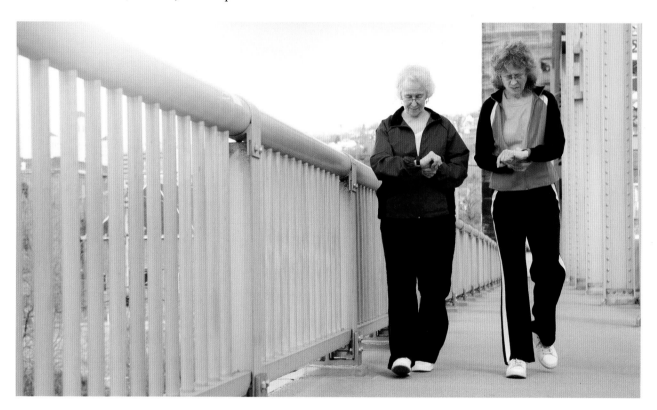

 JODY'S STORY: Build exercise into your work life

At work we have this thing called the Fit Wit: Fitness Wellness Initiative Team. We started using pedometers and having challenges. That was over a year ago. Now I know what it takes to walk at least 10,000 steps a day. I'm learning more about nutrition, and exercise. I'm just walking, and doing portion control with my meals. Just those two things can change your life. That gets me excited. When you see positive changes happening, it feels really good, and you want to keep doing it. You want other people to get involved too. If you've got information for them, it helps so much. Many people at work are doing things that they never did before — like taking the stairs instead of the elevator. We're in a four-story building. We have stair climb challenges regularly, where you mark off your flights. It's excellent, it's a team building thing. I haven't taken an elevator since we started. I'm just so happy about it. And I was someone who never really exercised before.

Carry essential eating utensils:

- A paring knife or pocket knife
- Your own cutlery
- A few reusable cups, bowls and plates

Seeds and nuts

A 1-cup (250 mL) serving of sunflower seeds with the shells on equals ⅓ cup (75 mL) of sunflower seeds without the shells. Each of these servings equals 240 calories.

Beware: 1 cup (250 mL) of ready-to-eat shelled nuts or sunflower seeds or trail mix, has about 700 to 800 calories!

Travel and still stay on track

If you enjoy recreational travel, or have to travel for work, here are some ideas to help you stay on track.

Make wise restaurant choices

Big meals mean big blood sugars! Try to choose smaller meals and space the meals out throughout your day.

Carry healthy foods in your vehicle.

- Have water or diet beverages handy. Forget the sweet drinks, desserts and junk foods.
- Pack an insulated bag with fresh fruit, raw ready-to-eat vegetables (such as carrots, celery sticks or edible snap peas), hard-boiled eggs, cheese slices, cheese strings or small containers of yogurt.
- Stop at a grocery store instead of sitting down at a restaurant. Buy buns and meat or sliced cheese and cucumbers to make a meal.
- For breakfast on the road, bring along small plastic containers that you have prefilled with unsweetened cereals or plain oatmeal and add milk. These are then ready-to-eat with a spoon. For oatmeal, add milk or yogurt to uncooked oats and let it sit overnight in your hotel room fridge. Top with nuts or fruit in the morning.
- Examples of easy travel meals or snacks:
  - A peanut butter or cheese sandwich
  - A can of tuna or salmon for a sandwich
  - Hard-boiled eggs with cherry tomatoes and sweet peppers
  - Cheese and crackers
  - Small package of almonds
  - Fresh fruit, packaged puddings or a few high-protein granola bars
- Most RVs or long-distance trucks have a fridge and freezer and microwave in the vehicle. You can heat up frozen leftovers brought from home or a frozen meal. A 700-calorie meal equals a large dinner from this book.

• When you are driving or trucking with a deadline, it can be hard to find time to stop regularly. Yet if you go too long without eating, you may get too hungry. Then you may overeat when you get to that all-you-can-eat buffet or restaurant. Try to have a couple of shorter stops, rather than one longer stop. This will give you the chance to eat meals at consistent times.

All-inclusive vacation and cruises

These vacations are not ideal for people with diabetes. The "free" food and drink is a temptation to overeat and over-drink because everyone else is doing it. While fun, these vacations can throw off your weight and blood sugar, and you'll be 5 pounds (2.5 kg) heavier when you return home. Remember, a weight gain like that, if not taken off soon afterward, can be considered a diabetes emergency. Remember the buffet rule: only go through the line once. Choose smaller amounts all along the way.

Exercise when traveling

When driving and you stop for gas, a coffee or meal, take an extra 10 minutes to walk briskly around the parking area. Long periods of sitting cause blood sugar to rise. Blood and fluid pool in your lower legs and feet. It's amazing how even 10 minutes of exercise can lower your blood sugar and improve your circulation. These short exercise breaks burn calories and give your back a break. Longer walks are even better.

When flying, get up and walk the aisles or do ankle rotations on long flights for better circulation to your feet. Between flights, walk in the airport.

When on holiday, bring along a bathing suit or pair of shorts and T-shirt. Stay at a hotel with a fitness room. Choose types of holidays that encourage walking and outdoor activity. Warm weather vacations provide an opportunity to do lots of walking, swimming and other exercise. Have fun!

 CAUTION

Low blood sugar can cause you to be confused or even pass out. This is dangerous if you are driving, for you and other drivers and pedestrians. Read page 336 for low blood sugar safety guidelines.

High blood sugar can also be dangerous, as it can make you feel tired and less alert.

If you are on diabetes or heart medication, talk to your diabetes educator or doctor about adjusting your medications if flying through one or more time zones.

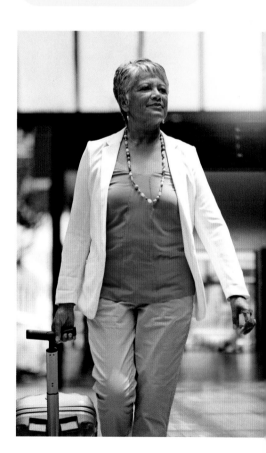

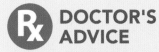

DOCTOR'S ADVICE

What's the secret to getting fit? Take time to do it. Every little bit counts. The goal is to do at least 150 minutes of aerobic exercise each week. That means at least 20 minutes of exercise such as walking each day.

Try not to use exercise as a reason to eat more. Have you ever said to yourself, "I went for a walk so I can eat a second helping." That defeats the purpose of the walk.

Keep moving

Open the front door, not the fridge door. Make exercise a part of your daily life. If you have kids, get active outdoors with your kids. Indoors, walk up and down stairs and hallways, dance, or use your stationary bike or treadmill. Start with 5 minutes of continuous exercise and work up to 15 to 30 minutes or more a day. Watch less TV — those cooking shows and ads make you hungry. Screen time takes away from time spent moving around and being active. When your weight plateaus, or levels off, and you don't seem to lose any more weight, doing more exercise is crucial to boost your metabolism and help you burn extra calories.

Walking gives you energy

Studies show that people are more productive at work and home with exercise breaks. If you get into work early, try a short walk first thing in the morning, or go for a walk at lunch or in the evening. Your daily walk will be a great start to feeling fit and taking off a few pounds.

Many of us live busy lives. It's difficult to make health a priority. Yet exercising your body will give you more energy for everything else in your life.

DOROTHY'S STORY: How her dog motivates her

I am a widow from Thunder Bay, in northern Canada. I experienced a terrible loss and, at that time, I turned to food for comfort. I gained over 30 pounds (13.5 kg). I was introduced to the Diabetes Meals for Good Health Cookbook, *and it became like a bible to me. As of today, I have lost this weight and my blood levels are normal. I am keeping the weight off with the help of healthy eating, drinking my water and exercises. I have a dog now and we walk every day; I dress for every kind of weather. I am much happier and able to move on with my life.*

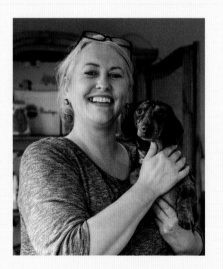

Hang out with healthy eaters

Do you have friends and family who encourage you to overeat with them? This can be a challenge. Surprisingly, when you start making positive lifestyle changes, it can rub off on those around you. Look for a support group or support persons who can provide positive reinforcement for your good efforts. Even finding one new friend or support outside of your usual circle of friends or families can make a big difference.

Studies show that your eating companions make a difference. If your family tends to eat a lot, that encourages you to be a big eater. Men eat more when eating with their male friends than they do when eating with a spouse or girlfriend. Women often try and "outdo" each other at parties and get-togethers, which encourages overeating. Some people eat alone. Some look for companionship while eating. When you are trying to cut back on food, changing the company you keep may help.

There is strength in unity. Having others in your home or in your community participate with diet and exercise changes will give all of you positive benefits.

Believe in yourself and your ability to make changes.

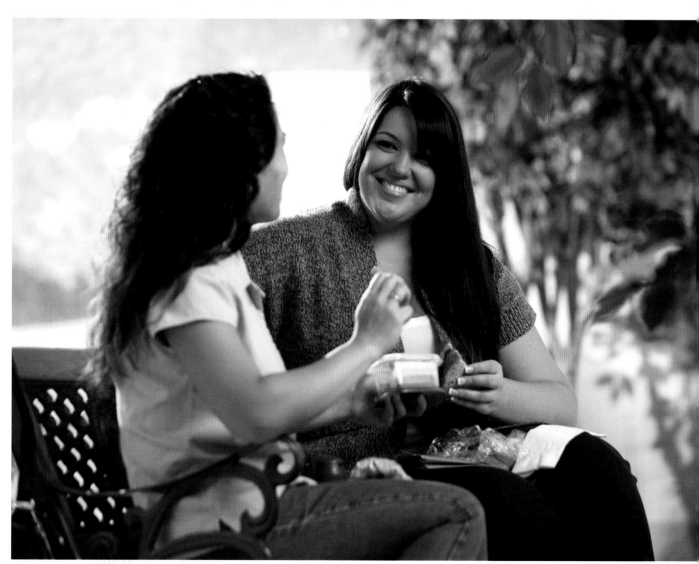

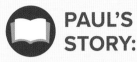

PAUL'S STORY:

Phone supports helped

My health insurance company has a counselor who calls every three months since the doctor diagnosed me with diabetes. It's very helpful. The nurse answers any questions I have about my blood sugars and my food and diet, too. It helps because it's positive reinforcement.

Join the team

Guidance and "cheerleaders" are essential for us all

You may benefit from sharing your commitment for change with others. Your journey of weight loss and diabetes management is lifelong. Developing a support team is important. This gives you motivation to keep on track and rewards you for your hard work and progress.

You choose your team. Visiting or communicating by phone, email or text with a dietitian, an insurance nurse, a diabetes educator or a doctor on a regular basis acts as important incentive to keep on track. They can help you monitor your weight, blood pressure or lab test results. A friend, family member, coworker, a walking buddy or an online or in-person support group, such as a weight loss support group, can also help. Search out an online weight support or diabetes group. Key search words are "weight loss support."

Make one change at a time. With each change, you'll move closer to your goals.

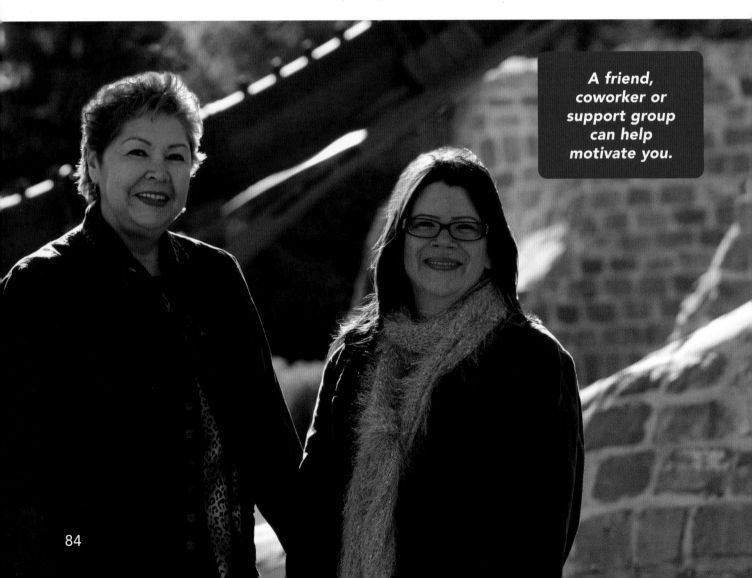

A friend, coworker or support group can help motivate you.

2. Carbohydrates and Your Blood Sugar

This section explains how different carbohydrates affect your blood sugar. Carbohydrates (carbs) come from starches, sugars and desserts, fruits, milk and vegetables.

On pages 85–89, you'll learn how eating less table sugar, sweet drinks and rich desserts will reduce excess carbs — and will reduce your blood sugar.

Starches, vegetables, fruits and milks are essential parts of a healthy diet. On pages 90–93, you'll learn about carbohydrate foods that have a low glycemic index. These raise blood sugar more slowly.

Limit sugar and sweet drinks

Added table sugar, sweet drinks, desserts and candies quickly turn into blood sugar. Fruit juice does have vitamins but is a liquid form of fruit sugar, and also needs to be limited.

When you eat a lot of sweet foods and drinks, your pancreas can't release enough insulin. Your blood sugar can be high for several hours.

Table sugar

- White or brown sugar, honey, corn syrup or maple syrup, jam and jelly are all forms of sugar.
- Eating a *small* amount of added sugar at some meals or snacks is acceptable. Only eat 1 to 2 teaspoons (5–10 mL), or what would fit in the end of your thumb.

Rule of thumb:
At each meal, limit added table sugar, honey or jams to an amount that would fit in the end of your thumb.

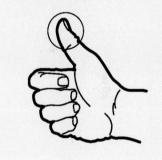

Words that mean sugar on food labels			
• cane sugar	• fruit juice	• honey	• sorghum
• corn sugar	concentrate	• maltose	syrup
• corn syrup	• glucose	• maple syrup	• sucrose
• dextrose	• high-fructose	• molasses	• sugar
	corn syrup		• syrup

Sorbitol, mannitol and xylitol are types of sweeteners used in some diet products. These raise your blood sugar just half as much as regular sugar.

Limit or avoid these sugary foods

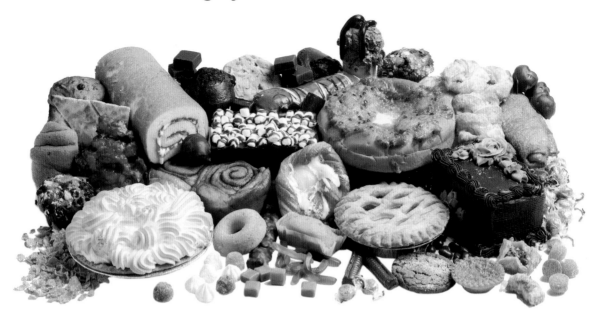

Remember, mega-sized desserts and muffins are extra high in sugar and fat.

Choose the light desserts shown in the meal section of this book and in the other two books in this *Health & Wellness Series* (see page 416).

Also see pages 100–105 for ideas on adapting recipes.

Limit or avoid these sweet drinks and juices

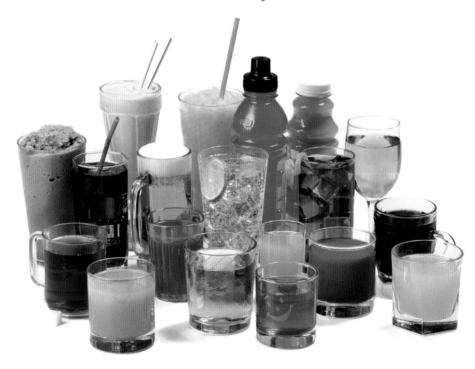

Skip the regular soft drinks

Each North American drinks about 26.5 gallons or 100 liters of soft drinks each year. That's equal to 42,800 calories per person. It takes about 3,500 extra calories to gain a pound (0.5 kg) of weight. This amount of soda can contribute to gaining more than 10 lbs (4.5 kg) in a year.

Portions are larger today.
In the 1960s, a 6-oz (175 mL) cola was the most common soft drink. This used to be an occasional special treat. The 32-oz (1 L) size is a common portion today. These are "empty calories" — sugar with no good nutrition.

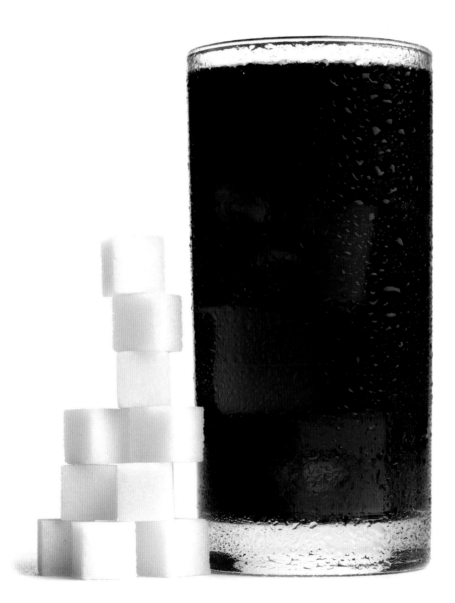

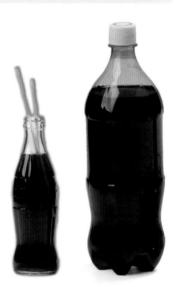

6-oz (175 mL) cola	32-oz (1 L) cola
4½ tsp (22 mL) of sugar	25 tsp (125 mL) of sugar
80 calories	430 calories

Every time you drink a 12-oz (355 mL) can of soda, you get **10 tsp (50 mL) of sugar** that you don't need.

Unsweetened juices have a lot of sugar

You may be surprised to learn that a 12-oz (355 mL) glass of unsweetened orange juice has the same sugar as a cola (10 tsp/50 mL of sugar). Apple juice has even more. Large bottles of juice make your blood sugar go up quickly.

Juice does have vitamin C and other nutrients from fruit, but you should have only a small glass (4 oz/120 mL of apple, orange or cranberry juice, or 2 oz/60 mL of grape or prune juice). Have this small glassful only occasionally (and not more than once a day) or replace all juice with water and fresh fruit. When thirsty, choose water, diet beverages, diet iced tea, sugar-free drink mixes, or unsweetened tea or coffee instead.

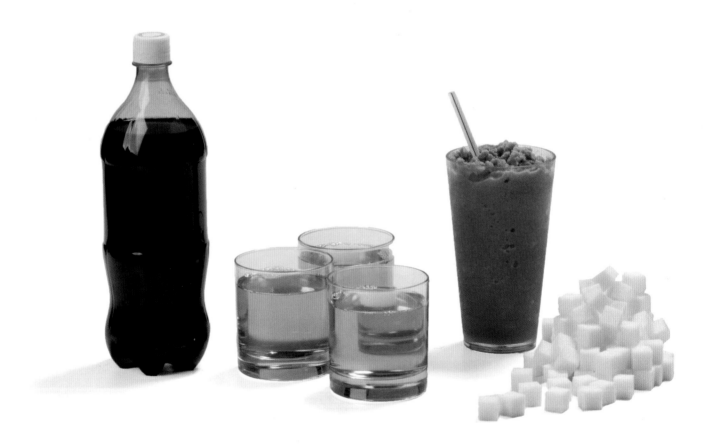

One 32-oz (1 L) bottle of cola, three 8-oz (250 mL) glasses of unsweetened apple juice and a 16-oz (475 mL) iced cappuccino. In these beverages, there are 60 teaspoons of sugar or 1,200 calories. This equals 240 grams of carbohydrates.

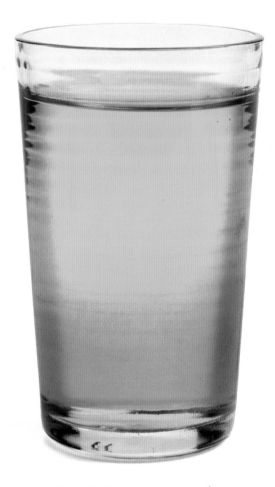

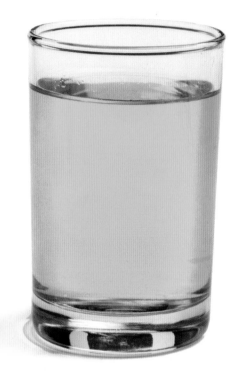

12 oz (355 mL) — too much!

4 oz (120 mL)

Every time you drink a 12-oz (355 mL) glass of unsweetened juice, you get 10 or more teaspoons (40 grams) of sugar that you don't need. Choose only the small glass on the right and count it as a fruit serving. Better yet, choose a fresh fruit and get all the benefit of fiber.

This larger glass of apple juice has the equivalent of three or four apples' worth of sugar. You wouldn't eat this many apples at once, but it's easy to drink that much sugar in one glass of juice.

Don't be fooled into thinking that juices with herbs or other products added are healthier. They still have the same amount of sugar as regular juice.

89

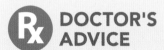

DOCTOR'S ADVICE

To determine if a food causes a sustained blood sugar spike, you need to measure your blood sugar both before you eat and two hours after you eat. Wearing a continuous glucose monitor (see pages 342–343) is a way to assess your blood sugar on a frequent basis.

Ways to slow down carbohydrate absorption

Control your portions.
Use the meal plans on pages 149–200 as a guide.

Divide your carbohydrates throughout the day.
Choose three meals a day and snacks in moderation, if needed.

Eat less of quickly absorbed carbohydrates.
This means eating less table sugar, sweet drinks, juices, desserts and sweets. Also limit any food that you have found causes a spike or a sustained rise in your blood sugar when you check your blood at home.

At a meal or large snack, include some protein or fat with your carbohydrate.
For instance, if you have crackers with cheese, the protein in the cheese slows down the absorption of the carbohydrate in the crackers. The carbohydrates will be absorbed more slowly than if you ate the crackers on their own.

Choose low glycemic index carbohydrates daily.
Keep reading to learn more information about this.

Glycemic index (GI)
Glycemic index is a rating of how quickly a carbohydrate food raises your blood sugar. We call this GI for short. Low GI foods raise your blood sugar slowly so are good choices. **See photo on opposite page.**

Eat slowly.
This slows down the absorption of your carbohydrates.

Go for a walk half an hour to an hour after eating.
This uses up blood sugar from the food you just ate.

Certain diabetes medications help.
Insulin and some medicines can help reduce blood sugar rise that happens after you eat. See pages 307–328.

Low GI carbohydrates — choose these!

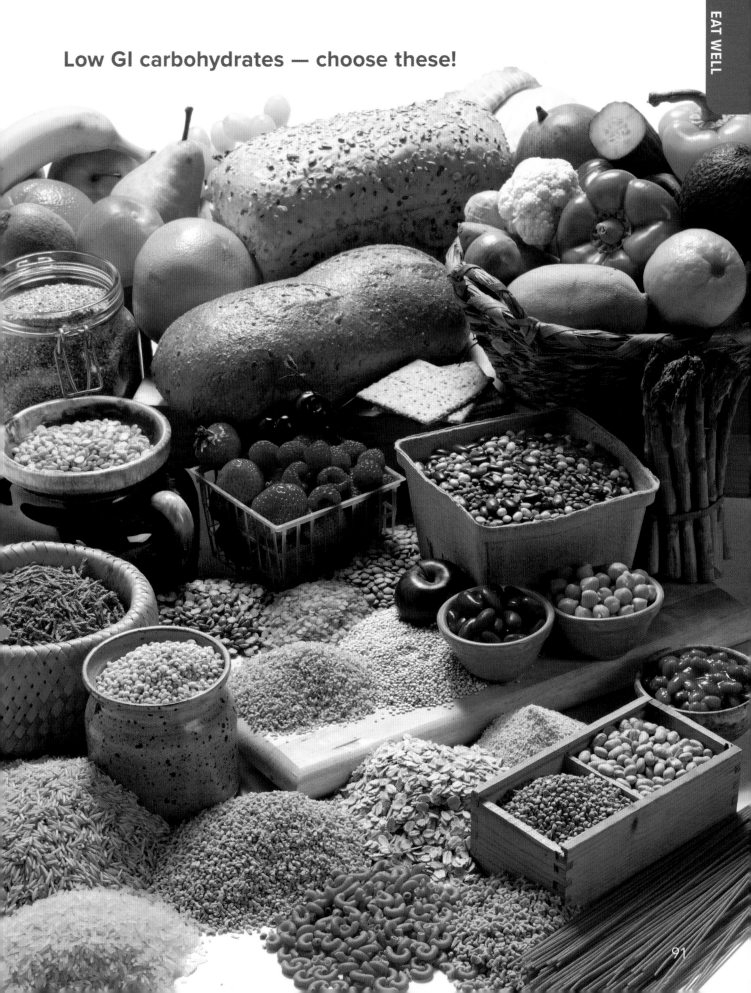

Inulin is a type of soluble fiber

Inulin — not to be confused with insulin — is added to some food products to increase their fiber.

One of the main sources of inulin used by food manufacturers is chicory root. Try chicory coffee as a change from regular coffee! Other sources of inulin are onions garlic, asparagus, bananas, dandelion roots and Jerusalem artichokes. Note: Inulin in large amounts, as with all fiber, can cause some bloating and gas. To avoid or limit this, add inulin products gradually to your diet.

A food that has a low GI ingredient doesn't mean the food will be low GI. For example, a granola bar made with oats and barley could have a lot of sugar added to it. This raises its glycemic index.

What makes a carbohydrate low GI?

Lots of fiber helps make a carbohydrate food low on the glycemic index. There are two main types of fiber.

- **Insoluble fiber** is in whole wheat, grains, fruits and vegetables. These foods have acids, such as phytic acid, that help slow down the absorption of carbohydrates. Phytic acid is also found in some foods high in soluble fiber, such as beans and lentils.
- **Soluble fiber** is in oatmeal, barley, chickpeas and lentils, beans, and some fruits and vegetables. These fibers grab on to carbohydrates, slowing down their absorption. They also remove some cholesterol from the body.
- Look for food products with more fiber listed on the label.
- Have cooked barley or quinoa instead of potato or rice for a change.
- Choose thin slices of rye, whole wheat or whole-grain bread (about 30 grams or 70 calories per slice).

Tartness or acidity: In addition to the acid in high-fiber foods, other acids that slow down the absorption of carbohydrates include lemon or vinegar, or tannins such as in tea.

- Enjoy a cup of tea with your meal.
- Add lemon or vinegar on your vegetables (instead of added fat). Lemon is also nice on fish and in tea.
- Try vinegar and dill added to canned beets or sliced cucumbers for a low salt pickle.

Less processing: Blood sugar spikes less when the carbohydrate is raw versus cooked, lightly cooked as compared to overcooked, whole rather than ground and firm fruit versus over-ripe fruit.

- Eat whole-grain breads more often than white bread.
- Choose fresh potatoes instead of instant mashed potatoes.
- Make porridge out of slow-cooking oats instead of instant oatmeal.
- Enjoy mostly raw fruits and vegetables instead of juices or over-cooked fruit.
- Make homemade meals from whole, fresh ingredients.

Fructose (fruit sugar) and **lactose** (milk sugar) convert more slowly to blood sugar than some other sugars or even some starches. Enjoy fresh fruit and milk or milk products as snacks or with meals.

Keep portions reasonable. A *large portion* of even a low GI carbohydrate can make your blood sugar rise because of the total amount of carbohydrate. For example, eating a big serving of a low GI food such as whole-grain bread can cause the same blood sugar rise as eating a high GI food such as white bread in a *smaller portion* or thinner slices. Portions are critical. Choose the meal and snack portions shown in this book as a guide.

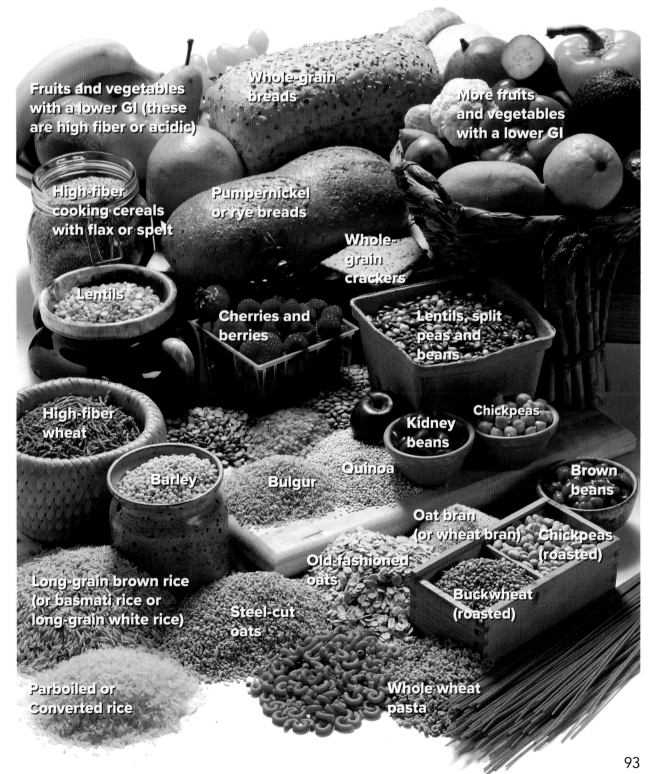

Fruits and vegetables with a lower GI (these are high fiber or acidic)

Whole-grain breads

More fruits and vegetables with a lower GI

High-fiber cooking cereals with flax or spelt

Pumpernickel or rye breads

Whole-grain crackers

Lentils

Cherries and berries

Lentils, split peas and beans

Chickpeas

High-fiber wheat

Kidney beans

Brown beans

Barley

Bulgur

Quinoa

Oat bran (or wheat bran)

Chickpeas (roasted)

Old-fashioned oats

Buckwheat (roasted)

Long-grain brown rice (or basmati rice or long-grain white rice)

Steel-cut oats

Parboiled or Converted rice

Whole wheat pasta

3. Food Labels

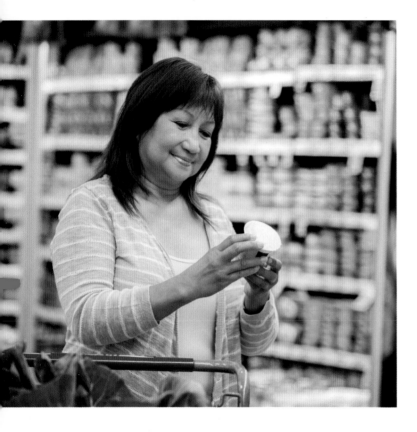

Healthy eating begins with what you bring home to eat. The foods you buy, garden or harvest are what you and your family will eat at home.

- When grocery shopping, bring a list and stick to it.
- Bring your reading glasses to read food labels.
- You don't need to try every new food.
- Choose familiar foods that you know are good choices.

If you are trying to lose weight, it is important to look at the total calories and serving size of each product. Calories come from carbohydrates, protein and fat. Food products are a poor choice if they have too much added sugar, fat (especially saturated fat) or salt. Foods that are higher in vitamins and minerals are more nutritious.

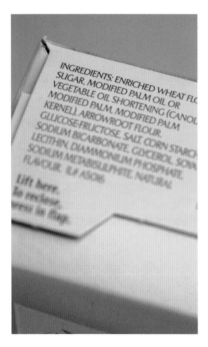

Ingredient list

Manufacturers are required to list ingredients in their products in order, from the heaviest to lightest. If you see sugar, fat or salt listed first, this is usually a bad choice.

The ingredient list can be hard to understand. Sometimes the list includes similar ingredients with each one mentioned separately. For example, a label for canned fruit might list "peaches, water, sugar, syrup and cane sugar." At first glance it looks like sugar is the third ingredient. However, sugar, syrup and cane sugar are all different types of sugar. In fact, if you add up these three types of sugar, the total sugar might actually be the second ingredient. This is why it's a good idea to also look at the Nutrition Facts table, which gives you more information. Compare the amount of sugar per serving between different brands.

Nutrition facts table

Serving size

Look at the amount in a serving size. Companies measure calories and other nutrition information based on this. The serving size listed isn't necessarily the same amount as you might eat...it's often smaller! For example, a chocolate bar may list the nutrition facts for only three squares, but most people eat the whole chocolate bar. So if you eat more, you get more calories, fat and sugar than shown on the label. A cereal box might list 1 cup (250 mL), but you might have 2 cups (500 mL) for breakfast. If you eat double the serving size, then you double the calories and nutrients.

The nutrients listed and their amounts

The nutrition information for a processed food is listed as a percentage that an average person might need in a day. This amount is listed on food labels as "% Daily Value," which means the percentage of your daily intake.

Sodium example: If a food serving such as a cup of canned soup has 30% sodium, that means it's salty and eating that serving will give you 30% (about one-third) of the sodium you need for the whole day. Consider choosing foods with a lower percentage.

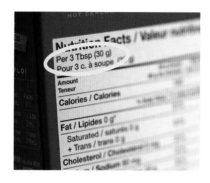

As a general rule:
- 5% Daily Value or less is *a little* of your daily intake
- 15% to 20% Daily Value or more is *a lot* of your daily intake from one product

Fudge bar, fat-free (ice cream)

Nutrition Facts	
Per 1 bar (66 g)	
Amount	**% Daily Value**
Calories 50	
Fat 0 g	0 %
Saturated 0 g	0 %
Trans 0 g	
Cholesterol 0 mg	0 %
Sodium 70 mg	3 %
Carbohydrate 13 g	4 %
Fiber 6 g	24 %
Sugars 4 g	
Protein 0.2 g	
Vitamin A	6 %
Vitamin C	0 %
Calcium	8 %
Iron	0 %

Get enough of these:
- Fiber
- Vitamins and minerals
- Monounsaturated fat and omega-3 fat

Get less of these:
- Calories, if you are trying to lose weight
- Fat
- Saturated fat
- Trans fat, now mostly removed by manufacturers
- Cholesterol
- Sodium
- Sugars, especially if they are added sugars

To help with weight loss: Look for food products with fewer calories.

To help with lower blood sugar: Look for products lower in carbohydrates, including starch and sugars, especially added sugar such as table sugar or honey. Fiber is also a carbohydrate but it doesn't increase your blood sugar.

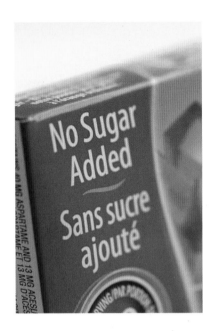

Nutrition health claims

What it says on the label	What it means
Low in sugar	Has no more than 2 grams of sugar per serving (equal to just $\frac{1}{2}$ tsp/2 mL of sugar), which is a good choice. **Caution:** If you eat more than one serving, the amount of sugar increases.
No sugar added or unsweetened	This doesn't have table sugar added to it. **Caution:** This food may have naturally sweet products added, such as concentrated grape juice.
Sugar-free	This is very low in added table sugar (0.5 grams or less). **Caution:** It may contain sugar alcohols like sorbitol (see page 102), fat, protein or salt.
Calorie-reduced	The food will have at least 50% fewer calories than the original product made by the same company. **Caution:** It may still have a lot of calories, if the original product had a lot.
Low-calorie	It has 15 calories or less per serving. This is very low in calories. It will have little effect on your weight or blood sugar. **Caution:** It may be high in sodium (salt).
Low in fat	Less than 3 grams of fat. One serving would be a good choice. **Caution:** If you eat several servings, the fat adds up.
Fat-free	This is very low in fat with no more than 0.1 gram of fat per serving. **Caution:** It may be high in sugar or sodium.
Low in cholesterol	This product has little cholesterol. **Caution:** It may still have a lot of calories, and cause weight gain. Weight gain can increase cholesterol.

Bottom line: Read the Nutrition Facts table and compare products! The nutrition health claim doesn't always tell you the whole story.

Healthy food tips

Cereals, per serving

Fiber: A high-fiber cereal will have at least 3 grams of fiber.

Added sugar: Choose cereals with 4 grams of sugar or less. This means each serving contains no more than 1 tsp (5 mL) of added sugar.

Added fat: Choose cereals with 2 grams of fat or less.

Compare labels: Read different cereal labels. If you're trying to lose weight, compare equal serving sizes. Try to choose the one with the lowest calories.

Bread and bagels

- "Whole grain" means the entire grain kernel (the outside fiber and the inside wheat germ), with all its health benefits, is in the bread. This is a good choice.
- Whole wheat (60% or 100%), rye, or multigrain breads are usually good choices for fiber, although they may not include the wheat germ.
- If you choose white bread or a bagel at a meal, complement the meal with high-fiber foods. For example, eat raw vegetables with your sandwich.
- Enriched means the manufacturer adds extra vitamins and minerals to the food.

Bread: Choose bread that has about **70 calories per slice**. This would equal 140 calories for two slices.

Bagels: Bagels are made from a dense dough, so are higher in carbohydrates and calories than bread.

- A small bagel (about 3 inches/7.5 cm across) will have about 160 calories. That's equal to about two slices of bread.
- A large bagel (about 5 inches/12.5 cm across) will have about 320 calories and is equal to four slices of bread.

**Foods with lots of fiber
are usually good choices.**

Healthy cereal

Nutrition Facts Per 1 cup (30 g)		
Amount	Cereal Only	Plus skim milk (125 mL)
Calories	**120**	**160**
		% Daily Value
Fat 2 g Saturated 0.2 g Trans 0 g	**3 %** **2 %**	**3 %** **2 %**
Cholesterol 0 mg	**0 %**	**0 %**
Sodium 270 mg	**11 %**	**13 %**
Carbohydrate 22 g Fiber 3 g Sugars 1 g	**7 %** **12 %**	**9 %** **12 %**
Protein 4 g		

Fiber on labels

Fiber goes through you without being absorbed. Therefore the calories and carbohydrates in fiber do not affect your blood sugar or weight.

Net carbs

If you take the carbohydrate number and subtract the fiber, you get the net carbs. (Net carbs may also be called available carbs.)

Net carbs example

Look at the cereal label above. The 3 grams of fiber means that there are 19 grams of net carbs (22 – 3 = 19). This is the amount that will mostly affect your blood sugar.

Non-dairy beverages

Soy beverage with added vitamin D and calcium is a nutritional alternative to milk. Beverages made from cashew, almond, rice, hemp or oats are lower in protein and are usually lower in carbohydrates if unsweetened. Compare the labels to milk labels to make sure they have equal amounts of calcium and vitamin D, and aren't sweetened.

Reduced-salt canned tomato soup

Nutrition Facts	
Per ½ cup (125 mL)	
Amount	% Daily Value
Calories 80	
Fat 0 g	0 %
Saturated 0.2 g	0 %
Trans 0 g	
Cholesterol 0 mg	0 %
Sodium 360 mg	15 %
Carbohydrate 19 g	6 %
Fiber 2 g	8 %
Sugars 11 g	
Protein 2 g	
Vitamin A	4 %
Vitamin C	15 %
Calcium	2 %
Iron	4 %

Canned fruit

Buy water-packed or juice-packed cans of fruit. If you buy fruit in syrup, this has more sugar in it. Rinse off the syrup to reduce your sugar intake.

Juices

A half cup (125 mL) of juice counts as a fruit serving ($\frac{1}{4}$ cup/60 mL for grape or prune juice). Limit juice and choose fresh fruit most of the time. Light juices made with a low-calorie sweetener are a reduced-sugar choice.

Milk

Skim and 1% milk are low in fat and are high in calcium and vitamin D. Avoid or limit milk with table sugar added, such as chocolate and other flavored milk. 1 cup (250 mL) of chocolate milk has 3 teaspoons (12 grams) of extra sugar added. If you want to choose chocolate milk occasionally, you can reduce the sugar by mixing it half and half with white skim milk.

Cheese

Cheese labeled as 20% or less milk fat (MF) will be lower in fat and calories than regular.

Sour cream and yogurts

Look for 0–2% MF sour cream or 0–2% plain yogurt, as these are lower in fat. If choosing a higher-fat kind, choose less.

Soups, canned or packaged

These soups usually have a lot of salt added. Choosing a reduced-salt variety helps cut back on sodium. Keep in mind that some soups may also have a lot of added fat: check the label. Consider making homemade soups with little or no added salt and lots of vegetables.

All fats have similar calories

All fats have about 45 calories per 1 tsp (5 mL). If you are trying to lose weight, even a small amount of fat — even olive oil — gives you extra unwanted calories.

Butter versus margarine

Butter and margarine are both fats. If you eat too much of either, your total fat intake goes up. This can increase your weight, which then can raise your blood cholesterol and blood sugar. Go lightly with any fats that you use.

Eat less saturated fats

Check food labels for the amount of saturated fat. If a food product has more than 2 grams of saturated fat, then don't choose it for everyday eating. Food products high in saturated fats will likely have palm oils, butter, lard or cream added to them. Remember, saturated fats from dairy, meat and processed foods add up during the day.

Unsaturated oils include olive oil and canola oil

Other oils include sunflower, safflower, soybean, corn and peanut oil, and specialty oils made from avocado, pumpkin seeds, walnuts and flaxseeds. These unsaturated fats are healthy for you. If you're trying to lose weight, you need to remember they still have a lot of calories, just like all other fats. So if you add more oil to your foods, then you need to cut back on other foods in your diet.

Mayonnaise and salad dressings

Fat-free is the lowest fat choice. Choices with fewer than 30 calories per 1 tbsp (15 mL) are lighter choices than the regular varieties.

Remember the rule of thumb:

At most meals, limit your added fat to an amount that will fit in the end of your thumb. This is about 1 to 2 tsp (5–10 mL).

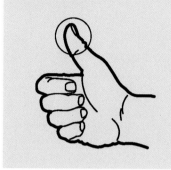

Banned trans fats

Trans fats are made from partially hydrogenated vegetable oils. Long-term studies show that these man-made processed fats clog blood vessels. In 2018, they were banned in food products in North America and they are still being phased out. Naturally occurring trans fats will still be listed on food labels.

Banning trans fats was a good decision, although governments did not ban the use of unhealthy saturated palm oils at the same time. Many food manufacturers replaced trans fats with palm oils, which continue to make processed foods unhealthy. Check ingredient lists on processed foods, and if the amount of saturated fat is high, it's probably made with palm oil. You will see palm oil also listed as coconut oil or vegetable oil.

Note: As a result of the increase in the demand for palm oil, tropical rain forests are being cut down and replaced with plantations of palm trees. This is a global environmental concern.

4. Light Desserts and Sweeteners

Q & A WITH KAREN GRAHAM: Taking charge of your sweet tooth

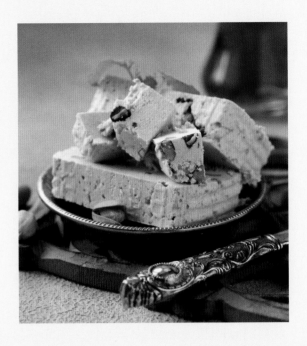

AMIR: I found out I had diabetes last year. Since then I have lost 8 lbs (4 kg) and my blood sugar has improved. But my wife has gone crazy about keeping me healthy and won't let me eat any sugar — no cake, no cookies, no halva, no jam, nothing. She's taken the fun out of eating. And, let's face it, I love eating, it's a big part of my life.

I know my wife is doing what she thinks is best, but this diabetes thing is frustrating both of us. Surely I can eat some sugar and desserts?

KAREN: Congratulations on your weight loss and improved blood sugar. Cutting out obvious forms of sugar has certainly helped you improve your diabetes. Your wife's concerns about your health sound genuine. You both need to know that having diabetes doesn't mean you can never eat dessert. It does mean switching to smaller portions and lighter desserts that are lower in sugar and fat.

First, it's not just extra sugar and desserts that give you high blood sugar. You gain weight from eating and drinking too much food over all, and then your blood sugar goes up. When you lose weight, your blood sugar goes down. And when you exercise, you use up the stored sugar in your body and your blood sugar goes down more.

So, I suggest you focus on eating the right portions of food. Use the meal plans in this book as a guide. I include small portions of regular or light jam at breakfast, and regular sugar in some light desserts. Desserts include fruits, puddings and other lighter desserts, plain cookies, smaller portions of ice cream or sherbet, or un-iced cake. Check out the dessert recipes in the other books in this *Health and Wellness Series* (see page 416). There are ideas on how to adapt your own favorite recipes (on pages 104–105). Consider choosing healthier foods, like the halva with tahini (sesame seed butter), and eat a smaller portion.

When you eat smaller portions of treats, then a reasonable amount of sugar can fit into your diet. Remember, a walk helps bring down blood sugar, especially an hour or so after a meal. A walk can also be a special time for you and your wife to spend together.

Using table sugar

Sugar is a source of carbohydrate in your diet. You don't have to avoid it completely; just limit it. For example, cut back on the amount of sugar you use in recipes. When you add sugar at a meal (such as honey, brown sugar or jam), use the tip of your thumb as a portion guide. For some people, having a small amount of honey or jam can help satisfy a craving for sugar. This is certainly better than depriving yourself and then binging.

Cookies

All cookies have sugar and fat! Look for ones that aren't too thick or large: 70 calories or less per cookie is reasonable. Limit yourself to two cookies.

Granola bars may seem healthier than cookies, but often they have lots of sugar and fat. Compare labels.

Yogurt

Choose:

- Yogurt with 100 to 120 calories per ¾ cup (175 g), which will be low in fat and have sugar replaced with a low-calorie sweetener
- Plain skim or 2% yogurt with no added sugar
- Plain skim or 2% Greek yogurt, which is lower in carbs and calcium and has more protein

Natural versus table sugar

Natural sugar comes from milk, fruits and vegetables. The Nutrition Facts table doesn't usually list natural sugar separately from added table sugar. Check the ingredient list to see if sugar has been added.

To tell if a boxed instant pudding has no sugar added, pick up the box. If it's very light, it's the low-sugar kind. The box of regular pudding made with sugar is a lot heavier. When you look at the label, you will see the low-sugar kind has zero grams of sugar and the regular kind has 15 to 20 grams of sugar.

Some people with diabetes choose to avoid as much added sugar as possible. Instead they use low-calorie sweeteners at the table and in baking. This is a personal preference. Either way works in a healthy eating pattern.

Cookies with 120 calories for two

Nutrition Facts	
Per 2 cookies (23 g)	
Amount	% **Daily Value**
Calories 120	
Fat 6 g	9 %
Saturated 2 g	12 %
Trans 0 g	
Cholesterol 0 mg	0 %
Sodium 70 mg	3 %
Carbohydrate 16 g	5 %
Fiber 1 g	4 %
Sugars 7 g	
Protein 1 g	

Ice cream

Nutrition Facts	
Per ½ cup (125 mL)	
Amount	% Daily Value
Calories 120	
Fat 5 g	8 %
Saturated 3.5 g	19 %
Trans 0.2 g	
Cholesterol 15 mg	2 %
Sodium 80 mg	3 %
Carbohydrate 17 g	6 %
Fiber 0 g	4 %
Sugars 15 g	
Protein 1 g	
Vitamin A	6 %
Vitamin C	0 %
Calcium	4 %
Iron	0 %

Most ice cream provides less than 5% of your daily calcium needs, so isn't a replacement for milk.

Some of these "sugar-free" products actually have more fat and more calories than regular candies or chocolates.

To determine the net carbs of a sugar-free candy, subtract any fiber and half of the sugar alcohol carbs from the total carbs.

Ice cream, frozen yogurt or sherbets

Choose brands that have 120 calories or less per ½ cup (125 mL). You may be shocked to know that some reduced-fat frozen desserts have more sugar, and some low-sugar ice creams have more fat than regular ice cream. The bottom line is that these are all desserts. Only choose them in a half-cup (125 mL) serving.

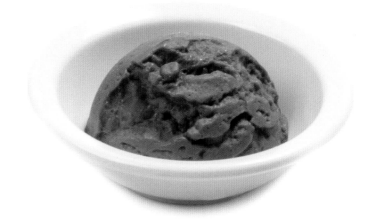

"Sugar-free" sweets

Beware: sugar-free candy or sugar-free chocolates have other types of sugar added. These other types may be sorbitol, mannitol or isomalt. These sugars are called "sugar alcohols" but are not actually alcohol. Sugar alcohols are only half absorbed by your body, so only half the sugar alcohol carbs affect your blood sugar and weight. However, since sugar alcohols don't taste as sweet as table sugar, the manufacturer may add more or may add more fat or salt to improve the flavor. Compare these sugar-free sweets to the regular products. Just because the label says "sugar-free" does not mean it is calorie-free and fat-free. Limit yourself to one or two pieces of candy or chocolate as an occasional treat.

Note: If you eat too many sorbitol candies, you might get diarrhea and bloating. This can happen if you eat 10 grams or more of sugar alcohols in a day. This is because the body isn't good at absorbing sugar alcohols. Some of it goes right through you.

Light syrups

Light syrups usually have less sugar and total carbohydrates than regular syrup, so are a good choice. Light syrups are made with less sugar and more water, and then are usually thickened with starch. They may also contain a sugar alcohol or a low-calorie sweetener.

Sugar-free jam

Some "sugar-free" jams can have as much sugar as regular jam. Concentrated grape juice sometimes sweetens sugar-free jam as a substitute for table sugar. When you concentrate grape juice, it's almost as sweet as regular sugar.

Other sugar-free jams contain extra fruit and less added sugar than a regular jam. You can also make homemade jams using reduced-sugar pectin or no-sugar recipes. These will have less sugar, and fewer calories per 1 tsp (5 mL), often as low as 5 to 10 calories per tsp (5 mL). However, as these jams don't taste as sweet as a regular jam, some people put more on their toast! Whether you eat 1 tbsp (15 mL) of this diet jam or 1 tsp (5 mL) of regular jam, the calories will be about the same.

Sugar-free and low-calorie drinks and snacks

Foods with a very low calorie level (of 20 calories or less per serving) will not affect your weight or blood sugar. Choose these as a low-calorie snack or addition to a meal (also see page 197). Examples are diet gelatin, diet (or "zero") soft drinks or diet gum. Water is always a good option, as it has no calories! Unsweetened black or herbal tea or coffee are also calorie-free.

Sugar-free gelatin

As with puddings, a box of sugar-free gelatin weighs very little compared to a box of gelatin that is made with sugar.

Make your sugar-free gelatin dessert fun: Use different color gelatins and, after you add the cold water, add different fruits.

Example of a good choice of no-sugar-added light syrup

Nutrition Facts	
Per 3 tbsp (45 mL)	
Amount	% **Daily Value**
Calories 30	
Fat 0 g	0 %
Cholesterol 0 mg	0 %
Sodium 75 mg	2 %
Carbohydrate 7 g	2 %
Sugars 6 g	
Protein 0 g	0 %

Remember the rule of thumb:

At most meals, limit regular jam, syrup (or honey) to what fits into the tip of your thumb; this will generally equal 1 to 2 tsp (5–10 mL), or if you have a larger hand, 1 tbsp (15 mL).

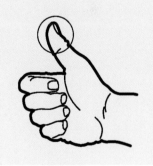

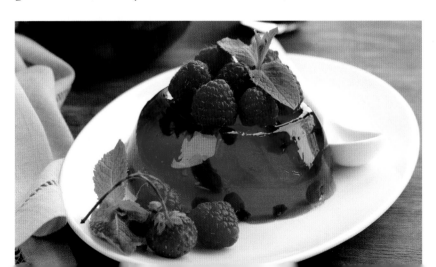

Note: "Light" recipes may already have the fat, sugar or salt cut back. These may not require any changes.

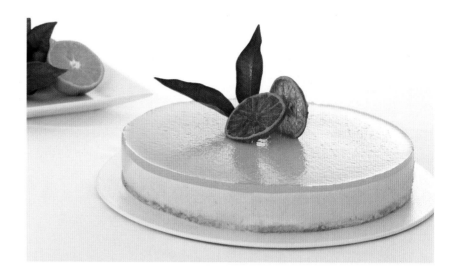

Making your dessert recipes lower in sugar and fat

Adapt your recipes

The substitutions listed in the chart on page 105 will help you change your own recipes so they are lower in sugar, fat or salt.

Make one change at a time

Make recipe changes gradually, one ingredient at a time. If you change several ingredients at once, your recipe may not work out.

Small changes count

For proper rising and browning of cakes and muffins, you often need fat, sugar and salt. Some recipes depend on a certain ingredient such as butter, whipping cream, honey or molasses for good flavor. The goal isn't to cut out all fat and sugar and end up with a product you don't like! Rather, make small changes in your recipes to make them healthier and have smaller portions. Over time, you will feel satisfied with desserts that are not as sweet or rich.

Boost flavor with spices and flavorings

Once you've cut back on sugar, fat and salt, it's time to boost the flavor in other ways. Now try adding:

- Spices such as nutmeg, allspice, cinnamon, cloves, cardamom or ginger
- Herbs like lemon balm or mint
- Lemon or lime juice
- Zest of lemon, lime or orange
- Flavoring extracts such as vanilla, coconut or peppermint

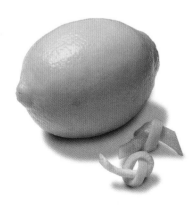

Recipe substitutions

If a recipe calls for:	Use this substitute or technique instead:
Sugar, honey, syrup or molasses	Sugar provides sweetness but is also important to keep the product tender and moist, and it allows cakes and muffins to brown nicely. *To reduce the sugar and still get a tasty result,* cut the sugar or sweetener in half. If you find the recipe is not sweet enough this way, replace all, or part of the sugar that you removed with some low-calorie sweetener. Some low-calorie sweeteners, like aspartame, lose their sweetness if baked at high temperature. Other sweeteners such as sucralose (Splenda) work well in baking.
Jell-O or pudding	Use sugar-free gelatin or sugar-free pudding mixes.
Whole or 2% milk (fresh or canned evaporated)	1% or skim milk *Here are four ways to make a lower-fat thickened milkshake or smoothie:* (1) put skim milk or canned evaporated skim milk in a bowl and freeze it for half an hour or until crystals form on the top. Then beat with electric beaters or in a blender until thickened, (2) add ice cubes to your milk and blend, (3) add frozen fruit, or (4) add Greek yogurt.
Half-and-half cream	Undiluted canned evaporated milk, or 2% milk
Fat: oil, margarine, butter, lard or shortening	Most cake-type recipes require some fat for a light texture, moistness and flavor. Start by decreasing the fat by half. Add an equal amount of applesauce, milk or yogurt in cakes and muffins. This will increase the carbohydrates slightly but decrease the fat and calories. Note: By reducing just 1 tbsp (15 mL) of fat in your recipe, you cut out 100 calories. Starch-thickened products such as soup, sauces and desserts do not usually need any fat added.
Regular mayonnaise or regular sour cream (14%)	Fat-free or light mayonnaise, fat-free (0%) sour cream or light sour cream (7%), or plain low-fat yogurt (or Greek yogurt), or 1% or 2% cottage cheese that you've blended until smooth
Regular fat cheese (over 28% MF)	Low-fat (20% or less MF) cheese
Regular cream cheese	Light cream cheese (14% MF or less)
Salt, baking soda or baking powder	To reduce sodium in your recipes, cut back on salt, baking soda and baking powder. Per teaspoon (5 mL), salt has 2,300 mg of sodium, baking soda has 1,300 mg and baking powder has 500 mg. For cakes, muffins or cookies to rise properly, you usually only need a small amount per cup (250 mL) of flour: $\frac{1}{8}$ tsp (0.5 mL) of salt and 1 tsp (5 mL) of baking powder. For soda breads or biscuits, use only $\frac{1}{4}$ to $\frac{1}{2}$ tsp (1–2 mL) of baking soda per cup (250 mL) of flour.
All-purpose (white) flour	Replace half of the white flour with whole wheat flour, or add 2 tbsp (30 mL) wheat bran or wheat germ to $\frac{7}{8}$ cup (220 mL) white flour to make a cup (250 mL). Try different kinds of flour marked "whole grain," such as spelt flour, amaranth flour, barley flour or oat flour.

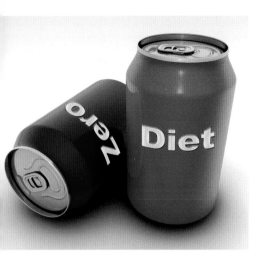

Most diet sodas are sweetened with aspartame.

Less common sweeteners:

- acesulfame-K (acesulfame potassium)
- saccharin
- neotame and advantame
- cyclamates (not approved in the United States, limited approval in Canada)

These sweeteners are sold as a variety of brand names. For example, saccharin is sold as Sugar Twin and Sweet 'N Low. Check the label ingredients.

Low-calorie sweeteners

Low-calorie sweeteners have been an amazing food product breakthrough because of their low calories and sweet taste. They make it possible to drink zero-calorie drinks other than water. Some low-calorie sweeteners can be used in baking.

Sucralose and aspartame

Both sucralose and aspartame are man-made chemicals that taste extremely sweet. The brand name for sucralose is Splenda. Aspartame is sold as Equal, NutraSweet and Sweet 'N Low. You need only small amounts to sweeten foods.

Stevia

This is a low-calorie sweetener that comes from a plant source.

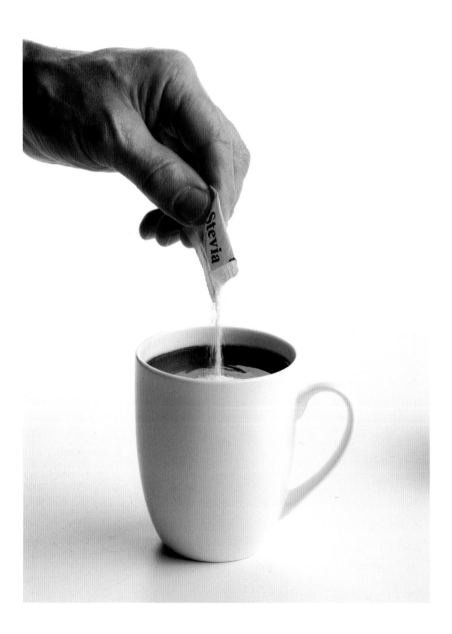

Sugar or low-calorie sweetener? Which is the best choice for a person with diabetes?

Too many sweet drinks and sweet foods will raise your blood sugar. If you are trying to choose between a can of regular cola that has 10 tsp of sugar (40 g of carbs) versus a diet cola with zero sugar, choose the diet cola. The diet cola won't raise your blood sugar. When your blood sugar is high, cutting out excess sugar helps bring it down as soon as possible.

If you drink 2 liters of cola daily, you would consume 50 teaspoons of sugar. That equals a full cup, or 250 mL, of sugar, or 200 g of carbs. The switch to 2 liters of diet cola will mean virtually no sugar. This will have a huge benefit on reducing your blood sugar.

The bigger question is *how many* diet products do we really *need* in the long-term? Do we need to be drinking diet soft drinks daily? Should we learn to drink more water? While diet soft drinks have no sugar, they have other ingredients that aren't good for us. In many cases, these include caffeine and phosphates (which draws important calcium out of our bones), and acids that are bad for our teeth.

As you get used to a healthy diet, you may not feel such a need for low-calorie sweetened products. Replace some of your diet beverages with water. Could you drink your tea or coffee with less or no sugar?

Consider eating your cereal without added sugar rather than adding a low-calorie sweetener. You may want to choose a smaller amount of a sugar-sweetened product instead of a larger amount of a diet product. For example, try eating ½ cup (125 mL) of regular yogurt rather than ¾ cup (175 mL) of yogurt with added aspartame or sucralose.

In some of my dessert recipes, I use low-calorie sweeteners. I also give an option to use sugar if you want, but to use less. I believe in moderation and balance in everything in life. This same common sense applies to low-calorie sweeteners.

Water is the best beverage to quench thirst.

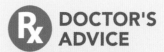

DOCTOR'S ADVICE

Do you actually lose weight using low-calorie sweeteners?

People can manage their diabetes and lose weight by making changes that include low-calorie sweetened products. These products provide variety to their diet and help them consume fewer calories.

However, some studies show that people who consume lots of diet products don't lose more weight. It may be that these people compensate by eating more of something else. One scenario might be: "I'm having a diet pop, so I can splurge and have the large fries." Other studies suggest that eating diet products regularly may make you crave more sweets. This is a possible disadvantage of these low-calorie products.

Moderation is always good advice.

Are low-calorie sweeteners safe?

The US Food and Drug Administration and Health Canada think aspartame and sucralose are safe. The American Diabetes Association and Diabetes Canada also say these are safe foods.

We still don't know the long-term effects of regularly consuming low-calorie sweeteners.

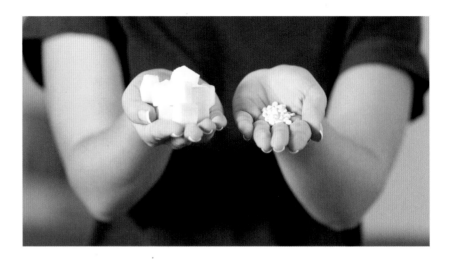

This sounds reassuring, but we may not have all the answers. The safety of people eating low-calorie sweeteners in larger amounts over many years is still unknown. When we gather new evidence, recommendations may change.

The case of trans fat is a good example (see page 99). Trans fat is a man-made product that was considered a "miracle" food by the food industry. Trans fats were first used commercially in the 1920s in England and more widely in North America after World War II. They quickly became part of nearly all processed foods. They were cheap, tasted good and could be fried and added to baked goods. Best of all, unlike vegetable oils and other natural fats, products made with trans fats could sit on the shelf for a long time and not go bad.

It was not until the late 1980s, nearly 30 years after we started commonly using trans fat in our foods, that red flags went up. Those studies linked excess consumption of trans fats to heart disease. It took another 10 years until comprehensive reviews of studies confirmed these effects. Then another 20 years passed before countries began banning them. This may not be what happens with artificial sweeteners. However, history has taught us that some caution and moderation is valuable.

5. Reducing Sodium

A small amount of sodium daily is essential to life

Salt, made up of sodium and chloride, is a mineral. Our body cells and tissues need salt. We use it for muscle and heart contractions, proper conduction of nerves and the transport of nutrients into body cells. Healthy kidneys efficiently get rid of excess sodium from the body. Athletes and manual laborers, especially those who work in hot and humid climates, need more sodium to replace what they lose in sweat. Table salt has iodine added. (It's not added to sea salt or coarse salt.) Iodine is essential for brain development and helps keep your thyroid healthy. Your thyroid has a role in a healthy body weight.

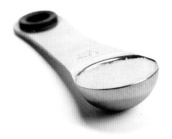

1 level teaspoon (5 mL) of salt is equal to about 2,300 mg of sodium. This amount of sodium is all you need each day (your Daily Value).

Too much sodium is not healthy

As with all good things in life, you can have too much of a good thing. This is certainly the case with salt. Most of us get too much sodium in our diet, mostly from processed and restaurant foods. The total upper limit of sodium recommended for the average person is 2,300 mg. This is about 1 teaspoon (5 mL) of salt a day. A teaspoon of salt may seem like a lot. However, some cans of soup have this much in one can!

How sodium affects a person with diabetes

Eating lots of salty foods doesn't cause your blood sugar to go up, but it may worsen your high blood pressure (hypertension). Evidence shows that people with diabetes may not get rid of extra sodium as efficiently as someone without diabetes. A person with diabetes can have higher blood levels of insulin and this will affect how kidneys respond to hormones responsible for sodium excretion. When your body holds more sodium, the sodium holds more water. Extra water in your body adds extra pressure inside your blood vessels. This damages your blood vessel walls, and puts you at risk for a heart attack or stroke. High blood pressure causes damage to your kidneys and eyes.

Sodium hides inside foods that are also high in fat, like fries and hamburgers, potato chips and bologna. Sometimes it's hard to tell whether sodium or fat is the greater villain. When you cut back on salty foods, you eat less fat too. Overall, you'll feel healthier.

Eating too much salt also contributes to osteoporosis, stomach cancer and kidney stones. Also, new research shows that a high salt intake might make it more likely for you to get dementia.

℞ **DOCTOR'S ADVICE**

The American National Institutes of Health has proven that diet can lower blood pressure as effectively as medication. They developed Dietary Approaches to Stop Hypertension, the DASH diet. This program helps prevent or treat high blood pressure; and prevent type 2 diabetes. We know from the DASH diet research that lowering blood pressure is more than just cutting out salt. The program is very similar to our meal plans and advice.

Here are other important steps to improve your blood pressure:

- Cut back on extra salt.
- Lose a bit of weight.
- Exercise every day.
- Limit or quit alcohol and cigarettes.
- Manage stress better.
- Eat potassium-rich and calcium-rich foods (including fruits, vegetables and milk).
- Take steps to improve the health of your blood vessels, such as eating foods low in saturated fat and high in antioxidants (see pages 118–121).
- Take your medications as prescribed.

How do I cut back on salt?

Restaurant and processed foods contain about three-quarters (75%) of the salt in our diet. Eat less of these salty foods!

Some food companies and restaurants are beginning to reduce the sodium they put in their products. This is because of consumer demand for lower salt and healthier food, but the change is slow. Compare food labels and restaurant nutritional lists. Look for the lowest amounts of sodium.

Five tips to reduce sodium

1. Cut your overall portions. As you eat less, you reduce your total salt intake.

2. Choose less of the high-sodium and very high-sodium foods listed on pages 116–117. These include prepackaged convenience foods and restaurant foods. Some of the saltiest foods are hot dogs, subs, hamburgers, pizzas, processed meats, soups, pasta dishes and potato chips. Also, consider whether the food item is part of a meal that includes other foods with salt. If you have a saltier food at one meal or snack, then choose lower sodium foods at your next meal.

3. Use less salt and salty seasonings at the table and when cooking. On certain foods, you may miss adding salt. If using salt occasionally, cut back. Limit it to a shake or two.

4. Replace salt with pepper, unsalted seasonings, herbs and spices, and lemon and lime.

5. Rinse and drain canned salted foods such as canned kidney beans or canned fish or corn. This rinses off up to one-third to one-half of the added salt.

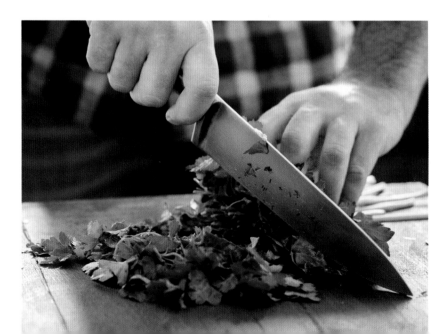

Check out the next few pages to see the amount of sodium in different foods. There are five groups, from lowest sodium to highest sodium. Very high-sodium foods are loaded with salt, ⅓ tsp (720 mg) sodium or more per serving.

The portions shown in the charts are based on typical diabetes food choices, except:

- Portions of some salty low-calorie "extras" are shown in smaller amounts.
- Some portions of meat or starch are shown in dinner meal sizes.
- Portions in the high-sodium and very high-sodium groups are based on standard restaurant or packaged portions.

When you look at a food label you will see sodium listed as a percentage. For example, under the column "% Daily Value" (which is the percentage of your daily needs) it might list sodium as 20%. This means that if you eat this food serving you will get 20% of the sodium that you need for the day. Other foods can contribute the other 80% of your sodium for the day.

A note about the sodium amounts listed on pages 112–117: Sodium amounts vary between manufacturers and restaurants, imported versus North American food products, and regular and "reduced-sodium" products. In some cases, sodium ranges are listed to reflect this variability. A few brand names are provided as examples.

Sodium foods	Amount of sodium in a food	
	milligrams (mg)	% Daily Value (% of your daily needs)
Very low-sodium foods	0–24	less than 1%
Low-sodium foods	25–140	1% to 6%
Medium-sodium foods	141–480	over 6% to 20%
High-sodium foods	481–720	over 20% to 30%
Very high-sodium foods	more than 720	more than 30%

Here's a packaged instant soup that has 20% of your daily sodium needs

Nutrition Facts	
Per 1 cup (250 mL)	
Amount	% Daily Value
Calories 90	
Fat 1 g	0 %
Saturated 0 g	0 %
Trans 0 g	
Cholesterol 0 mg	0 %
Sodium 482 mg	20 %
Carbohydrate 18 g	8 %
Fiber 1 g	
Sugars 3 g	
Protein 2 g	

Yes, you can do it! It's possible to eat healthy, delicious, everyday meals and eat less salt. Use the *Seven-Day Meal Plan* on pages 149–200 as a guideline.

EXCELLENT

100%

75%

50%

25%

These portions provide less than 1% of your % Daily Value.

Very low-sodium foods

These portions each provide 0 to 24 mg sodium. This is less than 1% of your daily needs. On labels, "sodium-free" or "salt-free" foods will have less than 5 mg of sodium per serving size shown.

1. Fresh or canned fruit
2. Dried fruit
3. Fruit juice or applesauce
4. Fresh vegetables, raw or cooked
5. Canned or frozen unsalted vegetables

6. Garlic, onions, herbs, spices, pepper and no-salt spice blends
7. NoSalt salt substitute is high in potassium — ask your doctor if it is safe for you to use (it can interact with some medications)

Choose unprocessed food

Nearly all unprocessed (natural) food is very low in sodium (salt). This includes fresh and dried grains and starches, vegetables and fruits, dried beans and lentils, unsalted nuts and seeds, and unsalted fats. It also includes most frozen or canned fruits and vegetables; choose the ones with no salt added. Meats have some natural sodium, but a 1-oz (30 g) portion is a very low-sodium food.

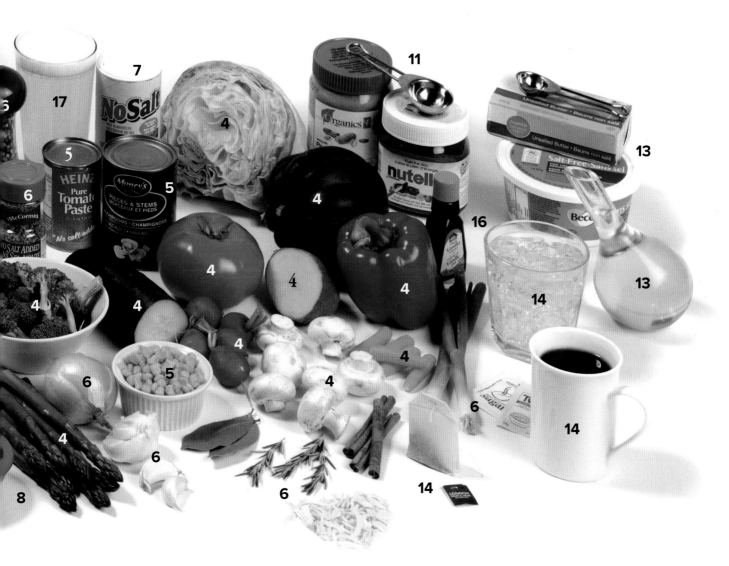

8. Grains and starches with no salt added (including wheat, pasta, quinoa, couscous, rice, oats, flour and popcorn)
9. Dried beans and lentils
10. Nuts and seeds
11. Unsalted peanut butter and nut butters

12. Unsalted meat, 1 oz (30 g)
13. Oils and unsalted butter or margarine
14. Water, tea and coffee
15. Jams, sweeteners and plain candies
16. Condiments such as cocoa, flavorings or vinegar
17. Beer, wine and alcohol (not mixed drinks)

GOOD

100%

75%

50%

25%

These portions provide less than 6% of your % Daily Value.

Low-sodium foods

These portions each provide 25 to 140 mg sodium. This is 1% to 6% of your daily needs.

Foods labeled "low-sodium" or "low-salt" will have less than 140 mg sodium per serving size shown.

Starches
Pancake, one 4-inch (10 cm): 110 mg

Vegetables
Carrots, 1 cup (250 mL): 85 mg
Celery, 2 medium stalks: 70 mg
Mixed vegetables, frozen, 1 cup (250 mL): 75 mg
Sweet potato, baked, ½ cup (125 mL): 45 mg
Vegetable juice, low-salt, 1 cup (250 mL): 140 mg

Milk and milk products
Hot chocolate mix, light, 1 package: 90 mg
Soy beverage, 1 cup (250 mL): 30 mg
Yogurt, low-fat, fruit with low-calorie sweetener, ¾ cup (175 mL): 110 mg
Yogurt, plain, low-fat, ¾ cup (175 mL): 115 mg

Meats and proteins
Chicken breast, baked, no skin, 4 oz (125 g): 85 mg
Egg: 60 mg
Fish, white, broiled, 4 oz (125 g): 65 mg
Hamburger, 4 oz (125 g) cooked: 75 mg
Peanut butter, regular (salted), 1 tbsp (15 mL): 65 mg
Peanuts, roasted and salted, 2 tbsp (30 mL): 35–55 mg
Tuna, canned in water, drained, ⅓ tin: 135 mg

Fats
Butter, salted, 1 tsp (5 mL): 40 mg
Margarine, non-hydrogenated, 1 tsp (5 mL): 35 mg
Mayonnaise, light, 1 tbsp (15 mL): 110 mg

Soups
Chicken noodle, low-sodium, canned, 1 cup (250 mL): 140 mg
Cream of mushroom, low-sodium, canned, 1 cup (250 mL): 60 mg

Desserts and snacks
Plain tea biscuits, 4: 115 mg
Chocolate bar, plain, milk chocolate, ½ bar: 35 mg
Ice cream, ½ cup (125 mL): 65 mg
LifeStyle brand cookies, 2: 70 mg

Beverages
Club soda, 12-oz (355 mL) can: 80 mg
Diet 7-up, 12-oz (355 mL) can: 45 mg
Diet ginger ale, 12-oz (355 mL) can: 120 mg

Condiments
Barbecue sauce, 1 tsp (5 mL): 50 mg
Ketchup, 1 tsp (5 mL): 50 mg
Mustard, ready-to-serve, 1 tsp (5 mL): 65 mg
Olives, green, stuffed, 4: 60 mg
Sour cream, 1% MF, 2 tbsp (30 mL): 35 mg
Worcestershire sauce, 1 tsp (5 mL): 55 mg
Bick's Yum Yum pickles, 7 slices: 100 mg

Salts
Add salts to your food occasionally and in tiny amounts.
1/16 tsp (0.3 mL) or about 4 quick shakes:
Table salt: 145 mg
Sea salt: 135 mg
Hy's without MSG: 105 mg
Garlic salt or celery salt: 75 mg
Half Salt: 65 mg
Accent (MSG): 40 mg

Medium-sodium foods

These portions each provide 141 to 480 mg sodium. This is 6 to 20% of your daily needs.

Low-fat products

Cheese and salad dressings labelled "low-fat" tend to be higher in salt. This makes it a challenge when choosing products. If your main goal is weight loss, choosing the lower-calorie product may be best. If your blood pressure is high or you have kidney problems, it's best to choose the lower-salt variety.

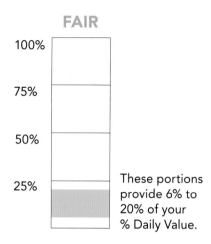

FAIR

100%

75%

50%

25%

These portions provide 6% to 20% of your % Daily Value.

Starches
Bagel, half 3-inch (7.5 cm): 155 mg
Bannock, half of a 3-inch (7.5 cm) piece: 85–170 mg
Bread, whole wheat, 1 slice: 170
Cereal, dry, bran flakes, 1/2 cup (125 mL): 130 mg
Cereal, dry, Special K or Cheerios, 2/3 cup (150 mL): 145–165 mg
French fries, fast food, no ketchup, small: 160–280 mg
Oatmeal, instant, plain or sweetened, 1 pouch: 225–300 mg
Pasta sauce mixes ("Side Kicks"), 1/4 package: 350–370 mg
Rice, converted, microwave (Bistro), flavored, 1/3 cup (75 mL): 140–200 mg
Soda crackers, unsalted tops, 7: 160 mg (salted: 275 mg)
Stuffing mixes, 1/4 pouch (30 g): 410–460 mg
Waffle, plain, frozen, 4-inch (10 cm): 260 mg

Vegetables
Beans, wax, canned, 1 cup (250 mL): 225–340 mg
Beets, canned, pickled, 1/2 cup (125 mL): 320 mg
Corn, kernel, canned, salted, 1/2 cup (125 mL): 150 mg
Mushrooms, canned, salted, 1/2 cup (125 mL): 350 mg
Peas, frozen, 1 cup (250 mL): 150 mg (canned with salt: 450 mg)
Salsa, 1/4 cup (60 mL): 300–480 mg
Spaghetti sauce, jarred or canned, 1/2 cup (125 mL): 360–480 mg
Tomato juice, 1/2 cup (125 mL): 325 mg
Tomato sauce, canned, 2 tbsp (30 mL): 195 mg

Milk and milk products
Milk, chocolate, 1 cup (250 mL): 200 mg
Milk, low-fat, white, 1 cup (250 mL): 125 mg
Pudding cup, no sugar, ready-to-eat: 180 mg
Pudding, light, made from a box, 1/2 cup (125 mL): 320 mg

Meats and proteins
Bacon, 1 slice: 185 mg

Baked beans, brown, canned, 1/2 cup (125 mL): 420–550 mg
Cheese, Cheddar, regular fat, 1 oz (30 g): 175 mg (low-fat: 205 mg)
Cheese, feta, 2 tbsp (30 mL): 230 mg
Cheese, processed, 1 slice (21 g): 310 mg
Corned beef, Klik or Spam canned, 1/12 can (28 g): 225–400 mg
Cottage cheese, 1% or 2%, 1/4 cup (60 mL): 205–215 mg
Pastrami or ham, deli, 1 oz (30 g): 330–375 mg
Salmon, pink, drained, 1/3 can: 310 mg
Sardines, canned in oil, drained, two 3-inch (7.5 cm): 240 mg
Sausage, Italian, 1/2: 455 mg
Sausages, pork and beef, 1 link (39 g): 315 mg
Veggie burger, 1 (75 g): 480 mg
Wieners, 1: 375 mg

Fats
Salad dressing, creamy, light, 1 tbsp (15 mL): 190 mg
Salad dressing, Italian, fat-free, 1 tbsp (15 mL): 210 mg

Desserts and snacks
Chocolate bar, such as Oh Henry (67 g): 160 mg
Corn chips or tacos, small bag (50 g): 335–430 mg
Donut, cake type, 3-inch (7.5 cm): 260 mg
Popcorn, microwave, 5 cups: 250–350 mg
Potato chips, lower-salt brands, 15 chips (25 g): 40–120 mg
Apple pie, 1/8 piece: 210 mg
Cake, from mix, 1/12 of a cake: 255–350 mg

Beverages
Hot chocolate, restaurant, 10 oz (300 mL): 360 mg

Condiments or salts
Baking powder, 1 tsp (5 mL): 300 mg
Barbecue sauce, 1 tbsp (15 mL): 150 mg
HP sauce, 1 tbsp (15 mL): 160 mg
Ketchup, 1 tbsp (15 mL): 140 mg
Mustard, ready-to-serve, 1 tbsp (15 mL): 200 mg

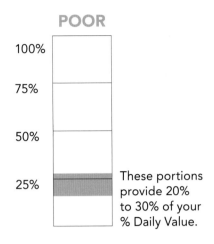

POOR

100%
75%
50%
25%

These portions provide 20% to 30% of your % Daily Value.

High-sodium foods

These portions each provide 481 to 720 mg sodium. This is more than 20 to 30% of your daily needs. Note: Two servings from this group will add up to about half of your daily sodium needs.

Products differ between brands

The amount of sodium differs between brand names, and between American and Canadian producers. Check and compare the amount of sodium in your usual food brands and other available brands in your supermarket.

Starches
Bagel: 6-inch (15 cm): 350–600 mg
French fries (fast food), large: 350 mg
   (570 mg with 2 ketchups)
Macaroni and cheese (Kraft Dinner), made without
   added fat, 1 cup (250 mL): 615 mg
Flavored rice, Spanish or other flavors in a box,
   1/3 cup (75 mL) cooked: 485 mg

Meats and proteins
Beef jerky, one 9-inch (23 cm) strip: 570 mg
Bologna, 2 slices: 550 mg

Soups
Chicken noodle, canned, made with water, 1 cup (250 mL):
   650–890 mg
Chicken noodle, canned, 25% less salt, 1 cup (250 mL):
   485–660 mg (some brands 410 mg)
Cream of mushroom, canned, made with water, 1 cup
   (250 mL): 850–930 mg
Cream of mushroom, canned, 25% less salt, 1 cup (250 mL):
   630–650 mg
Tomato soup, canned, made with water, 1 cup (250 mL):
   695–800 mg (some brands 480 mg)
Tomato soup, canned, 25% less salt, 1 cup (250 mL): 720 mg

Meal items
Cheeseburger (fast food): 640–750 mg
Chili, canned, 1 cup (250 mL): 650 mg
Hamburger Helper, 1/5 package made with meat and milk,
   1 cup (250 mL) prepared: 695 mg
Pizza, 1/6 of 12-inch (30 cm) pizza: 350–650 mg
Pizza, frozen, rising crust, 1/6 (128 g): 540 mg
TV dinners, light: 480–540 mg (also see very high-
   sodium foods)

Desserts and snacks
Cheezies/cheese puffs, 3/4 cup (175 mL): 440–520 mg
Popcorn, theatre, large: 530 mg or more
Potato chips, regular salt brands, 30 chips (50 g): 600 mg

Condiments
Dill pickle, 1 (60 g): 570 mg
Reduced-salt bouillon, beef or chicken, 1 sachet: 530 mg
Reduced-salt soy sauce, 1 tbsp (15 mL): 550 mg

Salts
Accent (MSG), 1 tsp (5 mL): 640 mg
Table salt, 1/4 tsp (1 mL): 580 mg
Baking powder, 1 tsp (5 ml) 520 mg

Sea salt, kosher salt and table salt are all salt!
Sea salt or kosher salt are typically coarse salts.
They aren't as finely ground as table salt.

Medications and sodium
Some medications contain sodium. Examples are some laxatives or antacids. Look for the word sodium in the drug name or ingredient list. Drugs that are effervescent (fizzy) also usually have sodium. Ask your pharmacist if any of your medications have sodium, and if so how much.

Very high-sodium foods

These portions each provide over 720 mg sodium. This is 30% or more of your daily needs.

Foods with over 1,000 mg are marked with an asterisk (*).
Foods with over 1,500 mg are marked with two asterisks (**).
Foods with over 2,000 mg are marked with three asterisks (***).

Restaurant food is very salty! Before you decide to eat out, search online for the restaurant's nutritional information.

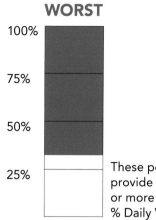

WORST

100%

75%

50%

25%

These portions provide 30% or more of your % Daily Value.

Soups
Chunky beef, canned, ready-to-eat, 1 cup (250 mL): 770 mg
Cream of mushroom made with water, 1 cup (250 mL): 800–850 mg
Soup in a cup, 1 pouch (11 g): 730–750 mg
Noodles in a bowl (110 g): 1,320–1,430 mg*
Noodles in a cup (64 g): 900–1,470 mg*
Soup, sub or coffee shop, 10-oz (300 g): 820–1,390*

Other foods
Corned beef or Klik, 4 oz (125 g): 900–1,140 mg*
Ham or Spam, 4 oz (125 g): 1,500–1,600 mg*
Pizza pop: 770 mg
Ravioli, mini, ½ can: 830 mg
TV dinner, light: up to 900 mg

Restaurant meals
Cheeseburger, double, with large fries and 2 ketchup: 1,720 mg**
Cheeseburger with small fries and 1 ketchup: 1,020 mg*
Chili, 10 oz (300 mL): 1,320 mg*
Chinese food, 10 oz (300 g) fried rice, 5 oz (150 g) BBQ pork and 1 veggie spring roll: 2,750 mg***
Grilled chicken salad (fast food) with dressing: 990–1,350 mg*
Hamburger (Whopper or Big Mac type): 930–1,020 mg*
Fried chicken breast: 1,050–1,310 mg* (grilled = 440 mg)
Fried chicken, big box meal (drumstick, 2 crispy strips, popcorn chicken, 2 homestyle sides and 32 oz/ 896 mL diet drink): 2,970 mg***
Macaroni and cheese, or store bought ready-to-eat, 1 cup (250 mL): 880–945 mg
Penne, baked, 3-cheese, small: 1,030 mg*
Pita, flat baked, extreme: 1,115–1,660 mg**
Pizza, Hawaiian, 6-inch (15 cm): 1,180 mg*
Popcorn chicken (KFC), large: 1,600 mg**
Poutine, 1 serving fast food: 2,720 mg***

Sandwich with fries: 1,370–4,200 mg***
Sandwiches, deli: 780–1,730 mg**
Sub, 6-inch (15 cm): 1,160–2,850 mg***
Taco salad: 1,400 mg*
Wings, Boston Pizza, breaded barbecue, single order: 3,770 mg***
Wraps, breakfast (Subway): 1,260–1,750 mg**

Snacks
Muffin, large, coffee shop: 510–790 mg
Potato chips, 350 g bag: 2,640 mg***
Potato chips, lower-salt brands, regular, 235 g bag (117 chips): 300–960 mg
Potato chips, ripple, 235 g bag (117 chips): 1,270 mg*
Potato chips, salt and vinegar, 235 g bag (145 chips): 2,915 mg***
Pretzel twists, 12 (50 g): 720–1,000 mg*

Condiments
Oyster sauce, 1 tbsp (15 mL): 750 mg
Sauerkraut, ½ cup (125 mL): 825–1,650 mg**
Soy sauce, 1 tbsp (15 mL): 1,030 mg*

Salts and salt substitutes:
Baking soda, 1 tsp (5 mL): 1,285 mg*
Garlic salt or celery salt, 1 tsp (5 mL): 1,170 mg*
Half Salt, 1 tsp (5 mL): 1,040 mg*
(contains half potassium chloride instead of sodium chloride).
Hy's seasoning salt without MSG, 1 tsp (5 mL): 1,700 mg**
Sea salt or kosher salt (coarse ground), 1 tsp (5 mL): 2,130 mg***
Table salt, 1 tsp (5 mL): 2,325 mg***

6. Lowering Cholesterol Levels

Q & A WITH KAREN GRAHAM: Improve your diet to lose weight and lower cholesterol

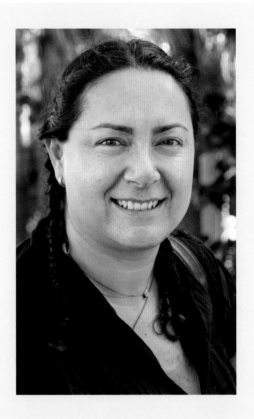

ROSITA: I have had prediabetes and high blood pressure for several years. My doctor recently did some tests and told me that now I also have high cholesterol and high triglycerides. I was shocked when he told me this. Even though I have put on weight over the years (I am 5'2" and I weigh about 160 lbs/73 kg), I didn't think it was so bad. He is considering starting me on a cholesterol pill. I hate to have to take more pills, though, so he suggested I try and lose some weight and improve my diet to see if I can bring my levels down. He said I may still need some new medications at some point. He wants to reassess my levels in three months. I would like to do this without medications. What would you suggest? How do I cut cholesterol out of my diet?

KAREN: Good for you to choose a healthier diet instead of taking more medications. While medications are important, being healthy in the long-term means changing your lifestyle. Your doctor is absolutely right.

You need a certain amount of cholesterol in your blood. It's an essential part of your body's cells and nerves. It also has a role in making bile for digestion, certain hormones and vitamin D. When you have too much, though, it can block your blood vessels. There are many factors that can cause cholesterol to go up, not just the cholesterol in foods. Your liver makes the majority of cholesterol in your body. When you lose weight, this can reduce how much cholesterol your liver makes. Weight loss also improves your body's ability to remove excess cholesterol from your blood.

Complete the Checklist on pages 119–121. Learn about other factors that also help improve cholesterol, such as exercise, reducing stress and reducing saturated fats. Eating less added sugar and drinking less alcohol can improve triglycerides. Cutting back on salt is an important part of reducing high blood pressure. After you complete the Checklist, focus on improving the things you "never" do or only do "sometimes." One or two changes is a great start.

Do you need additional help with food planning?
Ask your doctor to refer you to a Registered Dietitian.

Checklist for cholesterol, triglycerides and blood pressure

Do You...

1. Eat smaller portions of food?

This will help you lose weight. When you weigh less, your heart doesn't have to work so hard. Your cholesterol, triglyceride and blood pressure usually come down. Your liver will make less cholesterol.

❑ most of the time
❑ sometimes
❑ never

2. Eat more soluble fiber?

This reduces your blood cholesterol. Find soluble fiber in foods such as oatmeal and oat bran, psyllium (added to some breakfast cereals), barley, peas, beans and lentils (such as lima beans, kidney beans, navy and black beans, soybeans and chickpeas), apples, pears, artichoke hearts, chicory and dandelion roots, onions, leeks and garlic.

❑ most of the time
❑ sometimes
❑ never

3. Eat less meat and unhealthy fats?

Choose smaller portions of meat and eat more vegetables. Have one or more meatless dinners each week. Add less fat to your meals. Eat fewer french fries, donuts, potato chips, cookies and fried chicken.

❑ most of the time
❑ sometimes
❑ never

4. Eat more healthy fats?

Choose foods that have omega-3 fats and monounsaturated fat. Have fish or seafood twice a week, or choose ground flaxseed (or flaxseed oil), wheat germ, or omega-3 eggs. In small amounts, choose foods such as olives, olive oil, canola oil, soybean oil, avocados, walnuts, almonds, hazelnuts, pecans, peanuts, pistachios, cashews, macadamia nuts, soy nuts, pumpkin seeds, sunflower seeds or sesame seeds.

❑ most of the time
❑ sometimes
❑ never

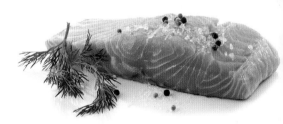

Note: An added benefit of these oils and nuts is that they have healthful plant sterols. These help remove some of the "bad" cholesterol from your blood.

5. Eat foods rich in B vitamins?

Some B vitamins, such as folic acid, reduce homocysteine. This is a harmful chemical which can build up in your blood vessels. You can lessen blood vessel damage and stroke by eating foods containing folic acid. Choose dark leafy green vegetables, whole grains, beans and legumes. Other sources of folic acid are flour, many dry cereals (check the label), orange juice, green peas, corn, beets, green beans, nuts and seeds.

❑ most of the time
❑ sometimes
❑ never

❑ most of the time
❑ sometimes
❑ never

6. Eat lots of antioxidants?

Antioxidants are plant compounds and vitamins that help reduce inflammation of your blood vessel walls.

- Dark green vegetables such as spinach, broccoli and kale
- Garlic and onions, broccoli, cabbage, Brussels sprouts, bok choy, cauliflower, turnip and rutabagas
- Peas, beans and lentils
- Orange and red vegetables and fruits such as carrots, squash, pumpkin, sweet potatoes, bell peppers, oranges, red grapefruit, mangos, watermelon and guavas
- Avocado, seeds and nuts, especially walnuts
- Herbs and spices such as rosemary, thyme, marjoram, sage, peppermint, tarragon, oregano, sweet basil and cinnamon
- Apples with the peel, cherries, plums, prunes and raisins
- All berries
- Grapes and pomegranate and their juices (limit to $\frac{1}{3}$ cup/75 mL a day)
- Fortified soy milk, soy protein, soy nuts and tofu
- Tea, especially green and black tea
- Hot cocoa, or an occasional small piece of dark cocoa-rich chocolate

❑ most of the time
❑ sometimes
❑ never

7. Eat less sodium and more potassium?

Less sodium: Limit restaurant foods, salty snack foods, processed meat, canned and packaged soups, and prepackaged convenience foods. Put away the salt shaker. Take out the pepper grinder, herbs and spices.

More potassium: Choose fruits and vegetables such as banana, melons, dried fruit, orange, kiwi, mango, pear, artichoke, avocado, beet greens, beets, Brussels sprouts, celery, mushrooms, parsnips, potato, pumpkin, spinach, carrots, yams, tomatoes and squash. Also eat potassium in bran cereals, beans, lentils, meat and milk.

❑ most of the time
❑ sometimes
❑ never

8. Include calcium?

Studies show calcium foods in your diet can help improve your blood pressure and reduce "bad" cholesterol. They also may play a role in improving blood pressure. For fewer calories, choose lower-fat milk and milk products. It is best to get your calcium from food, not supplements. Some studies show calcium taken by pill may build up in your blood vessels and is not healthy.

9. Limit sugars and sweet drinks?

Juice, soft drinks, other sweetened beverages, desserts and candies increase your blood sugar and triglycerides.

❑ most of the time
❑ sometimes
❑ never

10. Limit alcohol?

If you drink two or more drinks a day, this increases your blood pressure. Any amount can worsen triglycerides.

❑ most of the time
❑ sometimes
❑ never

11. Limit coffee?

Limit specialty coffees loaded with fat and sugar. Filtered coffee is the best choice for your cholesterol. The paper filter soaks up a natural chemical in the coffee called terpenes. Terpenes can raise blood cholesterol. Perked coffee, french press and espresso all have more terpenes than filtered coffee. There is some evidence that excess caffeine may increase heart arrhythmias and homocysteine. Limit to 3 to 4 cups (750 mL–1 L) per day. Replace some coffee with water.

❑ most of the time
❑ sometimes
❑ never

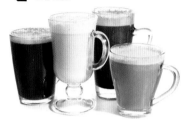

12. Keep active?

Exercise improves blood flow and increases your metabolism to help burn calories. Doctors recommend at least 25 minutes of exercise a day. Try walking or using an exercise bike. Start slowly and gradually do more.

❑ most of the time
❑ sometimes
❑ never

13. Avoid smoking?

Try to cut back or quit. You may have tried to quit before. Please think about trying again.

❑ most of the time
❑ sometimes
❑ never

14. Manage your diabetes?

Improving your blood sugar can improve your blood cholesterol, triglycerides and your blood pressure.

❑ most of the time
❑ sometimes
❑ never

15. Manage your stress?

Stress harms the inside lining of your blood vessel walls. Seek help from a friend or professional if your stress bothers you too much. Stay busy to take your mind off worries. When you exercise or laugh, "happy hormones" go through your body to help you relax. A walk in the evening will help tire you out and help you sleep better.

❑ most of the time
❑ sometimes
❑ never

How did you do? If you checked "most of the time" often, you are doing well.

If you checked "never" often, then consider trying to make some changes in these areas.

7. Herbs and Vitamins

Herbs and spices

Fresh or dried herbs and spices are nutritious additions to your diet. Buy them at a grocery store or grow them. Many are easy to grow in your garden or in a windowsill pot. The greatest benefit of herbs is their flavor. When you add them to other foods, you can cut back on your use of salt, sugar or fat as flavorings.

Healthful herbs and spices

These may be of benefit to blood sugar: cinnamon, allspice, black pepper and fenugreek. Enjoy these spices added to your foods. (At this time, buying and taking concentrated extracts of these is not recommended.)

These antioxidant foods protect against heart disease and cancer: garlic, onions and chives, rosemary, thyme, marjoram, sage, peppermint, tarragon, oregano, sweet basil, cinnamon, curry powder and paprika.

These herbs are mild blood thinners: garlic, onions and chives.

These may reduce inflammation in blood vessels: turmeric, ginger, rosemary, black pepper and chili peppers.

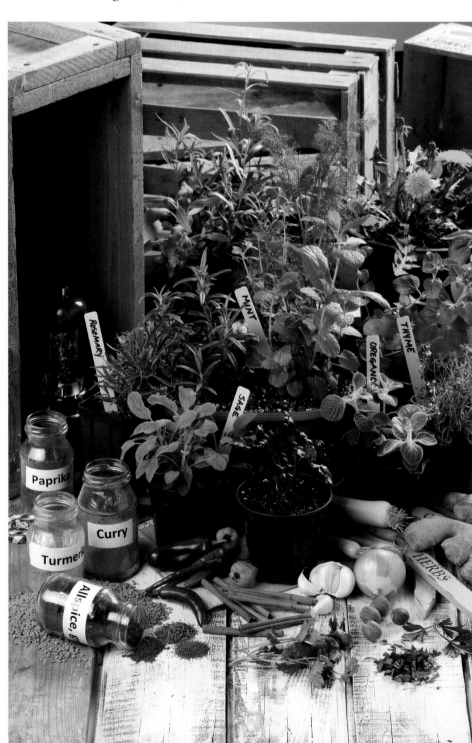

Tea

People around the world have been drinking black, green and oolong brewed teas for thousands of years. After water, tea is the second most common beverage in the world. Its antioxidants may help remove unwanted chemicals from the blood vessels. Tea contains polyphenols (a type of healthful plant chemical) which helps insulin work better. Tea without added milk has the most antioxidants (as milk proteins can partially bind with the polyphenols). Tea has tannins in it. Tannins are the dark color of tea. Tannins help reduce the glycemic index of food. For many, the greatest benefit of tea is that it has a soothing taste and helps family and friends relax.

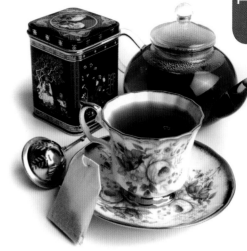

Go for brewed tea
Powdered tea and bottled ice tea contain lots of sugar (except for sugar-free varieties). Brewed tea, whether it's hot or cold, has more health benefits.

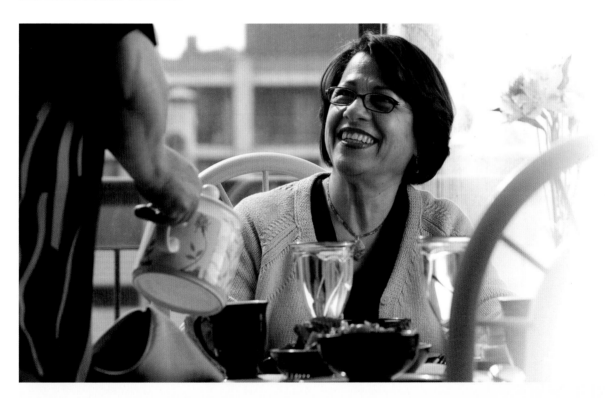

Herbal teas

Herbal teas are beverages made from any part of a plant except tea plant leaves. Herbal teas sold in grocery stores are safe, calorie-free and caffeine-free. Homemade herbal teas made directly from herbs, roots or leaves, and/ or steeped for longer, may be more potent. These homemade teas therefore may have medicinal health benefits, and risks, just like herbal supplements; seek your doctor's advice about safety.

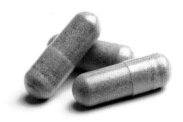

About a quarter of prescription medications have active ingredients that come from plants.

Researchers have found the following problems in many containers of imported herbal supplements:

- The bottle didn't contain the herbs as listed.
- The capsules were a stronger or lesser dosage than stated on the bottle.
- There were harmful contaminants, such as lead or arsenic, with the herbs.

Herbal supplements

What are herbal supplements?

They are herbs concentrated into a pill, liquid or powder form. People use them for medicinal purposes.

Herbal regulations

In the United States, herbal supplements are called "dietary supplements." Manufacturers don't have to get FDA approval in the way they would if they were selling prescription drugs.

In Canada, Health Canada regulates herbal supplements as natural health products (NHPs) or homeopathic medicines (HMs). Clinical safety trials using humans aren't required for most herbal supplements; the government approves them based on available information only. The government gives each herb a natural product number (NPN) or a drug identification number (DIN-HM). Look for these numbers on herbal supplements, including if you buy them online.

Concerns about herbal supplements

Not enough testing and regulation; benefits and risks vary

Governments don't test and regulate herbal supplements in the same rigorous way as prescription medications. Variable growing seasons, contaminants in the earth and water, and pesticides and fertilizers all affect a plant's growth. For this reason, it's hard to create standardized dosages in supplements. Some concentrated supplements may contain uneven amounts of beneficial or toxic components.

There are many herbal manufacturers that claim their supplements help lower blood sugar. The truth is there is not enough research to prove if this is true. There are thousands of herbs from around the world, and most have not been studied in a scientific way to measure benefits and risks. Their effects on your blood sugar can vary.

On the good side, more science-based research of herbal supplements is being funded. See pages 126–129 for information on some herbs that have been studied for benefits and risks.

If in doubt, don't take it.

Do not take these dangerous herbal supplements

These are commonly available herbs that can cause health problems from kidney, liver or lung damage, cancer, high or low blood pressure or a heart attack.

Beware of chaparral, coltsfoot, comfrey, ephedrine (ephedra or ma huang), germander, jin bu huan, lobelia, phenylalanine and sassafras, *Timospora crispa*, and L-tryptophan. *Note that this is not a complete list.*

Interactions with medications

Herbs can cause side effects or interact with other medications. Your pharmacist has access to herbal dictionaries. She can tell you of any known potential benefits and risks, and possible interactions with other herbs or drugs. You can get online information about herb-drug interactions from WebMD or the National Center for Complementary and Integrative Health.

Herbal supplements with known drug interactions:

- There is a risk of increased bleeding (for example in the stomach) if you take willow bark, devil's claw, alfalfa, chamomile, evening primrose oil, feverfew, ginkgo biloba, ginseng, red clover, reishi mushroom, or large amounts of garlic, ginger or cinnamon. If you are on a blood thinner such as warfarin or aspirin, the bleeding risk increases.

- St John's Wort interferes with antidepressants such as fluoxetine (Prozac). It also interferes with some cholesterol medications. It can worsen your chances of a bad sunburn if you also take glyburide.

- Dried aloe, cascara sagrada, senna or licorice can cause low potassium levels. This then causes interaction with some heart and blood pressure pills.

- Ginseng, licorice, yerba mate and yohimbine can make your blood pressure go up. For information on yohimbine, see page 399.

Natural does not necessarily mean safe.

If you take herbal supplements, please tell your doctor or pharmacist. Doctors do not recommend herbal supplements if you are pregnant. There isn't enough information about whether they are safe for your growing baby.

Herbs and kidney disease

If you have kidney damage, stop taking all herbs unless your doctor tells you to take them. Your kidneys filter out excess drugs and herbs into your urine. If your kidneys aren't working fully, herbs can build up in your body and cause more damage.

These herbs are not safe when you have kidney disease:

- bucha leaves
- juniper berries
- uva ursi
- parsley capsules
- *Artemisia absinthium* (wormwood)
- autumn crocus
- chuifong tuokuwan
- horse chestnut
- periwinkle
- sassafras
- tung sheuh
- *Vandellia cordifolia*

Note: Starfruit is a tropical fruit (not an herb), but be aware it has a toxin in it that is passed out of the body by healthy people, but remains in the body when you have kidney disease.

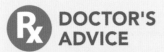

DOCTOR'S ADVICE

How to assess effect of herbs on your blood sugar

Take the same amount of herb on at least three occasions, before eating the same meal (and same size). Take your blood sugar before you eat and two hours after you eat. Now do the same without the herb. Measure the difference. Your physical activity and stress should be about the same on each occasion. While not conclusive, this might give you some idea of the effect of the herb. While you may be measuring a placebo effect, if it improves your blood sugar this is helpful.

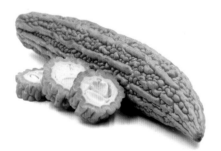

Bitter melon is a vegetable that grows in the tropics. It's also called balsam pear or karela. People cook this vegetable into stir-fries or make it into a juice.

Benefits of herbal supplements

Herbal supplements are generally not as strong as most prescription medications. For this reason, they may be your "drug" of choice. You may find the less potent over-the-counter herbal supplement of some benefit. For example, for a mild muscle ache, you may find resting and a cup of peppermint tea helps you feel better. You may not need a commercial pain killer.

What is the diabetes placebo effect? Imagine you take an herbal supplement (or vitamin pill) that your doctor feels is useless, but you believe it will help your blood sugar. This belief often helps you feel happier, less stressed and more in control of your health. This could actually help your blood sugar! How we think can have a role in keeping our bodies healthy.

Helpful diabetes herbal supplements
Bitter melon (Momordica charantia)

- **Potential benefits:** Bitter melon has been used as a traditional diabetes medicine in many parts of the world. Good long-term research has not yet been done in North America to give us clear evidence that it is helpful in people with diabetes. However it is very promising, as animal studies have suggested that it may (1) help the pancreas make more insulin, (2) help tissues pick up blood sugar more easily or (3) reduce how much sugar the liver makes.

- **Potential side effects:** If you are taking bitter melon, you may need to adjust your diabetes medications. Bitter melon may cause your body to lose too much potassium. This is a concern if you experience diarrhea or take laxatives or certain blood pressure pills that also pull potassium out of your body. Doctors don't recommend bitter melon if you are pregnant, as it might cause a miscarriage.

⚠️ **CAUTION**

Always tell your pharmacist or doctor what herbs and medications you are taking. Ask how much is safe for you. Herbs, like medications, can be good for you and can cause side effects if you take too much of them.

Berberine (Coptis chinensis)
- **Potential benefits:** Berberine could lower blood sugar at doses of 500 mg taken two to three times a day. It has some promising benefits, but it also has some risks.
- **Potential side effects:** Talk to your doctor about berberine's safety for you. It may cause stomach upset. It's not recommended if you are pregnant or breastfeeding, have heart disease, or if you take cyclopsorines, statins for cholesterol or blood pressure pills called calcium channel blockers.

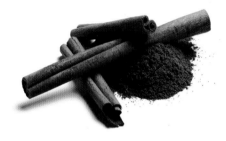

Chinese cinnamon, or cassia (Cinnamomum aromaticum)
This is the kind of cinnamon available in grocery stores.
- **Potential benefits:** Some studies show mild benefits to reducing blood sugar from eating about ½ to 1 tsp (1–2 g) of cinnamon daily. Doctors don't recommend you take more than 1 tsp (2 g). Other studies show no benefit.
- **Potential side effects:** More than 1 tsp (2 g) of cinnamon a day may increase blood thinning. Do not eat more cinnamon than this if you are on a blood thinner such as aspirin or coumadin.

Ginkgo biloba leaf extract
- **Potential benefits:** Some evidence suggests that ginkgo leaf extract may help protect blood vessel walls and improve circulation. It's used in Europe and sold as an approved drug, but not regulated as a drug in North America.
- **Potential side effects:** Ginkgo interacts with some antibiotics, cholesterol medication, and blood thinners. Gingko can cause bleeding if you take it in large amounts.

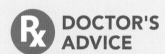

℞ DOCTOR'S ADVICE
Ginseng and ginkgo is not recommended by most doctors. More research of the herbs and drug interactions is needed.

Ginseng root or berry extract
- **Potential benefits:** Some studies show American ginseng root and Asian ginseng root or berry extract have benefits in decreasing blood sugar rise after a meal. However, other studies have not shown ginseng improves A1C levels. It may improve cholesterol and triglycerides.
- **Potential side effects:** Some ginseng species (but not American ginseng) have significant side effects at high doses, including high blood pressure. Ginseng can interact with your diabetes medications and can cause low blood sugar. Ginseng can also interact with pills you are taking for depression or to stabilize your mood, and with water pills, also called diuretics.

Ginseng's side effects are not clear because of the large varieties of ginseng used in different studies.

Gymnema grows in India and comes from the leaf of a woody plant.

Gymnema sylvestre

- **Potential benefits:** *Gymnema sylvestre* may help diabetes in three ways: (1) decrease the absorption of sugar from your gut, (2) improve how your body uses blood sugar, and (3) stimulate your pancreas to make more insulin.
- **Potential side effects:** As with some other herbs that may lower blood sugar, gymnema may also interact with other diabetes medications. We need to do more research to know more about its benefits and side effects.

Milk thistle (Silybum marianum)

- **Potential benefits:** The seed of the plant has a compound called flavonolignan which makes insulin work more effectively. Some studies have shown a daily dose of 600 mg has some benefit in reducing blood sugar.
- **Potential side effects:** In some people it can cause mild stomach upset. It is considered a safe herb although it can interact with some medications. Check with your pharmacist.

Prickly pear cactus and aloe vera

These are two different desert plants. The scientific name for prickly pear cactus is *Opuntia streptacantha*. You may know aloe vera as a common house plant. These herbs are usually sold as capsules.

- **Potential benefits:** Both plants have gel-like sap in their leaves. This sap contains soluble fiber. Soluble fiber can lower fasting blood sugar by slowing down the rate that you absorb carbohydrates.
- **Potential side effects:** Prickly pear cactus and aloe vera can interact with diabetes medications. If you take diuretics (water pills) such as lasix or hydrochlothiazide, or a heart pill called digoxin, you must talk with your pharmacist or doctor before taking this. Prickly pear cactus also may cause unwanted skin changes, like eczema. Aloe vera can cause diarrhea in some people.

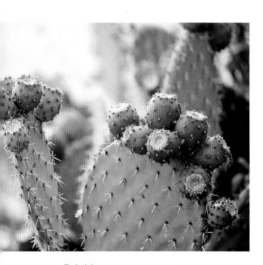

Prickly pear cactus

Reishi mushroom (Ganoderma lucidum)

- **Potential benefits:** Proteins and starches found in the mushroom may increase insulin levels and improve both blood sugar after meals and A1C. More research is needed to assess its benefit. A 500 mg capsule, no more than three times a day, is recommended to avoid side effects.

- **Potential side effects:** If you take antiplatelet or anticoagulant medications, daily doses of 3,000 mg or more of reishi mushroom may further thin the blood, increasing the risk of bleeding. Other side effects commonly seen at these higher doses are dry mouth and nose, itchiness and stomach upset.

White mulberry (Morus alba)

- **Potential benefits:** The leaves of the white mulberry have flavonoids and starches that can reduce the absorption of sugars in the intestine. This can help lower the blood sugar after a meal. The effective dose is 3–9 mg of the active ingredient deoxynojirimicin three times daily before meals.

- **Potential side effects:** White mulberry is generally well tolerated. However, more studies are needed.

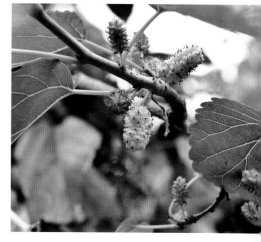

White mulberry

Vitamins and minerals

Food is the best source for vitamins and minerals

You will get all the vitamins and minerals you need if you eat a variety of foods. See *Hands-On Food Guide* on pages 55–57, and the healthy meal plans in this book. The chart on pages 132–133 shows you good food sources for common vitamins and minerals, and what they do for your body. These foods help you prevent and manage diabetes complications. When you eat whole foods, you eat vitamins and minerals in safe amounts. Also, in whole foods, they are combined with healthful fiber, antioxidants and plant chemicals (called phytochemicals). Food is the best way to get your nutrients in just the right amount.

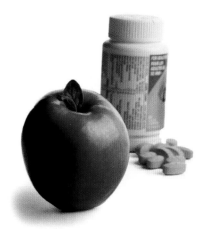

Vitamins don't replace healthy eating.

You do not need to take vitamin and mineral pills unless your doctor or dietitian prescribes them. If a doctor prescribes you a vitamin or mineral pill, ask why, and know how many you should take. Also, remember the importance of eating healthy foods and regular exercise.

For some people, taking supplements can be life-threatening

For example, people who have a rare genetic condition called hemochromatosis get a build-up of iron in their body. It gets worse if they take any iron pills. Hemochromatosis can lead to diabetes and heart disease and a variety of other problems. It is life-threatening if not treated.

Do you live in the north with low winter sunlight?

The Canadian and Alaskan governments recommend certain age groups take vitamin D. For example, as you get older, your skin doesn't make vitamin D as well.

Do researchers believe supplements work?

Research over the past 20 years has shown limited or no benefit to taking vitamin and mineral pills. A large study (Archives of Internal Medicine Journal, 2009) of women ages 50 to 79 showed that multivitamins didn't protect against heart attack, stroke, cancer or an early death. These results are a shock to many. Nearly half the population of women and nearly as many men take a multivitamin pill.

In other studies, taking vitamin C, E, beta carotene (which turns into vitamin A) and selenium didn't show conclusive benefits. The US Preventive Services Task Force looked at more recent research (up to 2013) and concluded there was limited evidence supporting any benefit from taking vitamins and mineral supplements for the prevention of cancer or heart disease. The American Diabetes Association (2019) concluded there was no benefit in taking a multivitamin pill for diabetes and heart disease.

For diabetes, chromium studies don't show any significant benefit for blood glucose levels except for those who are malnourished and lacking chromium. Vitamins B_1, B_6, and B_{12} don't show conclusive benefits in treating diabetic neuropathy. The American and Canadian Diabetes Associations concluded there was no benefit to blood sugars from taking vitamin D. However, there is new evidence of the benefit of magnesium.

When are supplements good for you?

A supplement can definitely help someone with a vitamin or mineral deficiency or who is malnourished. Here are some other examples of when supplements help:

- To help heal a foot or lower leg wound
- To offset the side effects of certain medications. For example, if you take metformin, you should be tested once a year to make sure your vitamin B_{12} level is normal.
- To try to slow down macular degeneration
- To boost nutrition during pregnancy
- To boost nutrition for those with dietary restrictions because of celiac disease or kidney disease
- For vegetarians or vegans, and others on restrictive diets

More is not better

Your healthy body looks after you, storing the vitamins and minerals that you need for later. For example, your body stores vitamins A, D, E and K and iron in your fat and liver. If you take vitamins or minerals in large amounts (mega doses), you may end up with more than you need. Vitamins A and D, folic acid and vitamin B_6, iron, zinc, calcium and selenium can make you sick or even kill you at high doses.

What is a mega dose?

A mega dose is a larger dose — more than what your body needs.

The Recommended Dietary Allowance (RDA) is the amount of each vitamin and mineral that you need for good health. If you take a dose of supplement that is at or above the upper limit (UL), you are more likely to have side effects. This is a mega dose. To determine the RDA and UL of each vitamin and mineral, search online for these words: "DRI tables." Multivitamin pills don't generally contain mega doses. However, when you buy vitamins or minerals individually, each pill will have a higher amount. If you take too many pills each day, your total intake goes up. You end up with a mega dose.

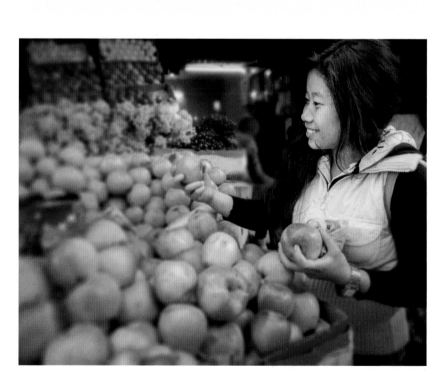

DOCTOR'S ADVICE

Mega doses aren't safe for anyone. If your kidneys aren't working well, it's particularly dangerous. Avoid doubling up on vitamin or mineral pills.

Food supplies what you need

You need tiny amounts of vitamins and minerals to be healthy. For example, you need 70 to 90 milligrams of vitamin C every day. You'll consume that in one large orange. If you also take a pill of 1,000 mg (or 1 gram) of vitamin C every day, your kidneys have to work harder to flush out the extra vitamin C.

131

Vitamin	What food is it in?	What does it do in the body?
Vitamin A (beta carotene can convert to vitamin A)	It's in organ meats, eggs, fish, milk, dark green and yellow and orange vegetables such as carrots, squash and sweet potatoes, tomatoes, mangos, pink grapefruit and cantaloupes. Manufacturers add it to milk, margarine and butter.	It's important for good vision, healthy teeth, nails, hair, bones and glands. Vitamin A helps protect your body cells against infection and is an antioxidant. This vitamin helps wounds heal.
Vitamin B_1 (thiamin)	B_1 is in whole bran (wheat and rice), enriched flour and cereals, wheat germ, meats, green peas, dried peas and legumes, and nuts.	B_1 helps your body use carbohydrates for energy and growth. It has a role in proper muscle coordination and the maintenance of nerves.
Vitamin B_2 (riboflavin)	B_2 is in milk, green vegetables, meats (especially organ meats), legumes, cheese, eggs, yogurt, cottage cheese, whole grains, enriched flour and cereal.	B_2 helps your body turn protein, fat and carbohydrate into energy. B_2 helps maintain healthy skin and eyes. B_2 builds and maintains body tissue.
Vitamin B_3 (niacin)	B_3 is in meats (especially organ meats), poultry, fish, peanuts, legumes, corn, whole grains, enriched flour and cereals.	B_3 helps to break down protein and turn food into energy. It helps keep your gut and skin healthy.
Vitamin B_6 (pyridoxine)	B_6 is in meats (especially organ meats), eggs, fish, legumes, walnuts, green leafy vegetables, bananas, grapes, watermelon, carrots, peas, potatoes, whole grains and wheat germ.	B_6 helps to make and to use certain proteins. It helps your nervous system work properly and protects you against infection. You need B_6 for a healthy heart.
Vitamin B_{12}	B_{12} is in meats (especially organ meats), shellfish, eggs, fish (particularly salmon and herring), milk and milk products, especially blue cheese. Some soy products have B_{12} added to them.	B_{12} helps make hemoglobin and healthy red blood cells, and helps maintain a healthy nervous system.
Folic Acid (folate)	Folic acid is in organ meats, beans and legumes, spinach, kale, parsley and other green leafy vegetables, asparagus, corn, green peas, fruits such as oranges, orange juice and melons, nuts, whole grains and yeast. It's also in flour, pasta and some rice marked "enriched."	Folic acid is necessary to make certain proteins and genetic materials for your cells and keeps your blood cells healthy. Folic acid taken during pregnancy reduces the risk of some birth defects. Both folic acid and vitamin B_{12} may help reduce your stroke and heart attack risk. In part, this may be because it helps reduce a chemical called homocysteine.
Vitamin C	Vitamin C is in fruit, especially citrus fruits and juices, strawberries, kiwi, cantaloupe and guava. It's also in tomatoes, cabbage, sweet peppers, potatoes, onions, broccoli and green leafy vegetables including dandelion greens.	Vitamin C helps in the production of collagen and is necessary for healthy skin, gums, blood vessels, muscles, teeth and bones. It aids in the absorption of iron. It works as an antioxidant and helps wounds heal.
Vitamin D	This is the "sunshine vitamin" — our skin makes vitamin D when we're in the sunshine. It's in fatty fish such as salmon or sardines, liver and eggs. Milk, margarine and butter contain added vitamin D.	Vitamin D works with calcium and phosphorus to build and maintain strong bones and teeth. It also has a role in muscle strength. Low vitamin D may be a risk for diabetes, hypertension, multiple sclerosis, cancer and arthritis.

| Vitamin E | Vitamin E is in vegetable oil, nuts and seeds, peanut butter, wheat germ, green leafy vegetables, avocado, legumes, eggs, margarine, butter, liver, milk, whole grains and fortified cereals. | Vitamin E is an antioxidant and helps protect your cell coverings. It is important in healthy blood cells and body tissues. |
| Vitamin K | Vitamin K is the "bacteria vitamin." In a healthy person, it's made in the gut by bacteria. It's high in green leafy vegetables and in fruit, cereals, dairy products, meat and vegetable oils. | Vitamin K is necessary for clotting of blood and healthy bones. |

Mineral	What food is it in?	What does it do in the body?
Calcium	Calcium is in milk and milk products, dates, blackstrap molasses, oysters, scallops, salmon and sardines with bones, fish heads, legumes, almonds, green leafy vegetables and broccoli. Manufacturers add it to some tofu, soy beverages and other non-dairy beverages.	Calcium is important for bone and tooth formation. Also, it helps in blood clotting. It's important for your nerve function, muscles and heart. It helps you keep a healthy weight and blood pressure.
Iron	Iron is in liver and organ meats, meats, eggs, shellfish (particularly oysters), nuts, sardines, legumes, broccoli, peas, spinach, prunes, raisins, bran, enriched cereals, blackstrap molasses and wheat germ.	Iron is important for healthy blood and muscle cells, and in the prevention of iron-deficiency anemia. Also, it helps in enzyme formation.
Magnesium	Magnesium is in green leafy vegetables, whole grains (such as quinoa), nuts and seeds (including peanut butter and other nut butters). Also, it's in legumes, peas, fish and seafood, yogurt, brown rice, oat bran and cocoa.	Magnesium helps in bone and tooth formation. It helps nerves, muscles and blood vessels work properly. Some studies have suggested magnesium may help improve fasting blood sugar and help insulin work. This is especially true for those who are low in magnesium.
Chromium	Chromium is in cereals and whole-grain bread, especially those with lots of bran. Some beer, red wine and grape juice contain chromium. It's also in meats, especially processed meats, poultry, fish, egg yolks and green vegetables.	Chromium helps insulin work. It may improve blood sugar, blood cholesterol and blood fat levels.
Potassium	Potassium is in fruit, particularly orange juice, bananas, pomegranates and dried fruits. Vegetables like carrots, potatoes, spinach and tomatoes, and meats and milk contain potassium.	Potassium is necessary for nerve and muscle function, and for maintaining acid-base and water balance in the body. It plays a role in a healthy blood pressure.
Selenium	Selenium is in brazil nuts, cashews, meat, seafood and poultry. There are smaller amounts in grains, dairy products and legumes.	Selenium is an antioxidant. It helps regulate thyroid hormones, which are important in weight maintenance.
Zinc	Zinc is in meats, liver, eggs and shellfish, specifically oysters, sardines, cheese, green leafy vegetables, oranges, prunes, strawberries, whole grains, and nuts and seeds.	Zinc is part of enzymes and insulin. It's also important for healthy skin and growth. It helps wounds heal. Zinc in combination with antioxidant vitamins might slow down advanced age-related macular degeneration (eye disease) for some people.

8. Alcohol

 Q & A WITH KAREN GRAHAM: Socialize without the high calories

MATTHEW: My partner and I have put on weight over the years. We like to sit out on our deck in the evenings and talk, have a few mixed drinks and eat peanuts. How should we change our routine now that I have diabetes?

KAREN: It is great that both of you are thinking about changing your evening routine. Here's some information to help you decide on your changes to make. All forms of alcohol including wine, liqueurs, coolers, beer, and hard liquor (spirits) have calories and can contribute to weight gain. Nuts are rich in nutrients but also are loaded in fat and calories. You might be surprised to learn that three drinks and half a cup of peanuts or mixed nuts can add up to 920 calories. In comparison, the large dinner meals in this book have 730 calories, and the large snacks have 200 calories.

Enjoy an alcoholic drink but reduce to one drink. Let your remaining evening drinks be a diet beverage or lemon water. Try different snacks found on pages 196 to 200, such as lightly oiled popcorn. The best thing about your evenings is that you're spending time together and talking. You have support from each other to change and be healthier because of your diabetes. Way to go!

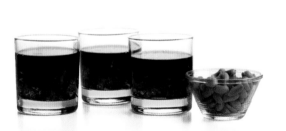

3 rum and cola (1.5 oz/45 mL rum and 4 oz/125 mL cola each) and ½ cup (125 mL) peanuts

920-calorie meal!

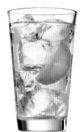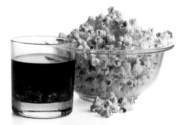

1.5 oz (45 mL) rum and diet cola, iced water with lemon and 4 cups (1L) lightly oiled popcorn

250-calorie snack

If you drink a glass of wine, a beer or mixed drink now and then, you don't have to give it up forever. Drink responsibly. On the following pages, you'll find more information about the risks, calories, health concerns and benefits of alcohol.

Risks of alcohol

Low blood sugar

Alcohol mixed with insulin or certain types of diabetes medications can cause low blood sugar (see pages 329–336). Overdrinking puts you at serious risk for dangerous low blood sugar that can occur up to 24 hours after drinking. If you drink too much, make sure you eat or drink some carbohydrate. Someone should stay with you and check your blood sugar every two to four hours, even during the night.

Avoiding low blood sugar when drinking alcohol:

- Limit drinks to one or maximum two.
- Do not drink on an empty stomach.
- If also exercising, for instance, dancing and drinking, have a snack with carbs to make up for the exercise.
- Do not mix alcohol with energy drinks, cannabis or street drugs.
- Have extra sugar handy to treat a low if needed.
- Tell your friends you have diabetes and how to treat a low.

Alcohol and energy drinks

Most energy drinks are high in caffeine. Both alcohol and caffeine are diuretics and both can make you lose a lot of fluid. They can cause dehydration and heart irregularities. You are particularly susceptible to dehydration when your blood sugar is high. Alcohol with energy drinks can conversely also cause low blood sugar.

Alcohol and cannabis (with THC)

Cannabis is now legal in many US states and in Canada. When you mix alcohol and cannabis with THC (the ingredient that makes you feel high), you could have significant issues with low blood sugar. See sidebar.

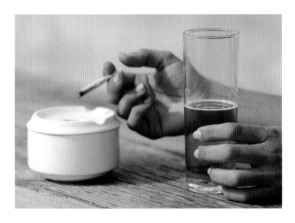

 DANGER

You have a risk of a dangerous low blood sugar when you drink too much alcohol. It's also dangerous when you mix alcohol with energy drinks or cannabis.

The high amount of caffeine in **energy drinks** can mask symptoms that you are drunk. This can lead to too much drinking, as your body doesn't give you signals to stop.

Cannabis, like alcohol, impairs, judgement. You may not realize you have low blood sugar. In addition, cannabis can keep you from throwing up. Your body won't get rid of the extra alcohol. This could lead to drinking too much. Your body won't be able to warn you to stop.

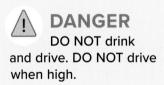 **DANGER** DO NOT drink and drive. DO NOT drive when high.

135

Bottom line

Alcoholic drinks add extra calories to your waistline. Plus, you may eat more when you drink. Just one bottle of beer or mixed drink a week can result in a 2-lb (1 kg) weight gain over the year. Five drinks a week can result in a 10-lb (4.5 kg) gain over the year.

Non-drinker:
Zero drinks

Occasional drinker:
A few drinks a week or a month

Moderate drinker:
One drink a day for women; two drinks a day for men

Heavy drinker:
More than three drinks a day

Alcoholic drinks are fattening

One and a half ounces (45 mL) of whiskey, rum or vodka has 100 calories. Beer, liqueurs, coolers and sweet wines contain alcohol plus sugar, boosting calories even more.

Alcohol can cause or contribute to many health problems

Alcohol is highly addictive. Some people are more likely to become addicted. Weigh any potential benefit of drinking alcohol regularly against the risk of addiction. Your liver can handle small amounts of alcohol. If you drink large amounts daily or on weekends, alcohol contributes to many health problems. These problems include:

- High blood pressure, high triglycerides and stroke
- Liver disease and pancreatitis
- Diabetes retinopathy, an eye disease
- Diabetic neuropathy, a nerve disease
- If pregnant, an increased risk of the baby getting fetal alcohol syndrome
- A greater risk for certain cancers, such as breast or liver cancer, even with low to moderate drinking
- If elderly and unsteady on your feet, an increased your risk of falling and breaking a hip or other bone

Do not drink alcohol if you:

- Are on medications or have a condition where alcohol is not recommended. Talk to your doctor.
- Plan to drive
- Are pregnant, trying to get pregnant, or breastfeeding
- Have pancreatitis, liver disease or very high triglycerides

Does alcohol have benefits?

Research shows that occasionally drinking alcohol, especially red wine, has some benefits in reducing heart disease. In part this may be due to an antioxidant called resveratrol. This is found in the skin and seeds of grapes, especially dark red and purple grapes. Some of these same benefits can come from eating grapes. Another possible benefit of occasional alcohol intake is that, for some people, it may help insulin work better.

Occasional consumption may help some people manage stress, by helping them relax. This is a good thing, but the key is *occasional.*

Alcoholic drink	Portion	Alcohol	Total carbs	Calories
Alcohol and nutrients vary between brands	In most common drink size	1 oz = 9.6 g 1 oz = 30 mL	Shown in grams and tsp (1 tsp = 5 mL)	
SPIRITS (hard liquor) (For example, whiskey, rum, brandy, vodka or gin. 40% alcohol by volume = 80% proof)				
On ice, or mixed with water or diet soft drink	1½ oz (45 mL)	1½ oz	0	100
Mixed with 4 oz soft drink, tonic water or juice	5½ oz (165 mL)	1½ oz	13 g (3¼ tsp)	150
Mixed with 4 oz tomato or clamato juice	5½ oz (165 mL)	1½ oz	5 g (1¼ tsp)	120
BEER				
Beer (7% alcohol)	12 oz (355 mL)	2 oz	10 g (2½ tsp)	185
Beer (5% alcohol)	12 oz (355 mL)	1½ oz	10 g (2½ tsp)	140
Light beer (4% alcohol)	12 oz (355 mL)	1 oz	4 g (1 tsp)	100–110
Ultra light/low-carb beer (3–4%)	12 oz (355 mL)	¾–1 oz	2–3 g (½–¾ tsp)	90–95
Flavored beer/radler (3–4%)	12 oz (355 mL)	¾–1 oz	2–3 g (½–¾ tsp)	90–95
Low-alcohol beer (0.5% alcohol)	12 oz (355 mL)	0.1 oz	10–16 g (2½–4 tsp)	65
WINE Alcohol content of wine can vary a lot. A light white wine may have 9%, a full-bodied red wine may have up to 12% and sherry and port have around 20% alcohol. Champagne might not have a high alcohol content but the bubbles in it cause it to be absorbed into your blood more quickly.				
Dessert wine, sweet (15–18% alcohol)	5 oz (150 mL)	1¾–2½ oz	16–20 g (4–5 tsp)	210–275
Dessert wine, dry (18% alcohol)	5 oz (150 mL)	2½ oz	2 g (½ tsp)	165
Table wine, red or white (12% alcohol)	5 oz (150 mL)	1½ oz	1–2 g (¼–½ tsp)	100–110
Champagne (8–14% alcohol)	5 oz (150 mL)	1½ oz	4 g (1 tsp)	105
Low-alcohol wine (8–10% alcohol)	5 oz (150 mL)	1–1½ oz	1–2 g (¼–½ tsp)	55–110
No-alcohol wine (0.5% alcohol)	5 oz (150 mL)	0.1 oz	14 g (3½ tsp)	65
CIDERS				
Sweet cider (6% alcohol)	12 oz (355 mL)	1¾ oz	14 g (3½ tsp)	170
Dry cider (6% alcohol)	12 oz (355 mL)	1¾ oz	12 g (3 tsp)	130
COOLERS				
Vodka cooler (5–7% alcohol)	12 oz (355 mL)	1½–2 oz	16–21 g (7 tsp)	220–250
Light cooler (3% alcohol)	12 oz (355 mL)	¾ oz	22–44 g (6–11 tsp)	170–250
COCKTAILS (made to standard recipes and sizes)				
Daiquiri	4 oz (125 mL)	2 oz	8 g (2 tsp)	140
Margarita	4 oz (125 mL)	2 oz	6 g (1½ tsp)	150
Mojito	4 oz (125 mL)	2 oz	6 g (1½ tsp)	160
Piña colada (also high in fat)	8 oz (250 mL)	2 oz	12 g (3 tsp)	325
No-alcohol drink — Bloody Mary	4 oz (125 mL)	0	8 g (2 tsp)	40
No-alcohol drink — strawberry daiquiri	4 oz (125 mL)	0	48 g (12 tsp)	200
LIQUEURS				
Cream-based (34–53% proof)	1½ oz (45 mL)	1 oz	12–24 g (3–6 tsp)	135–165
Non-cream based (80% proof)	1½ oz (45 mL)	1–1½ oz	6–10 g (1½–2½ tsp)	115–135

9. Taking Care of Yourself When Ill

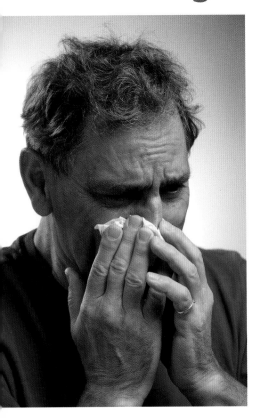

This section includes information about what to eat when you are ill. There are photographs to give you ideas of what to drink or eat when you are sick. It also includes information on medications and checking your blood sugar when you are ill. It is important to balance your food with your medications to ensure your blood sugar doesn't go low or really high when you are ill.

A brief illness might include the flu, a cold, food poisoning, or a bout of severe pain lasting one or several days. You may vomit, have diarrhea, a cough, sore throat, fever, pain or infection.

> ⚠️ **CAUTION**
> **Call your doctor, a medical help line or go to a clinic or emergency room if you have:**
>
> - **High blood sugar.** Your blood sugar is consistently above 270 mg/dL (15 mmol/L) and you feel very unwell.
> - **Low blood sugar.** You have continual lows, and are unable to keep your blood sugar above 70 mg/dL (4 mmol/L).
> - **Dehydration.** You feel very thirsty, with a dry mouth and skin. When you pinch your skin, it doesn't bounce back. You have muscle cramps, reduced sweat and urine, and you may feel dizzy or confused. Dehydration can happen because of vomiting, diarrhea, fever and high blood sugar.
> - **Fever.** You have a fever over 100°F (37.8°C).
> - **Bleeding.** You have blood in your urine, stool or vomit.
> - **Unusual symptoms** such as numbness or stiff neck.
> - **Concerns** that you are getting worse. You're worried about your illness and your symptoms worsen.

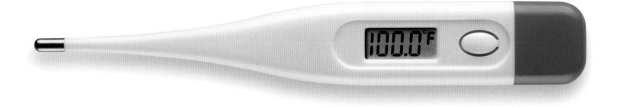

Take your insulin and medication

When you're sick, blood sugar usually goes up, even if you aren't eating much. The reason blood sugar goes up is that illness or pain increases stress hormones in your body. These hormones increase your blood sugar.

Occasionally, blood sugar can go low, especially if you aren't eating and have diarrhea or vomiting.

Adjusting insulin

- If you take insulin and adjust it yourself, then follow your adjustment guidelines.
- If you don't adjust your own insulin, contact your doctor or diabetes educator for recommendations.

Diabetes pills

- Don't change your diabetes pills dosage during a short illness.
- If your symptoms last more than 24 hours and you can't drink enough fluids, call your doctor or pharmacist about which medications to temporarily stop. This includes diabetes pills and other pills too.

Other medications

- If a doctor prescribes any medication for short-term illness, such as pain killers, antibiotics or decongestants, ask if it will affect your blood sugar. Also, over-the-counter medications can affect blood sugar or blood pressure. Ask your pharmacist or doctor about these.

Cough drops and syrups and cold medicines

- Check labels of cough or cold medicines for sugar. One teaspoon (5 mL) of sugar will equal 4 grams of carbohydrate. If you can't tolerate most foods, then take regular sugar-containing cough drops or cough syrup as part of your daily carbohydrate intake.
- If your blood sugar is high, use sugar-free cough drops or cough syrup.

Sugar-free products can cause diarrhea

Be aware that sugar-free products usually have sugar alcohols in them such as sorbitol or isomalt. These can cause mild diarrhea if you eat 10 g in a day, and worse diarrhea if you eat 20 g or more in a day. Just three or four sugar-free cough drops could cause or worsen diarrhea.

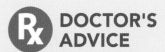

DOCTOR'S ADVICE

Take your medication

Keep taking your insulin or diabetes pills, unless your doctor or nurse tells you otherwise.

Plan ahead

Talk to your doctor or diabetes educator before you get sick. Learn how to adjust your insulin and other medications if you get sick.

If you live on your own

Tell a family member or friend that you're sick. They may need to come and stay with you, call or check on you periodically.

To help relieve a sore throat, gargle a salt and water solution.

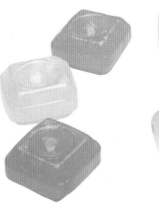

If you don't check your blood sugar at home...

Learn the signs and symptoms of high and low blood sugars; see page 18 and 331. Also see treatment of lows on pages 332–334.

 CAUTION
If you are not able to drink enough fluid, call your doctor.

Your doctor may tell you to stop certain pills to protect your kidneys.

Limit or avoid red liquids and foods

This includes red foods such as red Jell-O, cranberry juice, red Popsicles, cream soda, red cough candies or beets. These can be confused with blood if you are vomiting or have diarrhea.

Check your blood sugar

You may need to adjust the times when you check your blood sugar, depending on how sick you are. To be safe, check your blood sugar every four hours. Check more often if your blood sugar is too high or too low. Write down your numbers. Call your doctor or diabetes educator to help you adjust your insulin dosage.

Drink lots of water and sugar-free fluids

It's easy to become dehydrated when your blood sugar is high, or if you run a fever, vomit or have diarrhea. Therefore, extra sugar-free fluids are essential.

Limit coffee, strong tea and caffeinated colas to less than 4 cups (1 L) a day. Caffeine causes you to lose water.

Sick day rule: one cup an hour

Try to drink a cup (250 mL) of fluids every hour that you are awake. As a general rule, this would be 8 to 10 cups (2–2.5 L) in 24 hours.

Eat lightly

If you aren't up to eating your usual meals and snacks, substitute lighter foods or drinks. There are examples of light foods or drinks in this section. These will help provide you with some carbohydrate as well as electrolytes (sodium and potassium). Don't drink alcohol while sick. Alcohol can contribute to a serious low blood sugar.

Rest and sleep

If you can, walk around a little to help your circulation. If you feel sick to your stomach, keep your head and shoulders raised when resting. Wear loose clothing or pajamas. Put a cool cloth on your face and neck.

Sugar-free fluids

Try these throughout the day and evening.

1. Water
2. Mineral water or soda water
3. Crystal Light or Sugar-Free Kool-Aid
4. Diet soft drinks (caffeine-free)
5. Sugar-free Jell-O
6. Weak tea
7. If you can't keep anything down, try ice chips.
8. Herbal tea (such as ginger tea)
9. Sugar-free Popsicle or Freezee
10. Broth or consommé

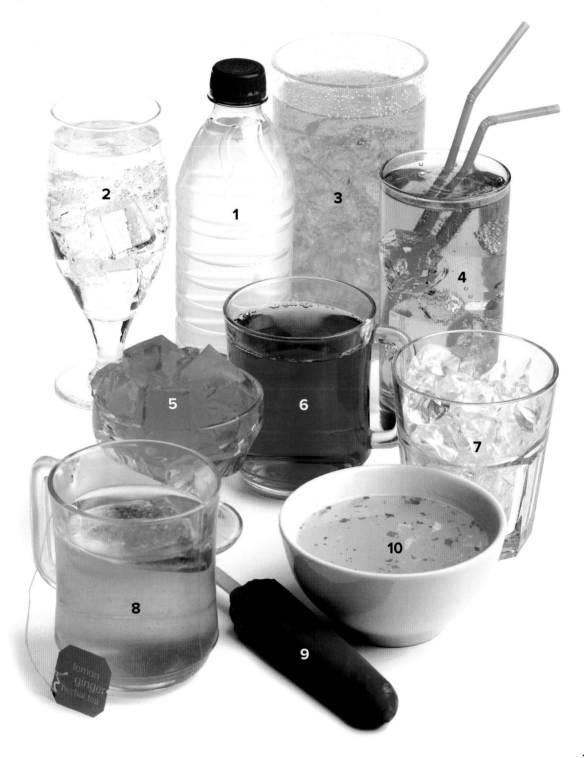

Lighter foods or drink ideas

Try to choose one of these every hour. Each of these has 15 grams of carbohydrate.

1. Kool Aid, 1 pouch ($\frac{3}{4}$ cup/175 mL)
2. Ginger ale or 7 Up (regular), $\frac{2}{3}$ cup (150 mL)
3. Pedialyte (pediatric), $2\frac{1}{2}$ cups (625 mL)
4. Gatorade (regular), 1 cup (250 mL)
5. Orange juice, $\frac{1}{2}$ cup (125 mL)
6. Nutritional supplement for diabetes, 1 cup (250 mL)
7. Yogurt (plain or diet), $\frac{3}{4}$ cup (175 mL)
8. Hot tea or lemon with 3 tsp (15 mL) of honey or sugar
9. Apple juice, $\frac{1}{2}$ cup (125 mL)
10. Ice cream, sherbert or frozen yogurt, $\frac{1}{2}$ cup (125 mL)
11. Cola, caffeine-free, 1 cup (250 mL)
12. Rice cake, 1
13. Toast or bread, plain or lightly buttered, 1 slice
14. Applesauce, $\frac{1}{2}$ cup (125 mL)
15. Soda crackers, 7
16. Melba toast, 4
17. Plain crackers (larger), 3
18. Fruit roll-up, 1
19. Chicken noodle soup, 1 cup (250 mL) or $\frac{1}{2}$ cup (125 mL) noodles
20. Cough syrup (regular), 1–2 tsp (5–10 mL)
21. Banana, 1 small
22. Plain biscuits, 3
23. Plain ginger cookies, 3
24. Plain digestive cookies, 2
25. Jell-O (regular), $\frac{1}{2}$ cup (125 mL)
26. Rice Krispies, Special K or Corn Flakes with milk, $\frac{1}{2}$ cup (125 mL)
27. Popsicle or frozen juice bar, 1 double stick
28. Candies, 3
29. Cough drops (regular), 4
30. Mints, 4
31. Jelly beans, 6

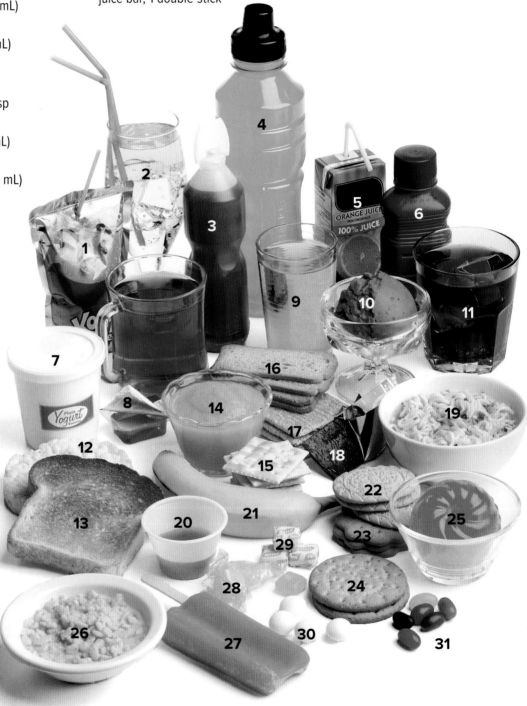

10. How to Gain Weight

If you are underweight, gaining some weight is good. Weighing too little can make you more likely to get an infection, have poor strength or break a bone. High blood sugar, poor appetite, or inadequate food intake can all cause weight loss. There may also be an underlying health problem that causes you to lose weight. Please talk to your doctor. This section provides guidelines on how you can gain weight without worsening your blood sugar. Eating more as well as taking insulin or diabetes pills may help you gain weight. Moderate exercise helps build muscle which also adds pounds.

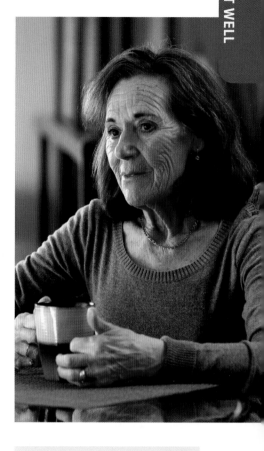

Have you had an unplanned weight loss?

Unplanned means you weren't trying to lose weight; it "just happened."

It can be unhealthy if you lost 5% of your weight in the past six months. A 5% weight loss means:

- A 6-lb (2.7 kg) loss if your weight was 110 to 125 lbs (50–57 kg), or
- An 8-lb (3.6 kg) loss if your weight was 150 lbs (68 kg)
- A 9-lb (4 kg) loss if your weight was 180 lbs (82 kg)

If you've always been a thin person, losing even a few pounds can be a concern. When you are sick or hospitalized you may lose weight, sometimes quickly. Talk to your doctor or dietitian if you don't put the weight back on and you feel unwell.

Diabetes medications may help

High blood sugar can cause weight loss. This happens because you lose large amounts of sugar in your urine. In order to stop losing weight and to regain lost weight, you need to bring down your blood sugar. It's likely you need diabetes medication or insulin. Talk to your doctor.

Starting today make some small changes

In this section, there are suggestions of what foods to eat to gain weight. There is a sample high-calorie meal plan to follow and, if your appetite is low, learn about ways to boost your appetite.

Body Mass Index (BMI)
You can also see if you are underweight or at a healthy weight by comparing your weight to a chart called the Body Mass Index (search "BMI calculator" on the internet). BMI is a measure of your weight compared to your height.

If your cholesterol level is high

Evidence shows that if you're 70 years or more, your low weight may be more of a health issue than your high blood cholesterol. Please ask your doctor or dietitian if you need to restrict extra fats.

Tips to gain weight

Spread out your calories: As with all people with diabetes, you will benefit from spreading your calories and carbohydrates across three small meals. You'll likely need small snacks in-between meals. It's helpful to add extra protein and fat to meals and snacks as this will give you calories with little increase to your blood sugar.

Sample meal plan, below: This chart shows you a healthy day's intake from the reduced-calorie Seven-Day Meal Plan, with ideas on how to boost the calories. This is just an example of a meal. Vary the portions and foods as necessary.

Ways to boost calories: Choose from lots of ideas and foods in this section. Foods high in saturated animal fat, such as whole milk and regular or high-fat cheese, are called extra fats. (See sidebar on pages 145 and 146.) If your cholesterol levels are good, choose these instead of the light varieties until you regain your lost weight.

Sample high-calorie meal plan Ways to increase calories at meals or snacks	
Breakfast 1 Oatmeal (pages 152–153)	• Use whole milk or cream instead of skim milk. • Add 2–3 tsp (10–15 mL) of oil, butter or margarine to your oatmeal. • Put extra chopped nuts on top.
Morning snack Small banana	• Spread some peanut butter on your banana.
Lunch 1 Deluxe Sandwich (pages 160–161)	• Put margarine on both slices of bread. • Add extra avocado or sliced olives to your sandwich. • Have a piece of cheese with your apple.
Afternoon snack	• Add a handful of peanuts to your small or medium snack.
Dinner 1 Minute Steak (pages 168–171)	• Add extra margarine or butter, sour cream and/or shredded cheese to your potatoes. • Use a high-fat gravy instead of a fat-free variety. • Choose a larger portion of meat. • Fry onion in extra fat. • Top your peas and carrots with some roasted sunflower seeds. • Use a regular fat pudding when making the English Trifle. • Add extra almonds to your serving of English Trifle.
Evening snack	• Supplement a small to large snack with a high-protein bar, diabetes nutrient bar or half a diabetes nutritional supplement beverage.

Boost calories with more protein and fat

- Increase your protein portions at all your meals and snacks. Protein includes lean meat, fish, skinless chicken, eggs, seafood, nuts and seeds.

- Add white beans or kidney beans to soup or casseroles. This will add some carbohydrate but will also boost protein.

- Try to always include a protein at breakfast. For example, an egg, a slice of low-fat cheese or lean meat, or chopped nuts on cereal.

- Add a slice of cheese to make meat sandwiches higher in calories.

- Use sockeye salmon, tuna or sardines canned in oil.

- Boil and peel a few eggs and put them in the fridge. Several times a week, grab one for a snack or with a meal. Scramble eggs with added fat and cheese.

- Swirl a beaten egg into soup or into macaroni and cheese while it is cooking.

- Add sliced or shredded cheese to soups, salads, sandwiches and casseroles, stews, mashed potatoes, ravioli and tacos. Have cheese as a snack with crackers or a muffin.

- Add a cheese sauce to vegetables.

- Have a spoonful of peanut butter straight from the jar! Add nut butter to fruit smoothies or milkshakes, or to a stir fry, tomato soup or casseroles. Try a spoonful of peanut butter stirred into $\frac{1}{2}$ cup (125 mL) of sugar-free vanilla yogurt or vanilla pudding.

- Add almonds, pistachios, walnuts, pecans, peanuts, hazelnuts, cashews or soy nuts, or pumpkin seeds or sunflower seeds, to casseroles, salads and desserts. Also choose these as snacks or on the side with your meals.

- Top pancakes or cereal with ground almonds.

- For a snack, have half of a sandwich or one piece of bread with protein on it: choose salmon, meat, cheese or peanut butter or even try peanut butter and cheese.

- Rather than eat fruit on its own, eat it with cheese, peanut butter or a few nuts. Try half a small banana spread with peanut butter, apple and cheese, or a pear spread with light cream cheese.

Extra fats
Choose extra fats if you want to gain weight and your cholesterol levels are normal.

Meats: Choose medium to fatty cuts of meat, and chicken with the skin on.

Cheese: Regular fat cheese.

Eggs: Eat eggs daily.

Yogurt: High fat yogurts with 5% or more MF. These yogurts are made with whole milk with some added cream.

Pudding: Make your pudding with whole milk or half-and-half cream.

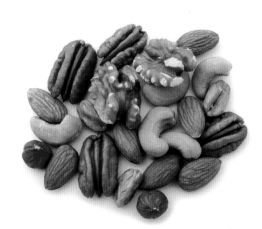

More extra fats

Butter or cream cheese: Choose butter or regular cream cheese instead of light cream cheese.

Milk: Drink whole 3% (homogenized) milk. Use whole evaporated milk.

Whole milk powder: Use a whole milk powder instead of skim milk powder.

Cream instead of milk: From the dairy case, buy half-and-half cream or whipped cream. Put it in your cereal, coffee or tea, puddings and canned fruit.

Cream drink: Drink a small glass of whipping cream flavored with a bit of vanilla or your own favorite flavoring.

Additions to recipes: Add butter, full-fat cream cheese, gravy, full-fat sour cream and whipping cream to recipes and foods.

- Olives have healthy monounsaturated fat; enjoy a few.

- Avocado is good for you. Slice it up and add it to a smoothie, sandwich, tortilla roll, tacos or in a salad. Try halving an avocado and eating it with a spoon. It is nice served with a dash of Worcestershire sauce, or lemon or lime juice.

- When eating sandwiches, toast or a slice of bread, crackers or a muffin, top it with margarine or another fat such as cream cheese.

- Drink 2% milk instead of skim.

- Greek yogurt (unsweetened) is high in protein. Some varieties are also high in fat, further boosting calories.

- You can also use low-fat evaporated milk full strength. A half cup (125 mL) will equal 1 cup (250 mL) regular milk. Add this to cereal, pudding, coffee or tea, or hot cocoa.

- Add skim milk powder to soups, stews, casseroles, mashed potatoes, cereals and scrambled eggs.

- Add $\frac{1}{4}$ cup (60 mL) of skim milk powder to each cup (250 mL) of milk to double the protein. Also, stir 1 tbsp (15 mL) of skim milk powder into a cup of yogurt or pudding. If using a plain yogurt, you can sprinkle in some sugar-free drink crystals for flavoring.

- Buy protein powder and add it to a variety of foods.

- Add dried unsweetened coconut to desserts, or coconut milk to curries or to beverages such as smoothies. New evidence indicates that coconut milk has a healthy type of fat, as long as it is not hydrogenated.

- Add extra oil such as olive, canola, corn, soya or coconut oil, margarine, mayonnaise, and salad dressings to recipes and foods such as mashed potatoes, rice or pasta, oatmeal, scrambled eggs, TV dinners or casseroles. Fry foods to get extra calories from the fats.

- Buy diabetes nutritional supplement beverages or snack bars at pharmacies or some large food stores, sometimes called "meal replacements." Look for brands that say they are especially for people with diabetes. These will be high in fiber.

Remember, these additions to your diet are just if you're trying to gain weight. Don't feed your family members extra fat if they do not need the additional calories.

Other things to help you gain weight

Eat three small meals plus snacks

- Have your meals and snacks at regular times. You may want to set an alarm to remind yourself to eat.
- Have a full meal at the time of the day when your appetite is best.

Slowly increase your food

Slowly increase your food intake. This allows your body some time to get used to the extra food.

Don't fill up on low-calorie foods

Limit plain coffee, tea, clear soup, diet drinks or raw, bulky vegetables. These fill you up but don't give you the calories that you need. However, drinking water is still important to help flush out your bladder, and to prevent constipation and dehydration.

If you get tired easily, use quick and easy foods

- Keep appealing, easy-to-make and favorite foods on hand and in sight.
- Buy ready-to-eat meals and foods such as ready-to-eat puddings or fruit cups. Try occasional frozen entrees or precooked foods, or salads from the deli.
- Cook meals in advance and freeze them in single portions.
- Order some extra meals to be delivered. Consider signing up for Meals on Wheels, or get take-out.
- Share a meal with a friend, neighbor or family member. Try eating somewhere new! It's nice to eat out at a restaurant, senior center, or a meal program at an apartment block or personal care home.

If you feel lonely, are disabled or a senior

Getting out more often may improve your appetite overall. Talk to friends or call the senior center to find out if there is anything going on that interests you. If you need a ride, call your local seniors' center or volunteer bureau. Ask them if they offer rides.

Take a multivitamin pill if you're not eating well

If you have lost a lot of weight or aren't eating well, a "one-a-day" vitamin and mineral pill may be helpful until you are eating better. Ask the pharmacist for a vitamin pill that does not interact with any other medications you take.

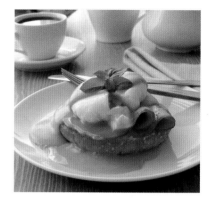

Boost the calories of your small breakfast meal by putting butter on the half bun and topping with ham, egg and cheese sauce.

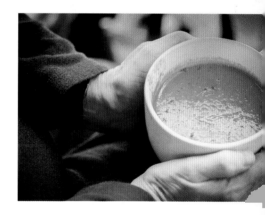

Boost your appetite

Dress it up. Make your meal look good. Use a colorful place mat, table cloth or napkin. Place a flower or candle on the table. Change these often. You deserve the best.

Flavor it up. Foods will taste better if you add herbs, lemon and spices. Ask your doctor or dietitian if it's okay for you to add a bit of salt to your food, as this also helps with flavor.

Sunlight helps. If possible, dine by a window to get some sunlight. Choose a comfortable chair to sit in when you eat. If you eat meals in your bed or in a big chair, prop yourself up with pillows so you can see your food and eat easily.

Fresh air is good. Try to get some fresh air every day. If you can't get outside, open a window briefly to allow stale smells to leave and to let in fresh air. When the weather is nice, try eating some meals outside on a deck, balcony or bench.

Freshen up your mouth. Some medications can cause a bad taste in your mouth and take away your appetite. Try chewing on a sprig of mint or parsley. Cinnamon or mint flavored sugar-free gum might also help.

Keep active

Do some physical activity. Even a short walk can help improve your appetite. Lifting small weights also helps you gain muscle as weight. This also brings down your blood sugar. Exercise is good for your overall health. Walking, swimming and biking build muscles and weight. Increase exercise gradually. Check out the Level 1 or 2 strength training and exercise program on pages 231–235.

Monitor your weight and request regular lab tests

- Get weighed at the doctor's office. Write down your weight. Also ask when you were weighed last and how much you weighed.
- Tell your doctor or dietitian if you have lost 5 to 10 lbs (2.2–4.5 kg) in the past six months.
- Have your blood sugar A1C done.

Seven-Day Meal Plan
with Recipes

Breakfast Meals

- All small breakfast meals have 250 calories.
- All large breakfasts have 370 calories.

Lunch Meals

- All small lunches have 400 calories.
- All large lunches have 520 calories.

Dinner Meals

- All small dinners have 550 calories.
- All large dinners have 730 calories.

Snacks

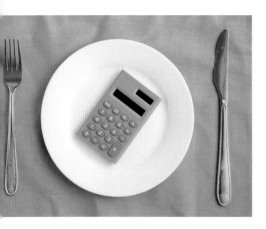

Nutrient Analysis

With total and net carbohydrate information at your fingertips, you can adjust your meals or insulin as needed.

Each carbohydrate choice has 15 grams of total or net carbohydrate. Carbohydrate choices are rounded. They are based on the following calculations:

Food Choices	NUTRIENTS PER CHOICE		
	Carbs	Protein	Fat
Carbohydrates			
Grains and starches	15 g	3 g	0 g
Fruits	15 g	1 g	0 g
Milk and alternatives	15 g	8 g	variable
Other choices	15 g	variable	variable
Vegetables (usually not counted)	< 5 g (most)	2 g	0 g
Protein	0 g	7 g	3–5 g
Fat	0 g	0 g	5 g

In this book, net carbs are used to calculate Food Choices, according to Diabetes Canada recommendations.

Net Carbs, or Available Carbs

Net carbs are also called available carbs. Net carbs is the total carbs minus fiber. Fiber is subtracted because it is mostly an indigestible carbohydrate and so it doesn't affect blood sugar.

Keep in mind that there are many factors that affect your blood sugar, not just carbs. For example, other foods at your meal, your portion size, the time of day you have your meal and your exercise can all affect blood sugar.

Cutting calories can help you stop weight gain or lose weight. This typically improves blood sugar, blood pressure and blood cholesterol.

There is more information on carbs in the *Diabetes Meals for Good Health Cookbook*; see page 416.

Should I choose the large or small meals?

If you choose a small breakfast, lunch and dinner, you will get 1,200 calories.

If you choose a large breakfast, lunch and dinner, you will get 1,620 calories.

Mix and match your meals. If you want, add in snacks to get a meal plan from 1,200 to 2,200 calories a day. See chart on the next page.

A. Daily Meal Plan Chart

Small meals with no snacks	1,200 calories
Small meals with two small snacks	1,300 calories
Small meals with one small and two medium snacks	1,450 calories
Small meals with one small, one medium and one large snack	1,550 calories
Large meals with no snacks	1,620 calories
Large meals with two small snacks	1,720 calories
Large meals with one small and two medium snacks	1,870 calories
Large meals with one small, one medium and one large snack	1,970 calories
Large meals with three large snacks	2,220 calories

Calories for the small meals:

- Breakfast has 250 calories.
- Lunch has 400 calories.
- Dinner has 550 calories.

Calories for the large meals:

- Breakfast has 370 calories.
- Lunch has 520 calories.
- Dinner has 730 calories.

Calories for the snacks:

- Low-calorie snack has 20 calories or less.
- Small snack has 50 calories.
- Medium snack has 100 calories.
- Large snack has 200 calories.

All the small and large meals in this book have the same calories as the 70 meals in the *Diabetes Meals for Good Health Cookbook.*

Calories and carbs of meals and snacks		
Breakfast meals	**LARGE MEALS have 370 calories** • total carbs 60 grams or less • net carbs 50 grams or less	**SMALL MEALS have 250 calories** • total carbs 50 grams or less • net carbs 40 grams or less
Lunch meals	**LARGE MEALS have 520 calories** • total carbs 90 grams or less • net carbs 80 grams or less	**SMALL MEALS have 400 calories** • total carbs 70 grams or less • net carbs 60 grams or less
Dinner meals	**LARGE MEALS have 730 calories** • total carbs 110 grams or less • net carbs 100 grams or less	**SMALL MEALS have 550 calories** • total carbs 90 grams or less • net carbs 80 grams or less
Snack groups	• Low-calorie snacks (20 calories or less)* • Small snacks (50 calories)*	• Medium snacks (100 calories)* • Large snacks (200 calories)*
		* Carbs vary between snacks

No matter which meal you choose, every dinner has either 730 calories (for the large meals) or 550 calories (for small meals). The same goes for breakfasts, lunches and snacks, only with fewer calories. Calories are consistent across each group — so you can pick and choose meals and snacks without having to count calories yourself!

BREAKFAST 1

Oatmeal

OPTIONS

- **Cranberries** may help reduce cholesterol. If you don't have cranberries, have chopped apple or another fruit instead.
- **Cinnamon** adds flavor, so you don't need as much sugar to sweeten food.
- **Pecans** provide protein to keep you feeling full through the morning. Pecans, almonds, peanuts, hazelnuts, walnuts, pistachios, and sunflower or pumpkin seeds are all a great source of healthy fats.
- **Bran.** Add a sprinkle for extra fiber.

All forms of oatmeal are good for you. Oats have soluble fiber which slows down blood sugar and helps lower cholesterol. Slower cooking types of oatmeal are in a more whole, unprocessed form, and are the healthiest. This includes steel-cut oats and large flaked oats. They take longer to digest, which means you have a slower rise in blood sugar. Follow the package directions for cooking your oatmeal.

Steel-cut oats (10 to 20 minutes)

These are whole oats (including the hull) chopped in pieces. Scottish oatmeal cooks a bit faster, as it has smaller chopped pieces of oats.

Large flaked oats (5 minutes)

These oats have been flattened by rolling. They look like flakes.

Quick-cooking oats (2 to 3 minutes)

These rolled oats are processed for longer than the large flaked oats. They are smaller flakes.

Instant oats (ready to eat with hot water added)

In processing, these oats are rolled and crushed. They will raise your blood sugar the fastest.

For a balanced breakfast, add milk to your oatmeal, and top with fruit and nuts.

Food Choices	Large Meal	Small Meal
Carbohydrate	3½	3
Protein	0	0
Fat	1	½

Your Breakfast Menu	Large Meal (370 calories)	Total Carbs	Net Carbs	Small Meal (250 calories)	Total Carbs	Net Carbs
Oatmeal or other hot cereal topped with:	1½ cup (375 mL) cooked (9 tbsp/135 mL)	35	30	1 cup (250 mL) cooked (6 tbsp/90 mL)	24	20
Cranberries (dried and sweetened)	1½ tbsp (22 mL)	9	8	1 tbsp (15 mL)	6	6
Cinnamon and bran cereal	sprinkle	–	–	sprinkle	–	–
Pecans or other nuts, chopped	1 tbsp (15 mL)	1	0	1½ tsp (7 mL)	0	0
Skim or 1% milk	1 cup (250 mL)	12	12	1 cup (250 mL)	12	12
		58 g	**50 g**		**42 g**	**38 g**

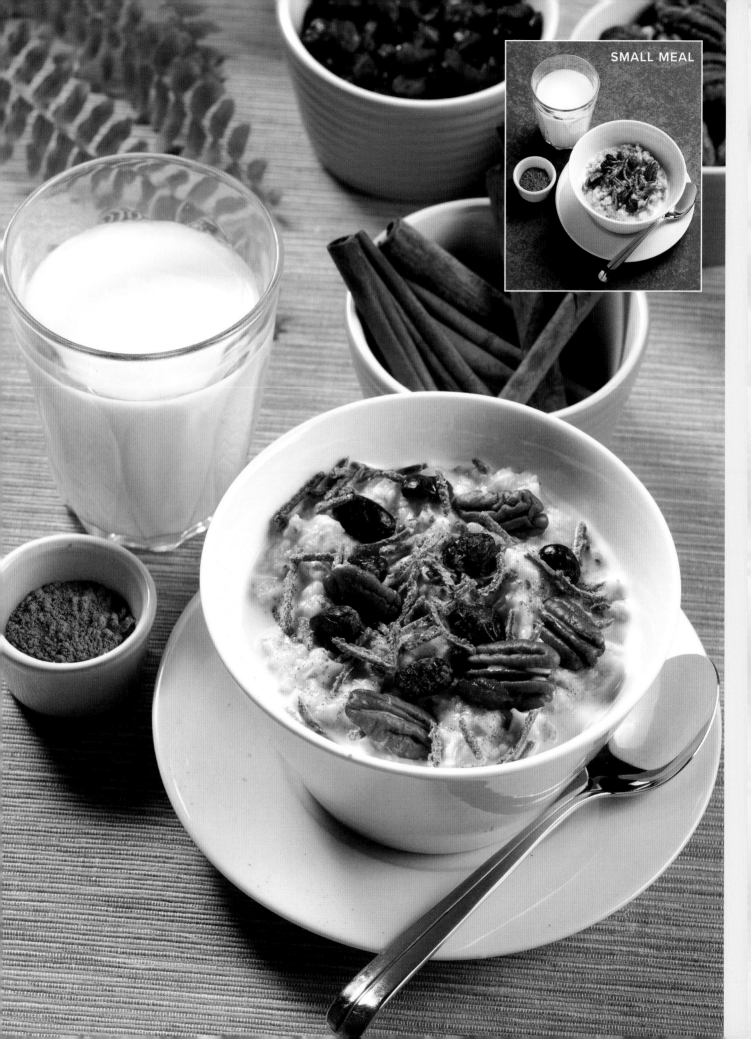

SMALL MEAL

BREAKFAST 2

Fruit Crepes

OPTIONS

Crepes are like thin pancakes. Fill them with a variety of fillings.

Crepe fillings:

- cottage cheese, shredded cheese or Greek yogurt
- fruit such as sliced peaches or pears, chopped apple, blueberries or strawberries, orange pieces or chopped banana, or dried dates or figs
- chopped peppers, mushrooms or salsa
- smoked salmon or shrimp

Crepes

Makes ten 8-inch (20 cm) crepes

1½ cups (375 mL) flour

½ tsp (2 mL) salt

1 tsp (5 mL) baking powder

1 tbsp (15 mL) sugar

2 eggs

1 cup (250 mL) skim milk

1 cup (250 mL) water

2 tbsp (30 mL) margarine or butter
  (for coating the pan)

PER CREPE	
Calories	117
Carbohydrate	17 g
Fiber	1 g
Net carbs	16 g
Protein	4 g
Fat, total	4 g
Fat, saturated	1 g
Cholesterol	38 mg
Sodium	193 mg

1. In a large bowl, mix together flour, salt, baking powder and sugar.

2. In a medium bowl, beat eggs with a fork or whisk. Add milk and water to the eggs, and mix well.

3. Add the egg mixture to the flour mixture. Whisk until smooth.

4. Heat a nonstick pan or crepe pan on medium to high heat. Using a pastry brush, lightly coat the pan with butter or margarine.

5. Ladle a thin layer of crepe mixture into the pan. For a 12-inch (30 cm) frying pan, you will need just under ¼ cup (60 mL) per crepe. Immediately tip the pan to even out the layer of batter. Cook until the edges are a little brown. Flip over and quickly cook the other side.

6. When making your next crepe, spread some more fat on the pan using your pastry brush.

7. Put some filling in your cooked crepes (see sidebar for examples), then roll or fold, and cut in half.

Food Choices	Large Meal	Small Meal
Carbohydrate	3	2
Protein	2	2
Fat	0	0

Your Breakfast Menu	Large Meal (370 calories)	Total Carbs	Net Carbs	Small Meal (250 calories)	Total Carbs	Net Carbs
Crepes	2	34	33	1	17	16
1% or 2% cottage cheese	¼ cup (60 mL)	2	2	¼ cup (60 mL)	2	2
Shredded Cheddar cheese	1½ tbsp (25 mL)	0	0	1½ tbsp (25 mL)	0	0
Peach	1	9	7	1	9	8
Tea	1 cup (250 mL)	1	1	1 cup (250 mL)	1	1
		46 g	**43 g**		**29 g**	**27 g**

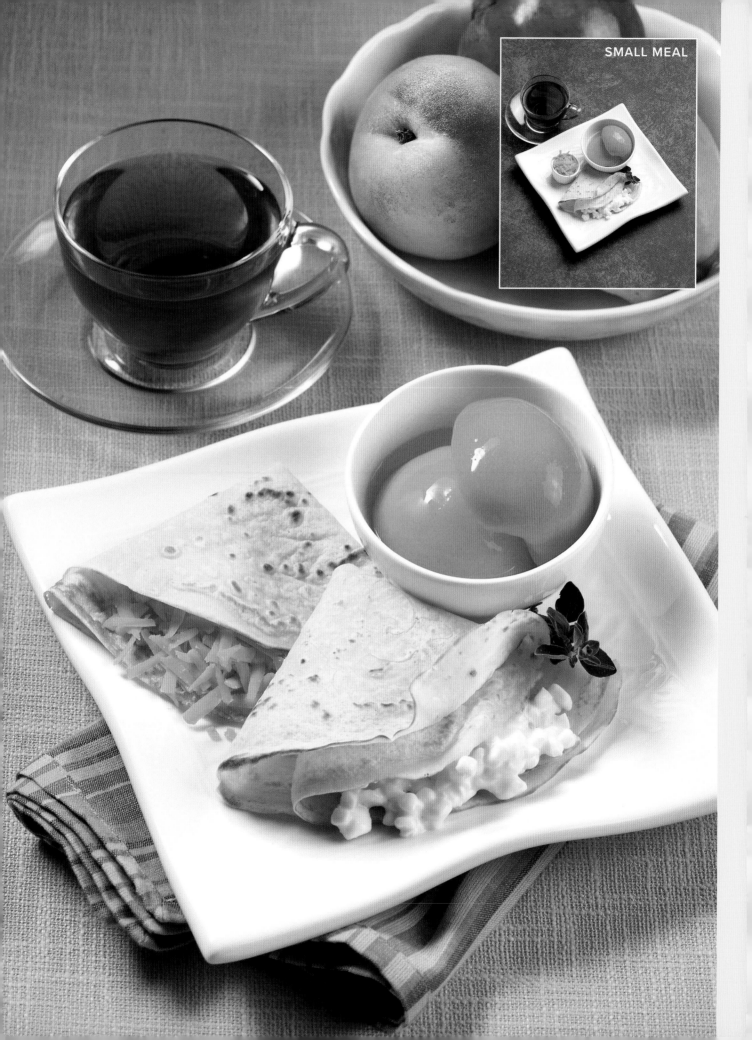

SMALL MEAL

BREAKFAST 3

Cereal with Berries

Shredded Wheat is an excellent cereal choice. It is a good source of fiber and has no added fat, sugar or salt.

Other examples of healthy dry cereals
- Wheatabix or Muffets
- Fiber 1
- Bran Flakes
- Kashi Heart to Heart

Rice Krispies, Puffed Wheat or Special K are also good choices, as they are low in added sugar (less than 1 tsp/5 mL or 4 g of added sugar) and low in fat. However, they are low in fiber, so if you want, you could top the cereal with a sprinkle of wheat germ bran or ground flax seed. Post Shreddies Original have an extra teaspoon (5 mL) of added sugar (9 grams total added sugar) but are low in fat, and an excellent source of fiber (6 g) and iron (50% of your Daily Value).

Tips when you are shopping
- When buying cereals, remember that:
  1 tsp (5 mL) of sugar = 4 g
  1 tsp (5 mL) of fat = 5 g
- For more label reading tips about cereals, go to page 95.

Are you looking for a caffeine-free hot drink to have with breakfast? Try a cup of herbal tea or a grain beverage with chicory (such as Caf-Lib). Chicory contains inulin, a type of soluble fiber that is good for people with diabetes.

OPTIONS
Half cup (125 mL) spoon-size shredded wheat equals 1 biscuit.

HEALTH TIP
Include a fruit with your cereal to start your day off right.
Blueberries and other berries have lots of antioxidants. These help keep your blood vessels healthy by reducing inflammation. Fresh and frozen (thawed) berries are equally nutritious.

Food Choices	Large Meal	Small Meal
Carbohydrate	3½	2
Protein	0	0
Fat	2	2

Your Breakfast Menu	Large Meal (370 calories)	Total Carbs	Net Carbs	Small Meal (250 calories)	Total Carbs	Net Carbs
Shredded Wheat or other cold cereal	1½ biscuit	28	23	1 biscuit	19	16
Skim or 1% milk	⅔ cup (150 mL)	8	8	½ cup (125 mL)	6	6
Blueberries or other berries	1 cup (250 mL)	21	17	½ cup (125 mL)	10	8
Chopped nuts (walnuts and almonds)	2 tbsp (30 mL)	2	1	2 tbsp (30 mL)	2	1
Coffee, tea or grain beverage with chicory	1 cup (250 mL)	1	1	1 cup (250 mL)	1	1
		60 g	50 g		38 g	32 g

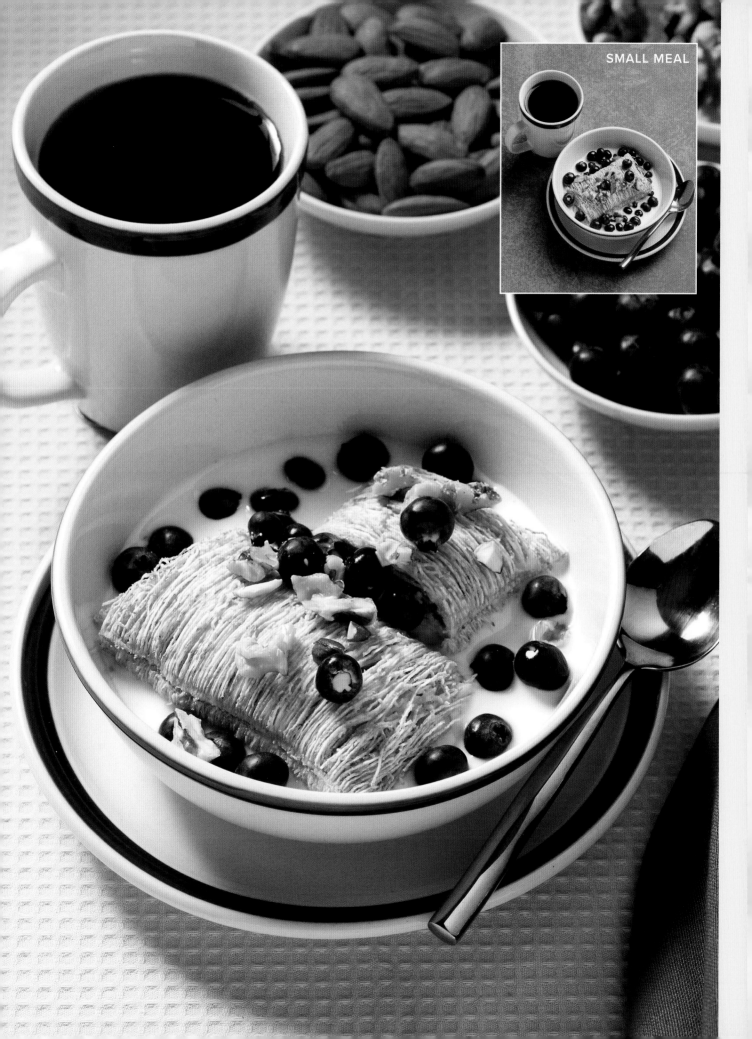

BREAKFAST 4

Poached Egg & Toast

HEALTH TIP

Mom was right all along!

Breakfast starts your engine (your metabolism) so you begin to burn calories and get energized. When you eat breakfast and other regular meals, you don't get as hungry and are less likely to eat more later. Less evening snacking means you wake up feeling ready for breakfast.

OPTIONS

Oregano

Fresh or dried oregano adds nice flavor to eggs!

Choose thin whole-grain bread

Thin sliced bread is best! If you want to decrease your carbohydrates and calories from bread, check the label for ones that have no more than 28 grams and about 70 calories per slice. Thin sliced bread (whether white, whole wheat or whole-grain) will have less effect on your blood sugar. Some breads that are marketed as "healthier" with lots of grains in them are actually cut very thick, and in some cases can have double the calories and carbohydrates of a regular sliced bread.

Now that you have your toast, top it with a protein

- 1 egg
- 1 oz (30 g) of cheese or cheese slice
- 1 tbsp (15 mL) of peanut butter
- 1 tbsp (15 mL) Nutella (hazelnut spread) can be chosen occasionally; it has more sugar, but less fat than peanut butter

Alternatives to 1 tomato

- $\frac{1}{2}$ cup (125 mL) tomato or vegetable juice
- 1 small mandarin orange
- $\frac{1}{2}$ peach, pear or apple

Food Choices	Large Meal	Small Meal
Carbohydrate	3	2
Protein	1	1
Fat	2	1

Your Breakfast Menu	Large Meal (370 calories)	Total Carbs	Net Carbs	Small Meal (250 calories)	Total Carbs	Net Carbs
Toast	2	26	22	1	13	11
Margarine or butter	2 tsp (10 mL)	0	0	1 tsp (5 mL)	0	0
Jam or jelly, or honey	1½ tsp (7 mL) (or 1 tbsp/ 15 mL if low-sugar jam)	7	7	1 tsp (5 mL) (or 2 tsp/ 10 mL if low-sugar jam)	5	5
Egg	1	0	0	1	0	0
Sliced tomato	1 medium	5	3	1 medium	5	3
Kiwi	1	11	9	1	11	0
Coffee	1 cup (250 mL)	1	1	1 cup (250 mL)	1	1
		50 g	**42 g**		**35 g**	**29 g**

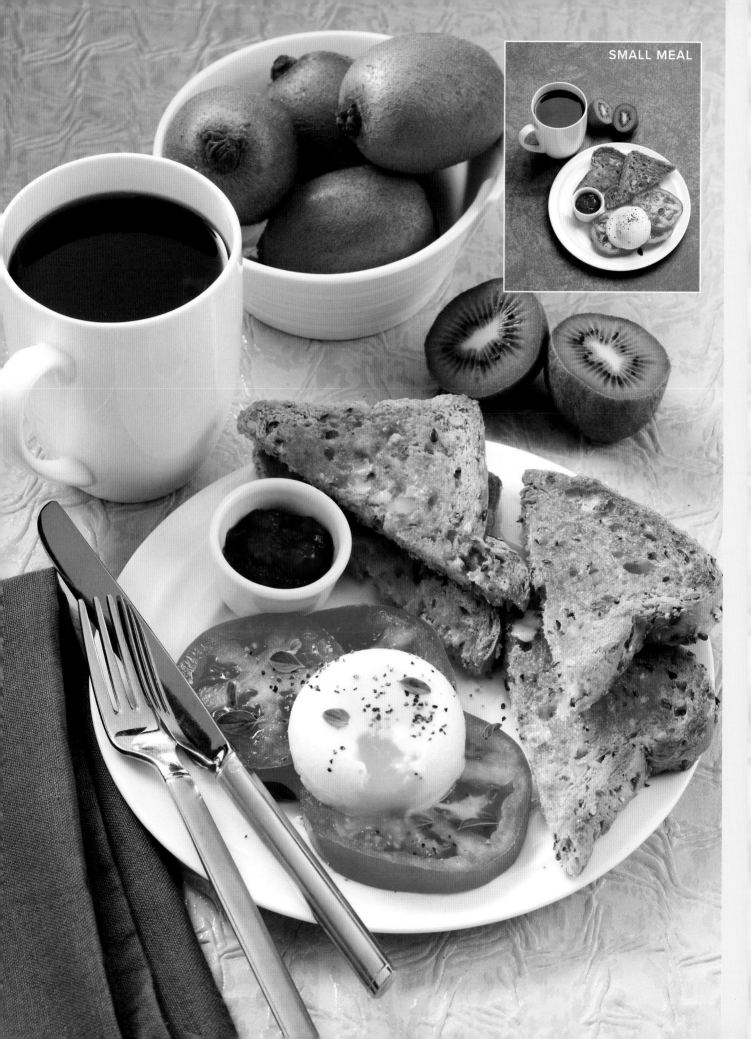

SMALL MEAL

LUNCH 1

Deluxe Sandwich

Here are three tasty sandwich fillings for two slices of bread. The large meal photo shows a half of each.

Grilled cheese

1 oz (30 g) cheese
2 tsp (10 mL) margarine spread on the outside of the sandwich

In a frying pan or sandwich grill, cook sandwich on both sides, until golden brown.

Avocado and turkey bacon

1 tbsp (15 mL) light ranch or blue cheese dressing
½ small avocado
1 to 2 slices red onion, thinly sliced
1 strip cooked turkey bacon or regular bacon

Ham and cheese

1 oz (30 g) ham or turkey
1 oz (30 g) your favorite cheese
1 tbsp (15 mL) light mayonnaise
lettuce and tomato

Other sandwich options

For protein: Choose leftover chicken, turkey, beef or pork, or tuna, salmon, shrimp, crab or sardines, peanut butter or sliced egg.

For toppings: Add slices of red onion, fresh mushrooms, thinly sliced peppers (or roasted peppers), lightly cooked asparagus spears, salsa, basil pesto, sliced olives or pickles, hot peppers or alfalfa sprouts.

Instead of salt on your sandwich: Use black pepper, fresh basil, dill, parsley or coriander, green onion or red pepper jelly.

OPTIONS

In a rush?
Pick up a hot, cooked rotisserie chicken, bring it home and remove all the skin. Slice it up for a fast filling for sandwiches or wraps. Also use it for your main course protein.

Food Choices	Large Meal	Small Meal
Carbohydrate	3½	3
Protein	1½	1
Fat	3	2

Your Lunch Menu	Large Meal (520 calories)	Total Carbs	Net Carbs	Small Meal (400 calories)	Total Carbs	Net Carbs
Sandwich of your choice	1½ sandwiches	47	39	1 sandwich	32	26
Celery	2 stalks	2	1	2 stalks	2	1
Apple	½	7	6	1	15	13
		56 g	**46 g**		**49 g**	**40 g**

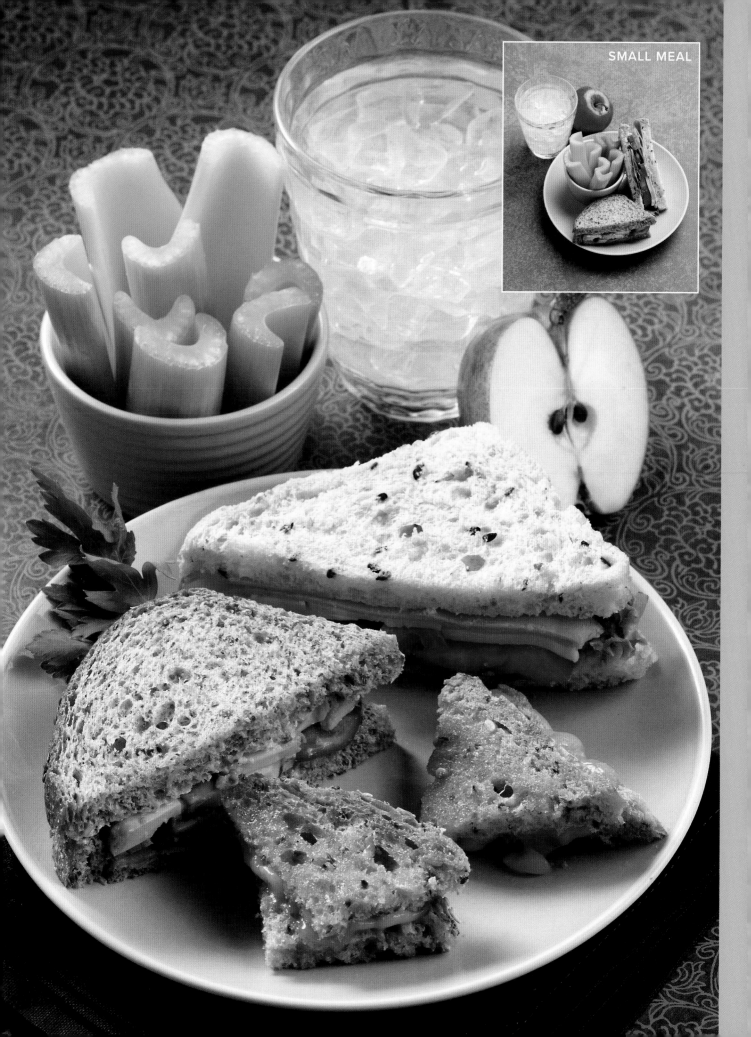

SMALL MEAL

LUNCH 2

Taco Soup

Your favorite hearty bowl of soup with crackers makes a great lunch on a cold or hot day! Make this taco soup ahead, and freeze any leftovers.

HEALTH TIP

Tips to reduce salt

- One-third to one-half of the salt is removed from canned vegetables when you rinse them in cold water.
- Commercial taco mix is salty, so the mixture of spices in this recipe is a great replacement.

OPTIONS

1 cup (250 mL) of almond beverage instead of milk has only 1 gram of carb.

Taco Soup

Makes 13 cups (3.25 L)

1 lb (500 g) lean ground beef
1 medium onion, chopped
2 large stalks celery, chopped
1 green pepper, chopped
28-oz (796 mL) can tomatoes, diced or whole
19-oz (540 mL) can kidney beans, rinsed
19-oz (540 mL) can black beans, rinsed
2 cups (500 mL) frozen kernel corn
2 tsp (10 mL) chili powder
1 tsp (5 mL) each cumin, oregano, paprika and garlic powder
½ tsp (2 mL) black pepper
2 cups (500 mL) water
Garnish: dollop of fat-free sour cream

PER CUP (250 ML)	
Calories	160
Carbohydrate	21 g
Fiber	5 g
Net carbs	16 g
Protein	12 g
Fat, total	4 g
Fat, saturated	1 g
Cholesterol	18 mg
Sodium	283 mg

1. In a large heavy pot over medium heat, cook beef, breaking it up with a spoon. Cook for 15 minutes or until no longer pink. Drain off any fat.
2. Add onions, celery and green pepper. Cook until soft.
3. Add the rest of the ingredients. Add water if soup seems too thick.
4. Bring to a boil, then cover and simmer for 30 minutes. Add extra water if getting too thick.

Food Choices	Large Meal	Small Meal
Carbohydrate	3½	3
Protein	2	1
Fat	0	0

Your Lunch Menu	Large Meal (520 calories)	Total Carbs	Net Carbs	Small Meal (400 calories)	Total Carbs	Net Carbs
Taco Soup (or other hearty soup)	2 cups (500 mL)	41	30	1 cup (250 mL)	21	15
Soda crackers	4	9	8	4	9	8
Carrot sticks	½ cup (125 mL)	6	4	½ cup (125 mL)	6	4
Almond beverage (unsweetened)	1 cup (250 mL)	1	1	1 cup (250 mL)	1	1
Grapes	15 (½ cup/125 mL)	14	13	15 (½ cup/125 mL)	14	13
		71 g	**56 g**		**51 g**	**41 g**

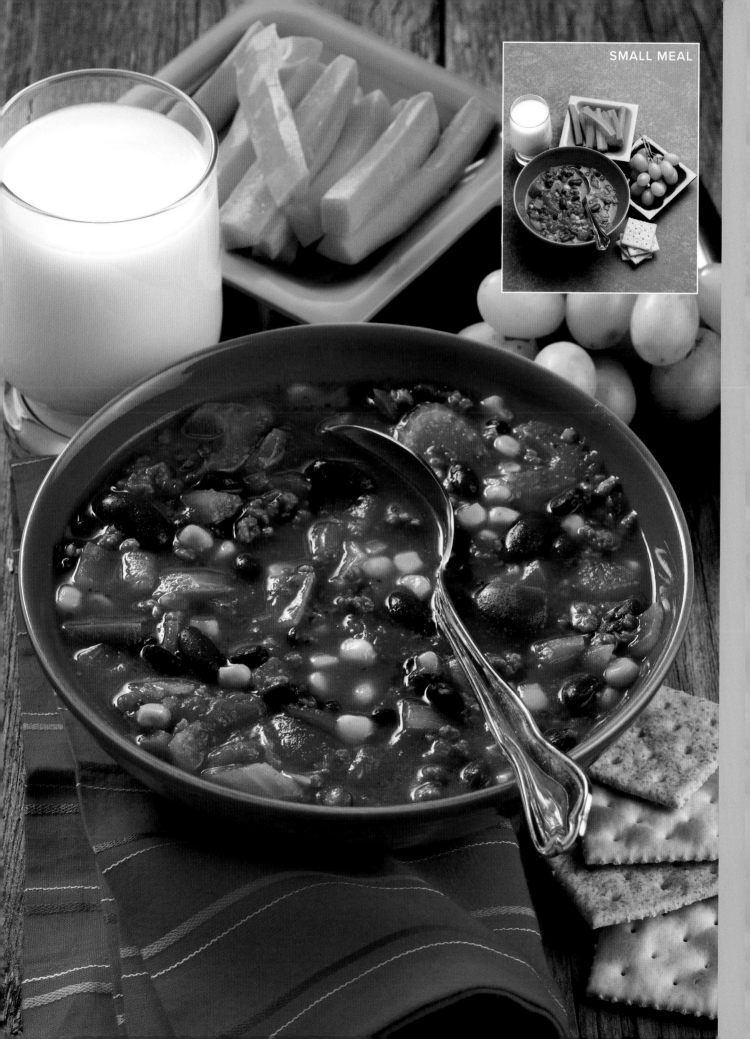

LUNCH 3

Luncheon Wrap

OPTIONS

Serve these wraps cold. Enjoy them fresh or make them a day ahead and store in your fridge. Different kinds of tortilla shells include plain, or spinach, dried tomato or cheese flavored. Fill your wrap with some protein such as fish or shrimp, egg, meat, chicken or cheese, and some vegetables.

Restaurant wraps

A variety of fast-food restaurants now carry wraps. If you are on the run for lunch, try to find a wrap that has 400 calories for the large lunch equivalent or 300 calories for the small lunch.

Here are the recipes for the three wraps shown in the photograph. The portions given below are for one 10-inch (25 cm) wrap, cut into three pieces.

Fish or seafood filling

½ cup (125 mL) tuna, salmon, crab or shrimp, drained
2 tbsp (30 mL) light mayonnaise or fat-free mayonnaise
1 green onion (or chives), sliced or chopped

Egg salad filling

2 eggs, hard-boiled, cooled and sliced or mashed
1 tbsp (15 mL) light mayonnaise or
    2 tbsp (30 mL) fat-free mayonnaise
½ dill pickle, chopped

Meat and cheese filling

1 tbsp (15 mL) light cream cheese herb and garlic spread
2 oz (60 g) precooked chicken, turkey or other meat
1 to 2 tbsp (15–30 mL) shredded cheese
red pepper strips (roasted or raw) or shredded carrots
several cooked asparagus spears

1. If using cream cheese, spread evenly on one side of the tortilla shell. If using mayonnaise, blend with your protein ingredient.
2. At one end of the tortilla shell, place the protein and vegetables. Add black pepper to taste.
3. Starting at the end with the filling, roll up the wrap into a tight roll.
4. Cut on an angle, in thirds, for a nice effect.

Food Choices	Large Meal	Small Meal
Carbohydrate	3½	3
Protein	2	1½
Fat	1	½

Your Lunch Menu	Large Meal (520 calories)	Total Carbs	Net Carbs	Small Meal (400 calories)	Total Carbs	Net Carbs
Wraps	1 wrap (3 pieces)	37	35	⅔ wrap (2 pieces)	24	23
Radishes	5	1	0	5	1	0
Skim or 1% milk	½ cup (125 mL)	6	6	½ cup (125 mL)	6	6
Pear	1	26	21	1	26	21
		70 g	**62 g**		**57 g**	**50 g**

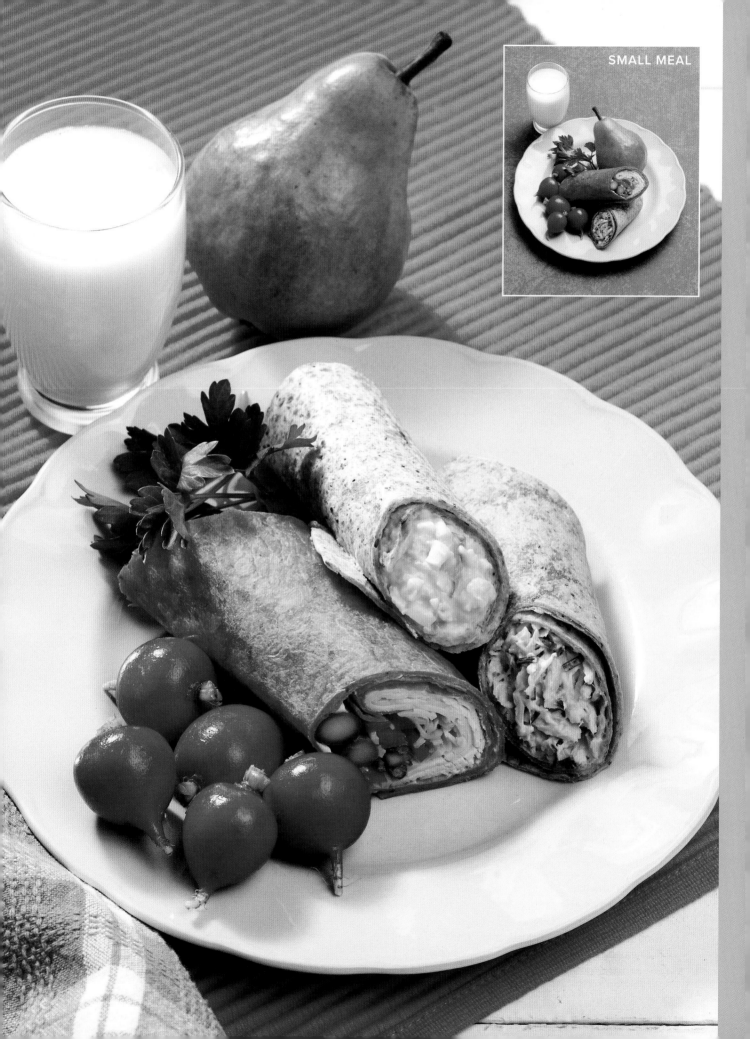

SMALL MEAL

LUNCH 4

Pizza Bun

HEALTH TIP

For a lower-salt option than tomato sauce, chop up a tomato and mix with a dash of oregano and basil.

OPTIONS

You can make your open-face pizza bun on a half hamburger or hot dog bun, half an English muffin or a slice of bread.

On one side of each half bun, add 1 tbsp (15 mL) of pizza or pasta sauce, tomato sauce or salsa. Then add your own favorite toppings. Try one of these varieties.

Additions for each half bun

Vegetarian Ranch

2 tbsp (30 mL) brown beans, black beans
     or kidney beans (drained)
corn (frozen or canned kernels), sprinkle
red pepper strips
1 tbsp (15 mL) shredded mozzarella or other cheese
chopped fresh cilantro or basil (optional)

Hawaiian

1 oz (30 g) chopped ham
chopped peppers and pineapple tidbits
1 tbsp (15 mL) shredded mozzarella or other cheese

Classic

½ oz (15 g) cooked lean hamburger, chicken or pepperoni
chopped peppers, mushrooms or other fresh or
     frozen vegetables
2 tbsp (30 mL) shredded mozzarella or other cheese

1. On a baking sheet, place cut bun and grill one side. Once toasted, turn bun over and spread with tomato sauce.

2. Top with the beans, chicken or meat, and cheese, vegetables and flavorings.

3. Broil in oven for a few minutes until the cheese bubbles.

Food Choices	Large Meal	Small Meal
Carbohydrate	4	3
Protein	1½	1
Fat	½	0

Your Lunch Menu	Large Meal (520 calories)	Total Carbs	Net Carbs	Small Meal (400 calories)	Total Carbs	Net Carbs
Pizza buns	3 halves	53	49	2 halves	37	34
Cucumber	½ medium	5	4	½ medium	5	4
Diet beverage	12 oz (355 mL)	0	0	12 oz (355 mL)	0	0
Pudding, no sugar added	½ cup (125 mL)	13	13	½ cup (125 mL)	13	13
		71 g	**66 g**		**55 g**	**51 g**

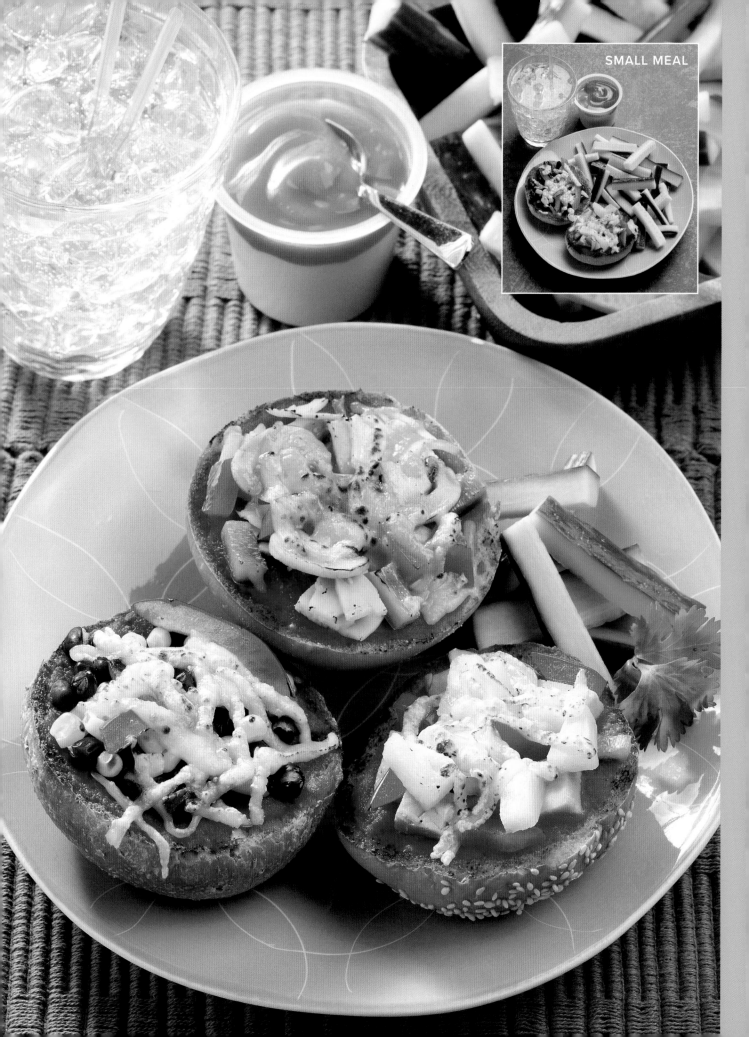

SMALL MEAL

DINNER 1

Minute Steak

Are you short of time? Is this one of your biggest challenges in making dinner? If so, this tasty, nutritious, quick meal is for you. Cook some potatoes, rice, quinoa or pasta to go along with it. Balance this meal out with some peas and carrots and bell pepper on the side.

This meal is so good that sometimes you might want to serve it to guests. Try the wonderful trifle for dessert. You can make trifle the night before, so it's ready to eat the next day. An alternative to the trifle is a $\frac{1}{2}$ cup (125 mL) of yogurt or pudding with one or two small plain cookies on the side.

FOOD FACT

Minute steak

Minute steak is outside or inside round steak that a butcher pounds until it's flattened. Also called tenderized frying steak, it cooks quickly, because it's a thin piece of meat.

OPTIONS

Hamburger patties

You can also make this recipe with thin hamburger patties instead of minute steak. Cook your hamburger through (until there is no pink color left) before adding the gravy.

Minute Steak

Makes 4 large servings (or 5 small)

1 small onion, sliced

2 tsp (10 mL) margarine or butter

1½ lb (750 g) minute steak or hamburger patties (1 lb/500 g for 4 small servings)

25 g package fat-free brown gravy (look for the brand with lowest sodium)

PER LARGE SERVING	
Calories	242
Carbohydrate	5 g
Fiber	0 g
Net carbs	5 g
Protein	39 g
Fat, total	6 g
Fat, saturated	2 g
Cholesterol	73 mg
Sodium	428 mg

1. In a large frying pan, melt margarine or butter, then add onions. Cook onions until soft at medium heat.

2. Move onions to the side, and add the meat to the pan and brown on both sides.

3. While meat is cooking, mix the contents of the gravy package with hot water in a glass measuring cup or bowl. Use the amount of water shown on the gravy package instructions (usually 1 cup/250 mL). Mix well with a whisk or fork.

4. Add the gravy to the pan with the onions and meat. Turn the temperature down to low-medium, cover with a lid, and simmer for 10 to 15 minutes.

Lady Vivian's English Trifle
Makes 5 servings

¼ of an angel food cake

2 tbsp (30 mL) light raspberry or other fruit jam (labeled as less than 20 calories per tbsp/15 mL)

1 tbsp (15 mL) sherry

1 cup (250 mL) frozen raspberries, unsweetened (or other frozen berries), thawed and well drained

1 ready-to-eat no-sugar-added vanilla pudding cup (106 g)

½ cup (125 mL) whipping cream (unwhipped measure)

1½ tsp (7 mL) icing sugar

1 tbsp (15 mL) sliced almonds, toasted

PER CUP (250 ML)	
Calories	160
Carbohydrate	18 g
Fiber	2 g
Net carbs	16 g
Protein	2 g
Fat, total	9 g
Fat, saturated	5 g
Cholesterol	31 mg
Sodium	152 mg

1. Cut the cake into 2-inch (5 cm) pieces. Place the pieces in a large bowl and add the jam. Mix gently with a spatula or spoon so that the jam coats the cake.

2. Drizzle sherry over the cake.

3. To drain berries, put in a sieve and, using the back of a spoon, push out all the juice.

4. Whip cream until soft peaks form. Add icing sugar at the end of the whipping.

5. Prepare the dessert in five individual dishes or in one large bowl. Layer the ingredients, starting with cake with jam and sherry on the bottom. Layer with raspberries, then pudding, and top with whipped cream.

6. Refrigerate for several hours so the flavors soak in.

7. Toast almonds by cooking at medium heat in a dry nonstick or cast-iron frying pan, stirring constantly, for 2 minutes or until golden. Let cool. Before serving the trifle, garnish with the toasted almonds.

RECIPE TIP

Angel food cake
Angel food cake is low in fat and calories compared to other cakes. Bake the angel food cake yourself using a boxed mix (make it ahead, so it has time to cool before you make the trifle) or buy it ready-made from the bakery. Freeze the rest of the cake to make another trifle or other dessert later (such as angel food cake with fresh fruit).

Sherry
A dry sherry gives trifle its distinctive flavor, but it still tastes scrumptious if you prefer not to add alcohol.

Food Choices	Large Meal	Small Meal
Carbohydrate	4	3
Protein	5½	4½
Fat	1	1

Your Dinner Menu	Large Meal (730 calories)	Total Carbs	Net Carbs	Small Meal (550 calories)	Total Carbs	Net Carbs
Minute Steak with gravy	large serving (¼ recipe)	5	5	small serving (⅕ recipe)	4	4
Potatoes with parsley	1½ medium	48	44	1 medium	32	30
Yellow or green beans	1 to 1½ cups (250 to 375 mL)	15	10	1 to 1½ cups (250 to 375 mL)	15	10
Bell pepper	¾ cup (175 mL)	7	6	¾ cup (175 mL)	7	6
English Trifle	1 serving	18	16	1 serving	18	16
		93 g	81 g		76 g	66 g

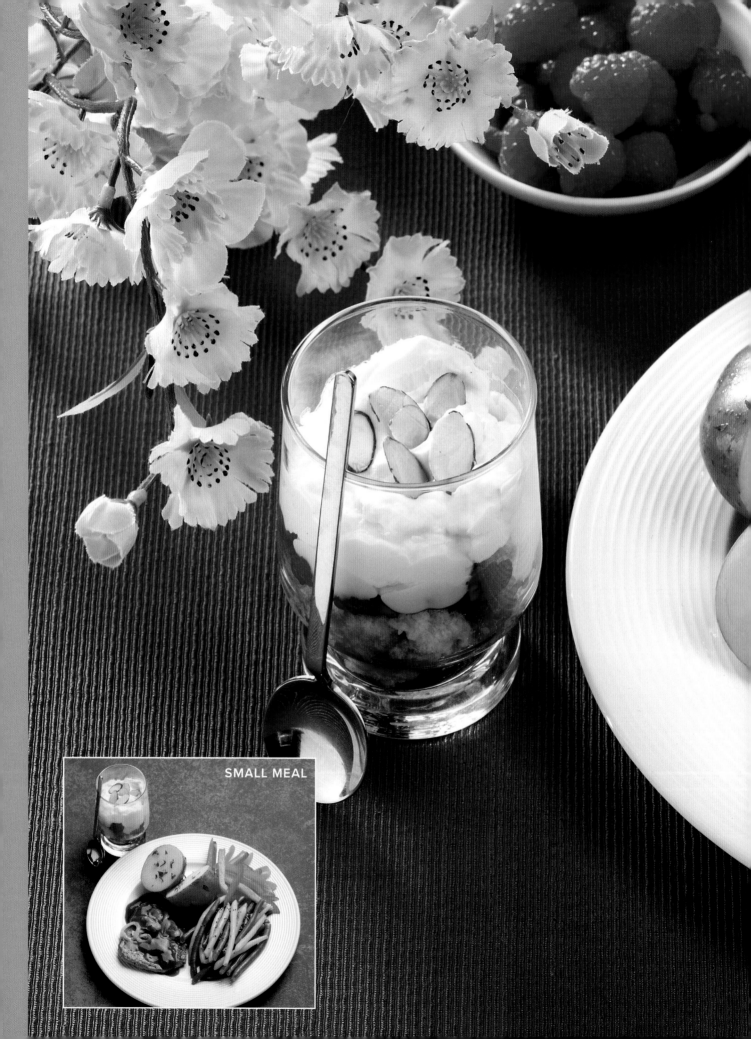

SMALL MEAL

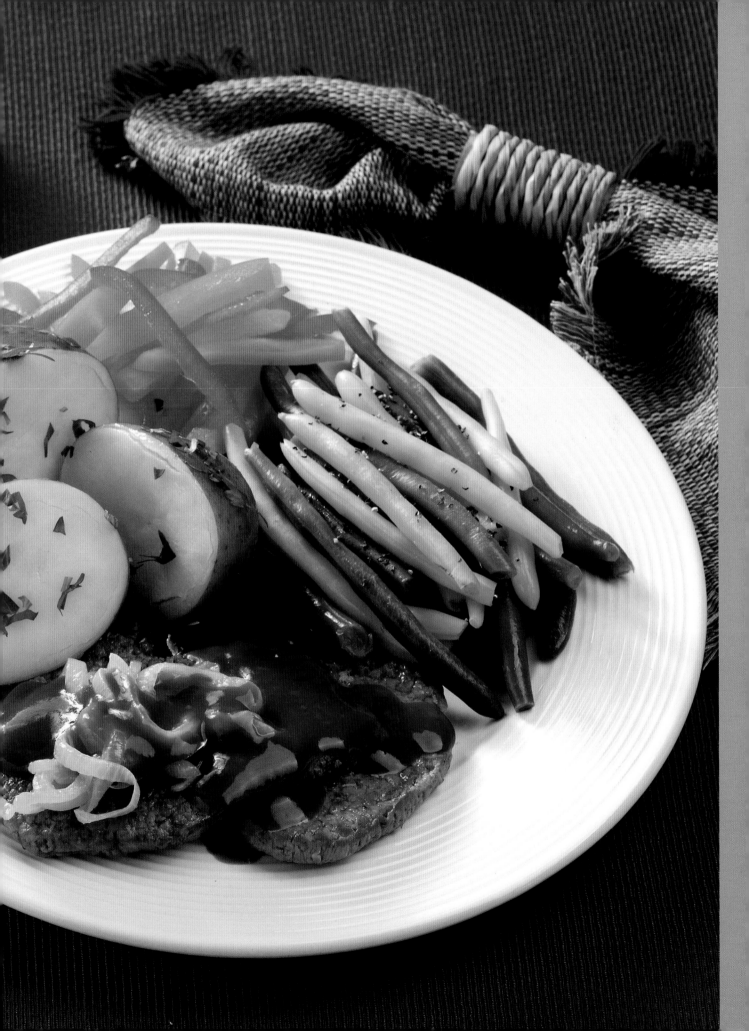

DINNER 2

Nuts & Bolts Stir Fry

Do you ever buy a package of pork chops or chicken breasts and end up with one extra piece? Keep the extra raw piece in your fridge for the next day to make a stir fry. This stir fry requires only a small amount of meat, as the protein is complimented with vegetable protein (nuts). The "bolts" in this meal are the red pepper sticks!

For dessert with this meal, enjoy yummy Peach Cobbler.

HEALTH TIP

Brown rice

Brown rice raises your blood sugar a bit slower than white rice and is a good source of fiber.

OPTIONS

If you want to make this meal vegetarian, you can add a few more nuts and omit the meat.

Use any combination of vegetables you have, such as asparagus, frozen mixed vegetables or cabbage.

Nuts & Bolts Stir Fry

Makes 4 large servings (or 5 small)

2 medium carrots, peeled and sliced

2 stalks celery, sliced

30 sugar snap peas or 45 snow peas, cut in half (or $\frac{1}{3}$ cup/75 mL frozen peas)

1 red pepper, cut into sticks

1 tsp (5 mL) vegetable oil

1 small onion, cut in small chunks

1 medium pork chop (or a 2-inch/5 cm piece of pork tenderloin), or 1 medium chicken breast (5 oz/150 g), all fat trimmed off, sliced thinly

$\frac{1}{4}$ to $\frac{1}{2}$ tsp (1–2 mL) hot pepper flakes, or few dashes of hot pepper sauce (optional)

1 tbsp (15 mL) oyster sauce (or soy sauce)

$\frac{1}{2}$ tsp (2 mL) ground ginger

1 cup (250 mL) cashews, peanuts or almonds, salted and roasted

1 tbsp (15 mL) sesame seeds, toasted

PER LARGE SERVING	
Calories	307
Carbohydrate	20 g
Fiber	4 g
Net carbs	16 g
Protein	15 g
Fat, total	20 g
Fat, saturated	4 g
Cholesterol	20 mg
Sodium	274 mg

1. Prepare your raw vegetables and place in a large bowl.
2. At medium heat, add oil to a nonstick frying pan or heavy pot. Once hot, add sliced meat and sear quickly until lightly browned. Add onions and gently sauté.
3. Add vegetables and hot pepper flakes to your meat. Cook, uncovered, until lightly cooked.
4. Add oyster sauce, ginger, nuts and sesame seeds and cook for another one or two minutes.

If you'd like, add a splash of milk or 1 to 2 tbsp (15–30 mL) of Greek yogurt or frozen whipped topping on your cobbler. It is also very good made with other canned fruit such as pears, apricots or fruit cocktail instead of peaches. However, this recipe does not work well with frozen fruit, which serves better in a crumble.

Peach Cobbler

Makes 8 servings

Preheat oven to 425°F (220°C)

three 14-oz (398 mL) cans sliced peaches, water or juice-packed, drained

⅛ tsp (0.5 mL) cinnamon

½ tsp (2 mL) almond extract

¾ cup (175 mL) flour

¼ cup (60 mL) sugar

1 tsp (5 mL) baking powder

¼ tsp (1 mL) salt

1 tbsp (15 mL) margarine or butter

⅓ cup (75 mL) skim milk

1 large egg

PER LARGE SERVING	
Calories	135
Carbohydrate	27 g
Fiber	2 g
Net carbs	25 g
Protein	3 g
Fat, total	2 g
Fat, saturated	0 g
Cholesterol	23 mg
Sodium	140 mg

OPTIONS

This dessert can be replaced with a couple of plain cookies or ½ cup (125 mL) of ice cream or frozen yogurt. Try a low-fat Greek yogurt.

1. Place peaches in an ungreased 8- by 8-inch (20 by 20 cm) pan or casserole dish. Add cinnamon and almond extract, and mix with peaches.

2. In a medium-sized bowl, mix together flour, sugar, baking powder and salt.

3. With a fork, blend margarine into the flour mixture. Then add milk and egg and continue to mix. Batter will be wet and gooey.

4. Spoon batter evenly over peaches.

5. Bake at 425°F (220°C) for 30 minutes or until lightly browned.

Food Choices	Large Meal	Small Meal
Carbohydrate	5½	4½
Protein	2	1½
Fat	2	1½

Your Dinner Menu	Large Meal (730 calories)	Total Carbs	Net Carbs	Small Meal (550 calories)	Total Carbs	Net Carbs
Nuts & Bolts Stir Fry	1 large serving (¼ recipe)	20	16	1 small serving (⅕ recipe)	16	13
Brown rice	1 cup (250 mL)	45	42	½ cup (150 mL)	30	28
Milk	1 cup (250 mL)	12	12	1 cup (250 mL)	12	12
Peach Cobbler	1 serving	27	25	1 serving	27	25
		104 g	**95 g**		**85 g**	**78 g**

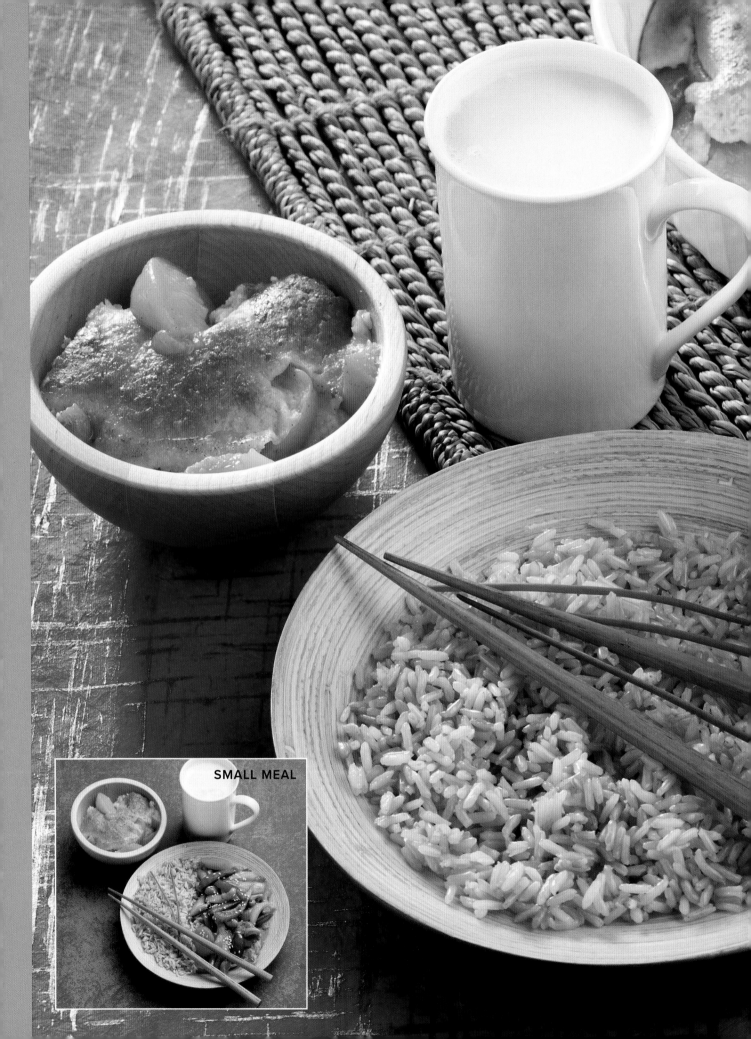

SMALL MEAL

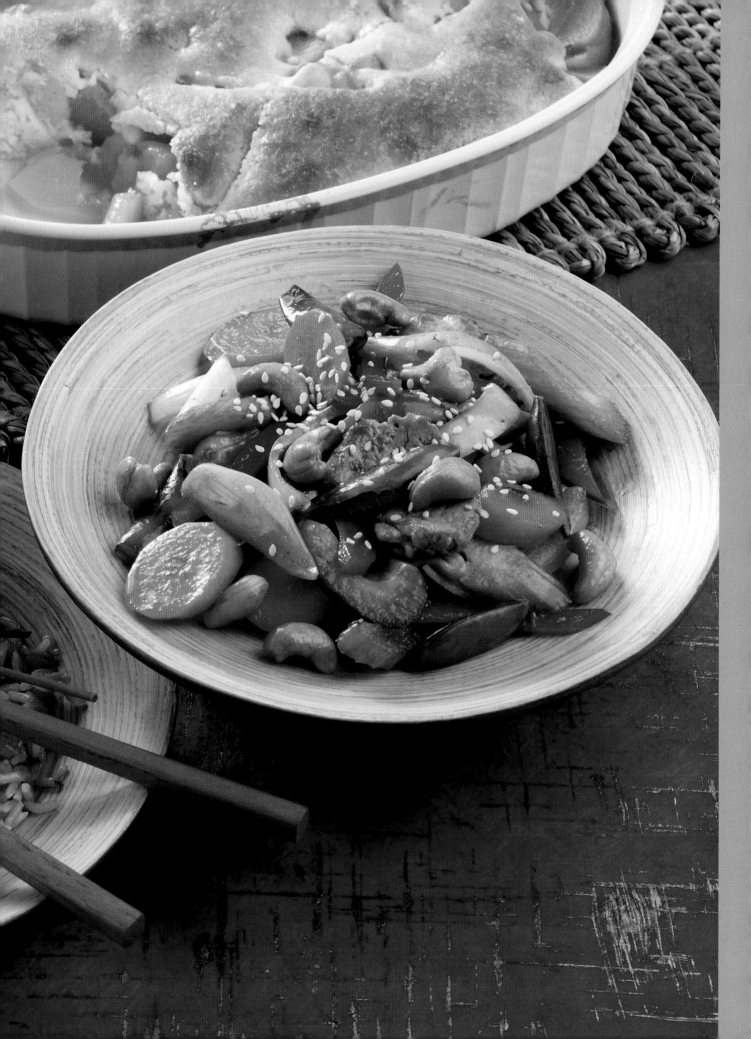

DINNER 3

Hot Chicken Salad

Enjoy Hot Chicken Salad with garlic bread and milk. Try Cinnamon Apple for dessert.

Green Salad

For each salad serving:

2 cups (500 mL) of greens
½ carrot, thinly sliced
2 large radishes, thinly sliced
½ medium tomato, chopped or wedges
2 tbsp (30 mL) shredded cheese

PER SERVING	
Calories	98
Carbohydrate	9 g
Fiber	3 g
Net carbs	6 g
Protein	5 g
Fat, total	5 g
Fat, saturated	3 g
Cholesterol	15 mg
Sodium	125 mg

1. Make the Homemade Chicken Strips (recipe below) and place in the oven to bake.

2. While the chicken strips are cooking, prepare a large green salad with tomatoes, carrots and radishes, or any combination of your favorite vegetables.

3. Remove the hot cooked Chicken Strips from the oven and put them on your salad, in strips or cut in pieces.

Homemade Chicken Strips

Makes 18 strips

½ cup (125 mL) bread crumbs
¼ cup (60 mL) dried Parmesan cheese
½ tsp (2 mL) oregano
1½ tsp (7 mL) dried parsley
2 to 3 tbsp (30 to 45 mL) milk
3 large (or 4 small) chicken breasts, skinned and fat trimmed off (14 oz/420 g total)

PER STRIP	
Calories	44
Carbohydrate	2 g
Fiber	0 g
Net carbs	2 g
Protein	6 g
Fat, total	1 g
Fat, saturated	0 g
Cholesterol	15 mg
Sodium	56 mg

1. In a bowl (or plastic bag), combine bread crumbs, Parmesan cheese, oregano and parsley.

2. Pour milk in another bowl.

3. On a cutting board, cut chicken breasts into strips (six per each large chicken breast or four per each small chicken breast). Flatten each strip with your hand or a meat pounder.

4. Dip each chicken strip into the milk. Then, one at a time, dip in the crumbs to coat evenly.

5. Place on a greased baking sheet and bake in a 400°F (200°C) oven. Cook for 10 minutes on each side, or until chicken is white inside.

OPTIONS

Try dandelion greens!

Add washed dandelion leaves and sliced roots to your salad. The leaves have vitamin C and the roots have soluble fiber. Don't use if they are sprayed with lawn chemicals.

OPTIONS

Homemade Chicken Strips are best as they are low-fat and salt-free.

If you are in rush, you can use instead:

- a commercial coating mix on your chicken, or
- commercial frozen breaded chicken.

These options will have more salt. The frozen breaded chicken will also have more fat.

Garlic Bread

Makes 1 slice (½ bun)

½ hot dog or hamburger bun,
    or 1 slice of bread
1 tsp (5 mL) margarine or butter
⅛ tsp (0.5 mL) garlic powder

1. In a small bowl, mix margarine
   or butter with garlic powder.

2. Toast your bread, and while hot,
   spread on the garlic margarine or butter.

PER SLICE	
Calories	106
Carbohydrate	13 g
Fiber	1 g
Net carbs	12 g
Protein	3 g
Fat, total	5 g
Fat, saturated	1 g
Cholesterol	0 mg
Sodium	153 mg

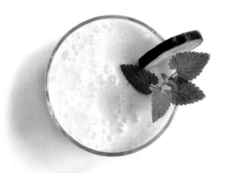

Buttermilk is rich in probiotic "good bacteria" that live in your gut and help keep you healthy. Other cultured milks include ayran (Turkish), doogh (Persian) and kefir (Russian).

Cinnamon Apple

Makes 2 servings

¼ tsp (1 mL) cinnamon mixed with
    1 tbsp (15 mL) sugar (or equivalent
    of a low-calorie sweetener)
2 small or 1 large apple, sliced

1. In a microwavable bowl, add
   cinnamon and sugar to the
   sliced apple.

2. Microwave for about 30 seconds until apple is slightly
   tender.

PER SERVING	
Calories	90
Carbohydrate	23 g
Fiber	2 g
Net carbs	21 g
Protein	0 g
Fat, total	0 g
Fat, saturated	0 g
Cholesterol	0 mg
Sodium	1 mg

Food Choices	Large Meal	Small Meal
Carbohydrate	4½	3½
Protein	5	3
Fat	1	½

Your Dinner Menu	Large Meal (730 calories)	Total Carbs	Net Carbs	Small Meal (550 calories)	Total Carbs	Net Carbs
Green Salad	1 serving	9	6	1 serving	9	6
Homemade Chicken Strips	5 strips	12	11	3 strips	7	7
Creamy salad dressing	1 tbsp (15 mL) (or 2 tbsp light)	3	3	1 tbsp (15 mL) (or 2 tbsp light)	3	3
Garlic Bread	1 bun or 2 slices of bread	26	25	½ bun or 1 slice of bread	13	12
Buttermilk or other cultured milk, low-fat	1 cup (250 mL)	12	12	1 cup (250 mL)	12	12
Cinnamon Apple	1 serving	23	21	1 serving	23	21
		85 g	**78 g**		**67 g**	**61 g**

177

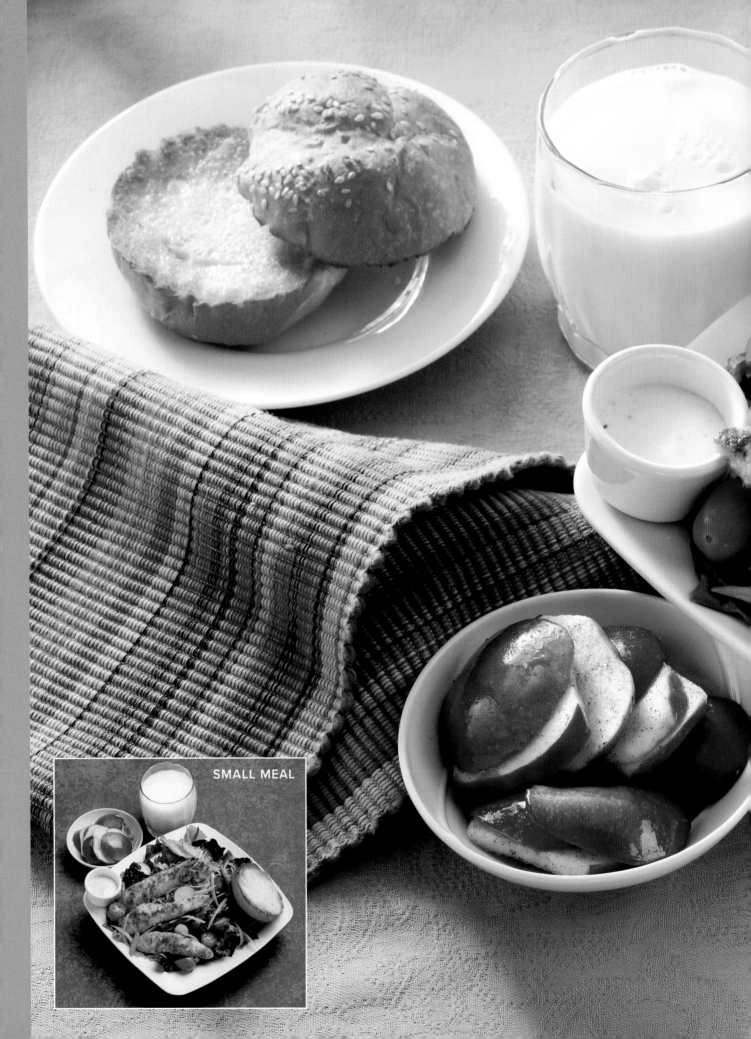

SMALL MEAL

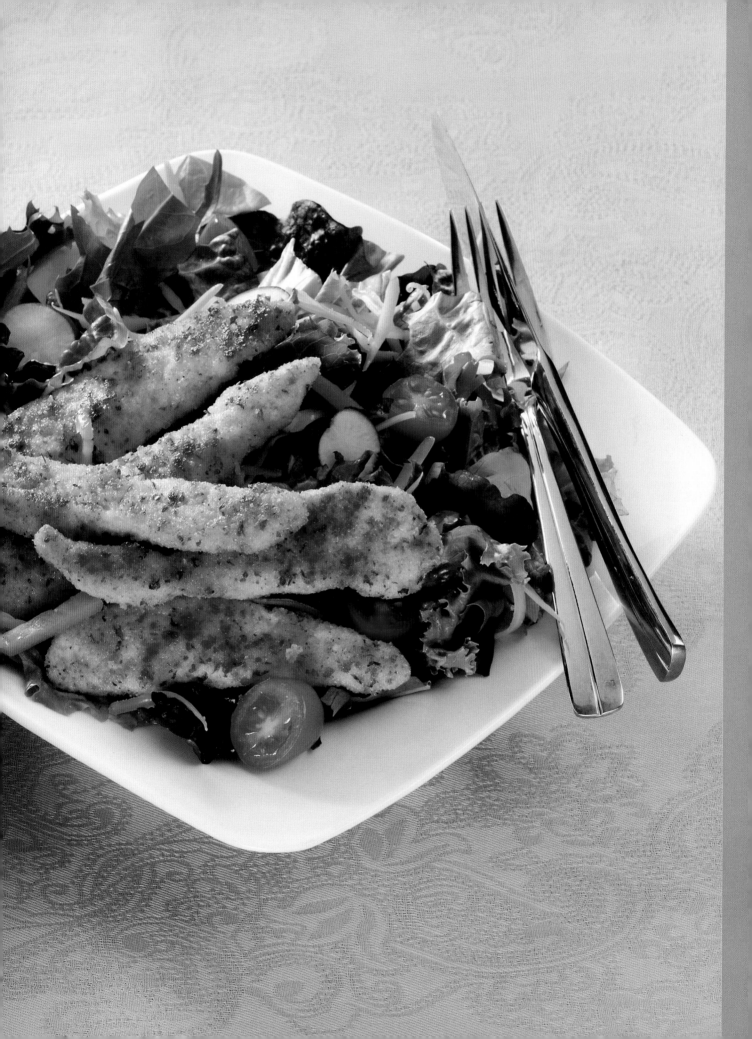

Vegetarian Sauce & Pasta

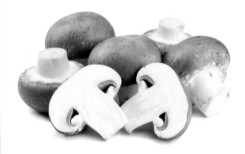

Serve the sauce over corkscrew noodles (rotini pasta). For a change, try whole wheat macaroni or spaghetti. Add a salad on the side, and have fruit and yogurt for dessert.

Vegetarian Sauce

Makes about 10 cups

PER CUP (250 ML)	
Calories	168
Carbohydrate	15 g
Fiber	4 g
Net carbs	11 g
Protein	7 g
Fat, total	11 g
Fat, saturated	2 g
Cholesterol	0 mg
Sodium	197 mg

2 tsp (10 mL) oil
½ cup (125 mL) water
1 large onion, chopped
3 large cloves garlic, finely
    chopped or minced
1 tsp (5 mL) oregano
¼ tsp (1 mL) each ground cloves
    and ground cinnamon
¼ tsp (1 mL) black pepper
¼ tsp (1 mL) hot sauce (such as Tabasco)
28-oz (796 mL) can diced tomatoes
1¾ cup (400 mL) of water
1 small tin (5½ oz/156 mL) tomato paste
3 large stalks celery, chopped
1 large green pepper, chopped
3 cups/750 mL (7 oz/200 g) fresh mushrooms
    (or 10-oz (284 mL) can mushroom pieces, drained)
½ cup (125 mL) shelled, unsalted roasted sunflower seeds
½ cup (125 mL) crunchy peanut butter

1. Place oil and water in a large heavy pot. Turn on heat to low-medium and add onion and garlic. Cook until soft, stirring occasionally. Add extra water if needed to keep moist.

2. Add spices and hot sauce to the onions. Cook for 1 or 2 minutes.

3. Add the other ingredients to the pot and stir well.

4. Cover pot with a lid and cook for 45 minutes to an hour on low-medium heat. Adjust temperature so it is just a simmer. Stir every 10 to 15 minutes, so it doesn't stick. If too thick, add extra water. If too thin, take the lid off and cook uncovered for the last 15 minutes.

Here's a delicious change from a cabbage-based coleslaw. Cabbage, cauliflower and broccoli are all excellent cancer-fighting vegetables. The salad dressing can also be used on lettuce-based salads.

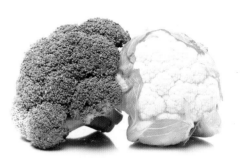

Cauliflower and Broccoli Slaw

Makes 4 servings

1 cup (250 mL) cauliflower, chopped
1 cup (250 mL) broccoli, chopped
¼ cup (60 mL) Mayo Parmesan
    Salad Dressing
1 small red apple, cored and chopped
2 oz (60 g) cheese, finely chopped (2 oz of cheese is a portion the size of four dice)

1. Combine ingredients.

PER SERVING	
Calories	90
Carbohydrate	10 g
Fiber	2 g
Net carbs	8 g
Protein	6 g
Fat, total	4 g
Fat, saturated	2 g
Cholesterol	11 mg
Sodium	268 mg

Mayo Parmesan Salad Dressing

Makes ¼ cup (60 mL)

¼ cup (60 mL) fat-free or
    light mayonnaise
1 tbsp (15 mL) parmesan cheese
1 tsp (5 mL) vinegar
1 tsp (5 mL) sugar
black pepper, to taste

1. Place all ingredients in a small bowl and stir or whisk until smooth, or place in a jar, seal with the lid and shake the jar.

PER TBSP (15 ML)	
Calories	24
Carbohydrate	4 g
Fiber	0 g
Net carbs	4 g
Protein	1 g
Fat, total	1 g
Fat, saturated	0 g
Cholesterol	3 mg
Sodium	150 mg

OPTIONS

If you choose low-fat Greek yogurt with no sugar added, rather than a regular yogurt, you would get 5 g fewer carbs in a ¾ cup (175 mL) serving.

Food Choices	Large Meal	Small Meal
Carbohydrate	5½	4
Protein	1	½
Fat	3	2

Your Dinner Menu	Large Meal (730 calories)	Total Carbs	Net Carbs	Small Meal (550 calories)	Total Carbs	Net Carbs
Vegetarian Pasta Sauce	1⅓ cup (325 mL)	20	14	1 cup (250 mL)	15	11
Rotini whole wheat pasta	1½ cups (375 mL)	55	49	1 cup (250 mL)	37	33
Cauliflower and Broccoli Slaw	1 serving	10	8	1 serving	10	8
Strawberries	1 cup (250 mL)	11	8	½ cup (125 mL)	5	4
Low-fat yogurt, no sugar added	¾ cup (175 mL)	14	14	¾ cup (175 mL)	14	14
		110 g	**93 g**		**81 g**	**70 g**

181

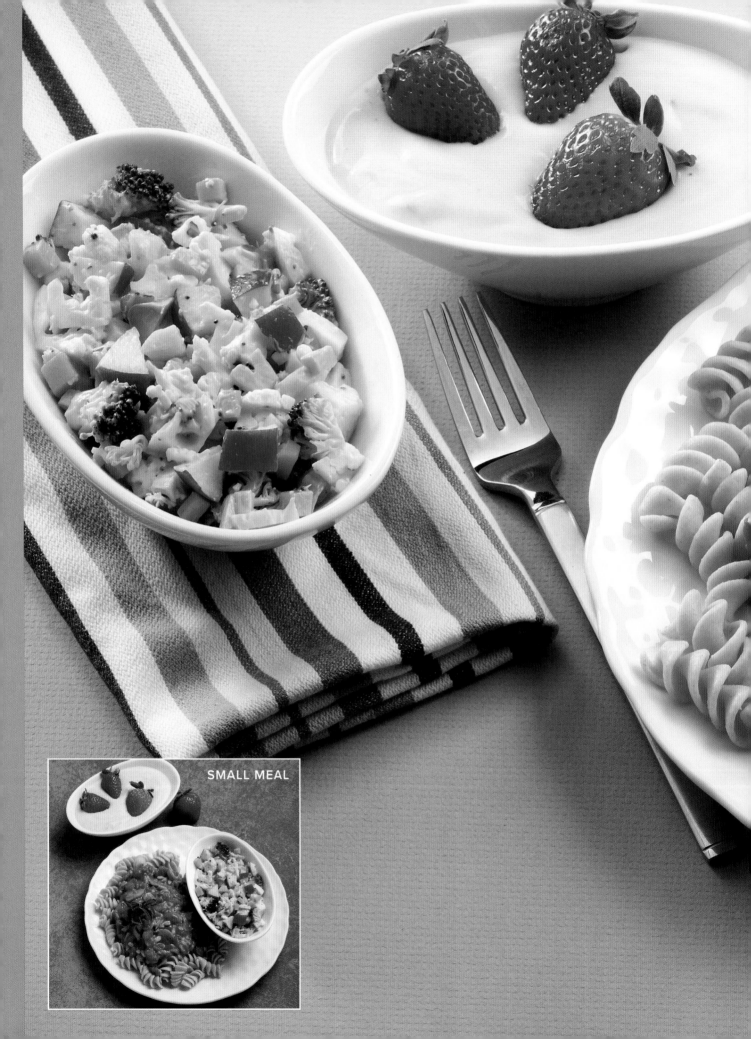

SMALL MEAL

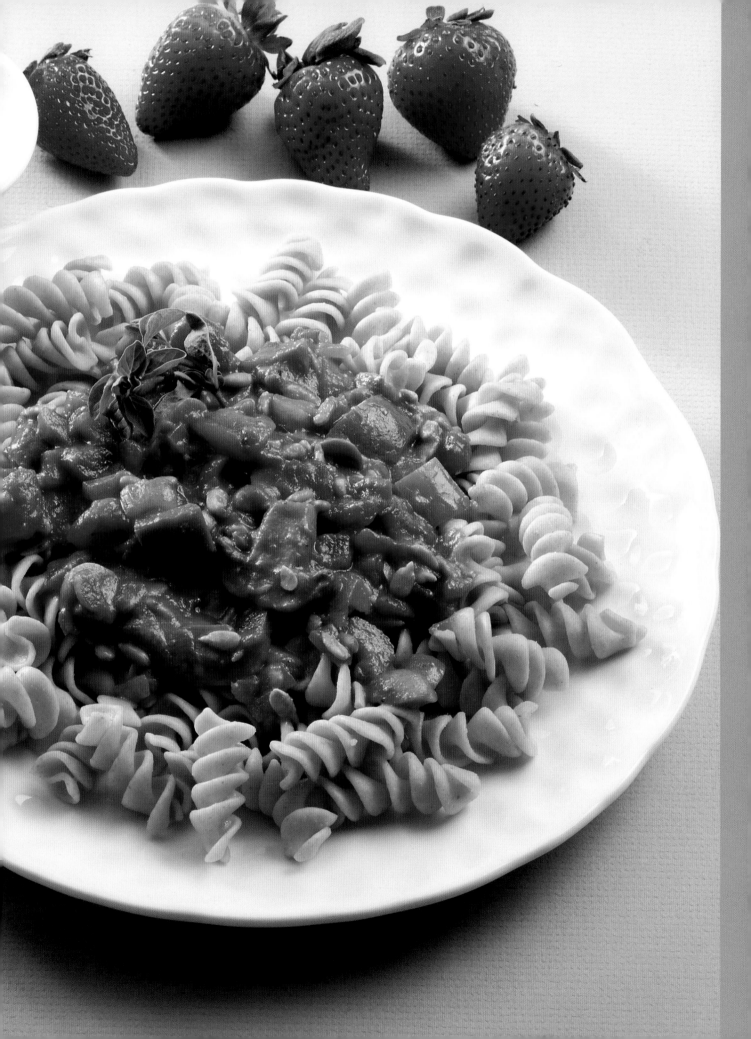

DINNER 5

Seafood Chowder

This chowder is an old-time favorite from the island of Newfoundland, on the Canadian East Coast. Fishing families make fresh chowder with whatever catch the fisherman brings home, and serve it with chunks of fresh hearty bread and butter. Enjoy this meal with a salad and for dessert, the delicious Lemon Zinger Pudding.

Karen adapted this recipe to use frozen fish and seafood, which is sometimes more readily available and less expensive than fresh. Using frozen fish, your soup will cook in half an hour. The soup is delicious the day you make it or next day. It also freezes well.

Seafood Chowder

Makes 8 cups (2 L)

1 tbsp (15 mL) margarine or butter

1 medium onion, chopped

3 cups (750 mL) water

2 medium potatoes, peeled
    and diced

1 medium carrot, peeled and chopped

7 oz (200 g) frozen salmon
    (about two 2- by 3-inch/5 by 7 cm fillets)

7 oz (200 g) frozen white fish
    (about two 2- by 4-inch/5 by 10 cm fillets)

1 tsp (5 mL) dried parsley or flaked savory (not ground savory)

1/4 tsp (1 mL) black pepper

7 oz (200 g) scallops, frozen

10 oz (300 g) shrimp, uncooked, or cooked, frozen, tails removed

PER CUP (250 ML)	
Calories	173
Carbohydrate	9 g
Fiber	1 g
Net carbs	8 g
Protein	22 g
Fat, total	5 g
Fat, saturated	1 g
Cholesterol	105 mg
Sodium	180 mg

1. In a large heavy pot, place butter and onion. At low-medium heat, sauté onion in butter until soft.

2. Add water, potatoes, carrots, whole pieces of salmon and white fish, dried parsley and pepper. Simmer uncovered at medium heat, stirring occasionally. The fish will gently break into pieces as cooking. Cook until potatoes are tender and fish is cooked (no translucence), about 10 to 15 minutes.

3. Add scallops and shrimp and continue simmering for another 5 to 10 minutes.

OPTIONS

If you would like to use thawed or fresh seafood or fish instead of frozen, simply reduce the cooking time by about 10 minutes. Add any fish juices to the chowder.

Scallops add a wonderful flavor and texture, but unfortunately they are expensive. Instead, you can increase your portion of white fish or shrimp and omit the scallops.

Yukon gold potatoes are nice in this recipe as they add a nice yellow color, but any potato will work!

RECIPE TIP

If the shrimp you buy have the tails on, remove the tails before adding to the chowder. To easily remove the tails from frozen shrimp, first soak them in cold water for a few minutes.

Lemon Zinger Pudding

Makes 6 servings

Preheat oven to 350°F (180°C)

3 large eggs, whites and yolks separated

3 tbsp (45 mL) sugar

2 tsp (10 mL) lemon peel, grated

¼ cup (60 mL) lemon juice (the juice from the lemon you just grated)

¼ cup (60 mL) sifted all-purpose flour

2 tbsp (30 mL) sucralose (Splenda)

1½ cups (375 mL) skim milk

2 tbsp (30 mL) margarine or butter (softened)

PER SERVING	
Calories	140
Carbohydrate	15 g
Fiber	0 g
Net carbs	15 g
Protein	6 g
Fat, total	6 g
Fat, saturated	1 g
Cholesterol	96 mg
Sodium	95 mg

RECIPE TIP

Egg whites beat better if they are at room temperature. Take the eggs out of the fridge when you start this recipe, and by the time you've completed step 2, the egg whites should be ready.

Cook the pudding in the oven inside a larger dish filled with some water. Cooking it this way allows this delicate pudding to cook without burning and to retain its lovely sauce.

1. Place egg whites in a medium-size glass mixing bowl. Place egg yolks in a second medium mixing bowl. Add sugar to the egg whites. Set egg whites aside.

2. To the second mixing bowl, with the egg yolks, add lemon peel and juice, margarine, flour, sucralose and milk.

3. Using an electric mixer, beat egg whites and sugar on high speed until soft peaks form.

4. Using the same beaters, beat egg yolk mixture at medium speed, scraping the sides with a spatula. Beat until blended; it will be a bit lumpy.

5. Fold egg whites into egg yolk mixture, turning it gently with your spatula.

6. Pour the batter into an ungreased 8-inch (20 cm) square baking dish. Then place this pan into a larger pan that is filled with about ½ inch (1 cm) of hot tap water.

7. Bake for 40 minutes, or until the top is lightly browned. Allow to sit in the pan with the water until the water has cooled, then remove the pudding dish. Serve warm.

Food Choices	Large Meal	Small Meal
Carbohydrate	4	3
Protein	6	4
Fat	1	1

Your Dinner Menu	Large Meal (730 calories)	Total Carbs	Net Carbs	Small Meal (550 calories)	Total Carbs	Net Carbs
Seafood Chowder	2 cups (500 mL)	17	16	1½ cups (375 mL)	13	12
Fresh bread	5 sticks (1½ thick slices)	27	25	3 sticks (1 thick slice)	18	17
Butter or margarine	2 tsp (10 mL)	0	0	1 tsp (5 mL)	0	0
Salad	1 large	6	4	1 large	6	4
Vinaigrette light salad dressing	1 tbsp (15 mL)	4	4	1 tbsp (15 mL)	4	4
Lemon Zinger Pudding	1 serving	15	15	1 serving	15	15
		69 g	**64 g**		**56 g**	**52 g**

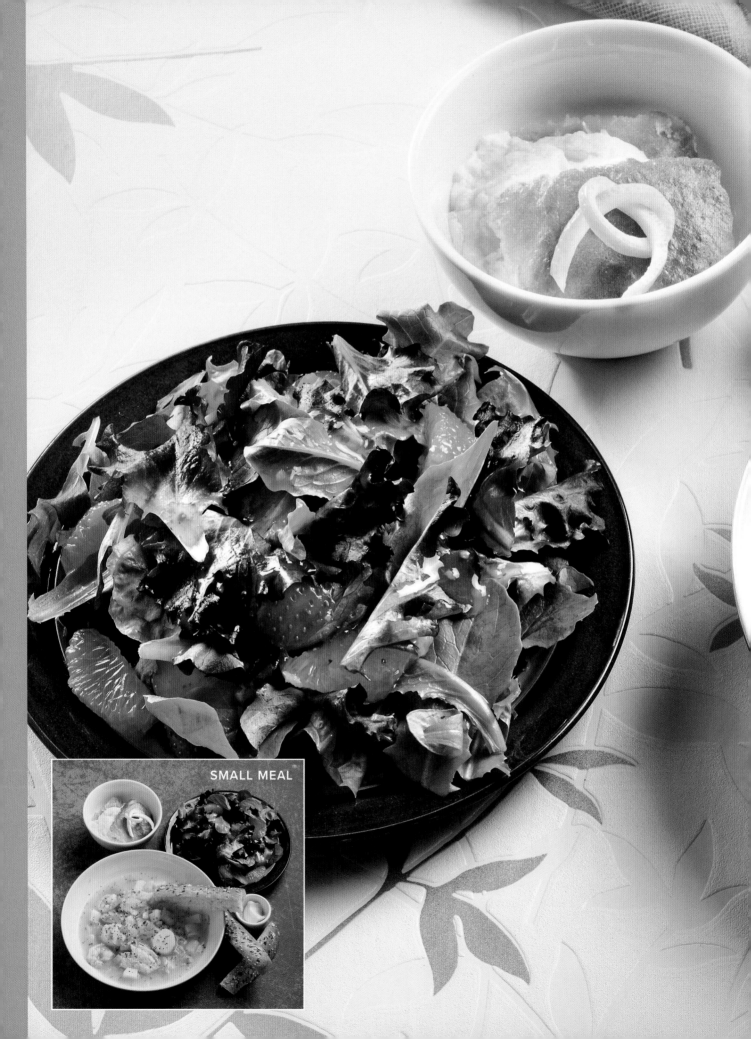

SMALL MEAL

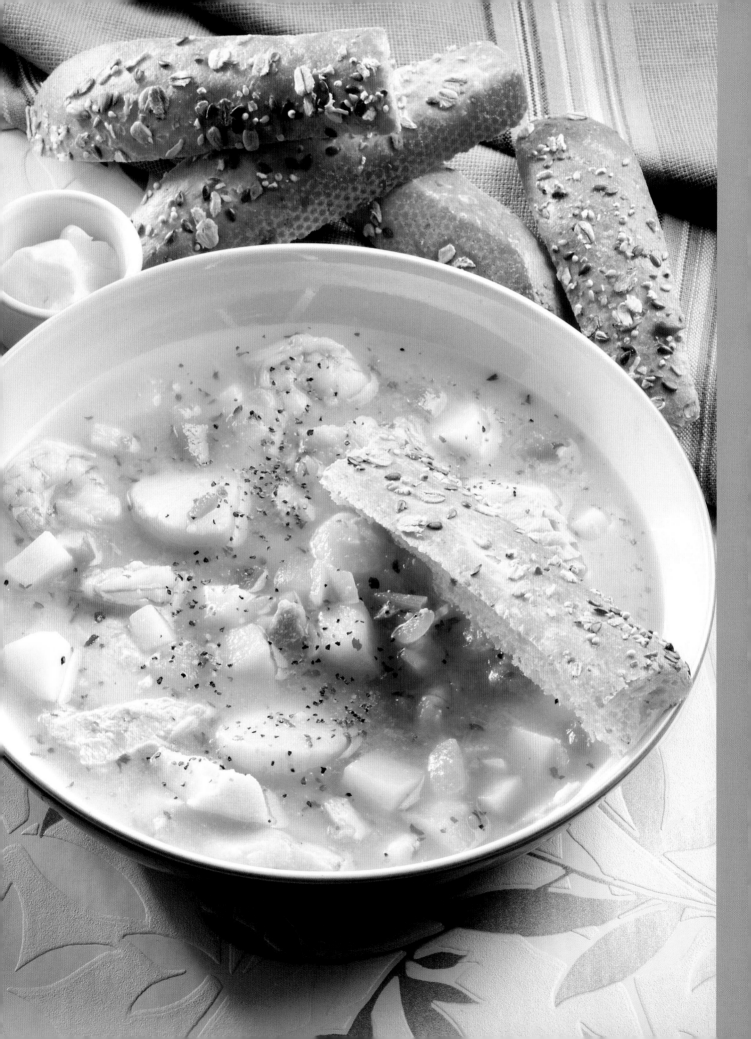

DINNER 6

Easy Chicken Curry

Make this curry the day ahead for the best flavor and thickness. As this is a large recipe, you can freeze the extra.

OPTIONS

Do you like it hot?

This is a flavorful curry but it is not spicy hot. If you like heat in your curry, add 1 tsp (5 mL) of chili powder or a few dashes of hot sauce.

Curry powder and garam masala are both fragrant Indian spice blends. Garam masala adds an important flavor to this recipe, but if it isn't available, replace it with curry powder (use 3 tbsp/45 mL in total) or an alternative Indian spice blend such as Korma or Biryani masala or vindaloo.

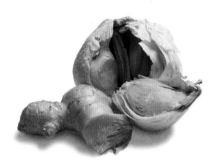

Easy Chicken Curry

Makes 6 large or 9 small servings

1 tbsp (15 mL) vegetable oil
¼ cup (60 mL) water
2 medium onions, chopped
6 cloves garlic, crushed or finely chopped
1 tbsp (15 mL) curry powder
2 tbsp (30 mL) garam masala
½ tsp (2 mL) salt
19-oz (540 mL) can of tomatoes (whole or chopped)
¼ cup (60 mL) packed fresh cilantro, finely chopped
1 cup (250 mL) unflavored low-fat yogurt
1 cup (250 mL) chicken stock
   (1 package reduced-salt bouillon + 1 cup/250 mL water)
18 skinned chicken drumsticks or thighs, skin removed
   (3½ lbs/1.7 kg weight with skin and bones or
   3 lbs/1.5 kg weight with skin removed)
¼ cup (60 mL) fresh cilantro, roughly chopped, for topping

PER LARGE SERVING	
Calories	352
Carbohydrate	14 g
Fiber	2 g
Net carbs	12 g
Protein	42 g
Fat, total	14 g
Fat, saturated	3 g
Cholesterol	145 mg
Sodium	581 mg

1. In a large heavy pot, heat oil and water over low-medium heat. Add onions and garlic to the pot. Cook until soft. Add spices and salt, stirring frequently, and cook for one or two minutes until the spices are well blended. Add a bit of water if too dry.

2. Add tomatoes, cilantro, yogurt and chicken stock. Blend together, then add chicken pieces.

3. Cover and simmer gently at low-medium heat. Stir periodically. Cook for 1 to 1½ hours, or until chicken is cooked. If too thick, add extra chicken stock or water if needed. If too thin, cook for the last 15 to 30 minutes without the lid.

4. After cooking, add chopped cilantro.

People often serve curries with a variety of condiments, such as mango chutney, chopped raw onions and tomatoes in an oil and vinegar mixture, pickles, marinated or curried vegetables, lentil dishes, dried coconut or fresh fruit. I've chosen three easy side dishes with this curry: raw grated carrots, shredded coconut and sliced bananas.

Basmati rice is always nice with a curry. Both white and a brown basmati rice are a good choice, as they have a lower glycemic index than short-grain rice. When cooked, the basmati rice grains have a wonderful flavor and don't stick together like many other kinds of rice. You can also use converted white rice, long-grained white rice, or brown rice.

Fruit and Cheese Kebabs

Go light for dessert with fruit kebabs. Combine a variety of fruits and cheese on a wooden skewer in the amounts shown in the photograph. This equals about half a fresh fruit serving and half an ounce (15 g) of cheese.

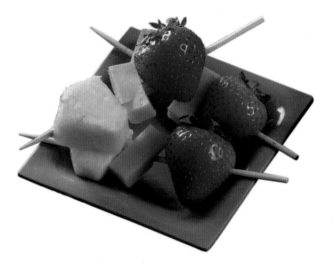

Food Choices	Large Meal	Small Meal
Carbohydrate	5	3½
Protein	6	4½
Fat	3½	2

Your Dinner Menu	Large Meal (730 calories)	Total Carbs	Net Carbs	Small Meal (550 calories)	Total Carbs	Net Carbs
Chicken Curry	large serving (3 drumsticks plus sauce)	14	12	small serving (2 drumsticks plus sauce)	9	7
Rice, basmati	1 cup (250 mL)	53	52	⅔ cup (150 mL)	36	35
Sliced banana	½ small banana	12	11	½ small banana	12	11
Shredded coconut, unsweetened	1 tbsp (15 mL)	1	0	1 tbsp (15 mL)	1	0
Grated carrots	½ cup (125 mL)	5	4	½ cup (125 mL)	5	4
Fruit and Cheese Kebabs	3 small skewers	8	7	3 small skewers	8	7
Tea	1 cup (250 mL)	0	0	1 cup (250 mL)	0	0
		93 g	86 g		71 g	64 g

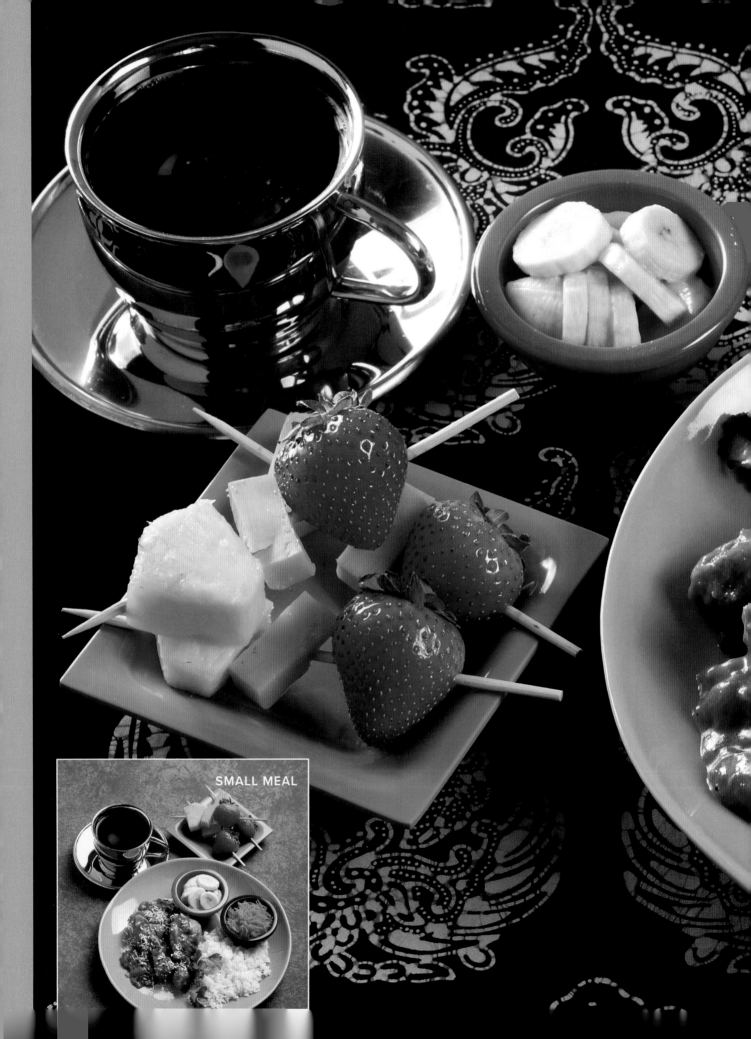

SMALL MEAL

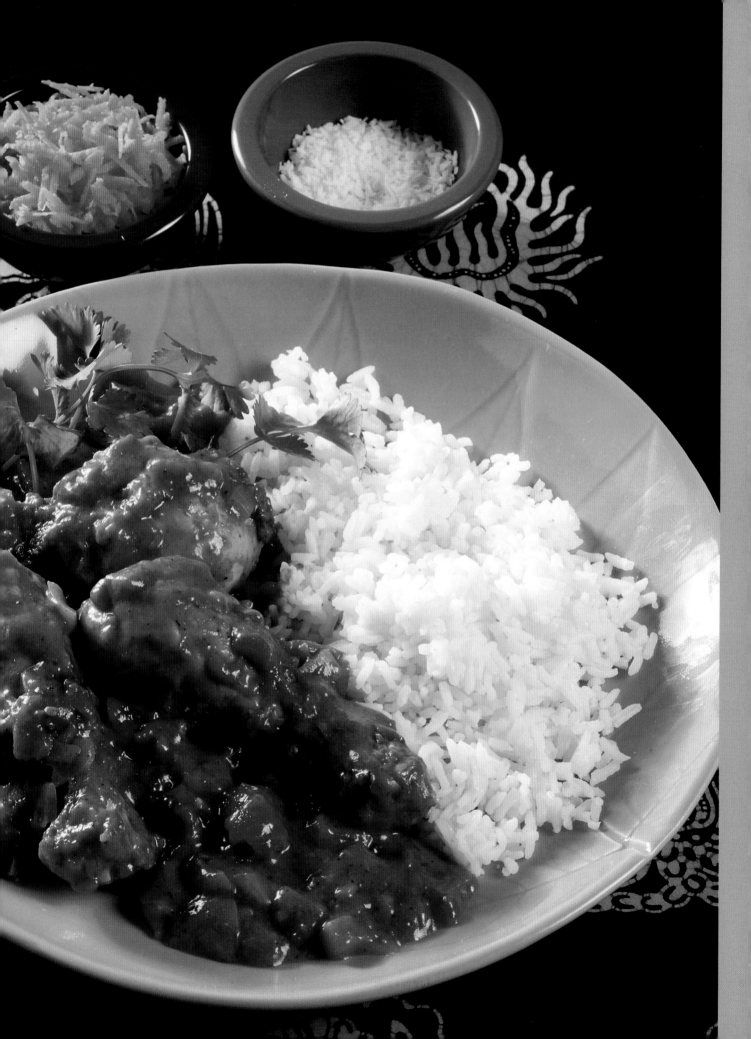

DINNER 7

Vegetable Omelet & Beans

RECIPE TIP

If serving two, double the omelet recipe, and use a larger nonstick frying pan if needed.

What could be easier than eggs and beans for a satisfying meal? This omelet is easy to make, but if you want an even easier meal, you can turn the omelet into scrambled eggs, using all the same ingredients. The toast with honey or jam becomes your dessert with this meal.

Vegetable Omelet

Serves 1

1½ tsp (7 mL) margarine, oil or butter

½ small onion or 2 green onions, chopped

1 cup (250 mL) raw vegetables (such as celery, peppers, cauliflower, broccoli or mushrooms), chopped

2 eggs

3 tbsp (45 mL) grated cheese

PER OMELET	
Calories	319
Carbohydrate	10 g
Fiber	2 g
Net carbs	8 g
Protein	20 g
Fat, total	23 g
Fat, saturated	8 g
Cholesterol	394 mg
Sodium	346 mg

1. In a small nonstick frying pan, sauté onions and vegetables in the margarine or other fat at low-medium heat.

2. While onions and vegetables are cooking, break eggs into a small mixing bowl. Beat eggs with a fork or whisk.

3. When onions and vegetables are soft, transfer the mixture into a bowl and set aside.

4. Pour egg into the greased frying pan. Immediately tip the pan to even out the layer of egg. As the egg is cooking, move any soft uncooked egg toward the edges of the pan, until all the egg is cooked.

5. Put the onion and vegetable mixture on one half of the omelet. Top with the grated cheese. Gently lift the other half of the omelet and fold on top. Lower the heat and cook it for another minute or two.

Beans, peas and lentils — an excellent choice!

Beans, peas and lentils, as compared to animal sources of protein such as meat, fish or chicken, are lower in saturated fat and a great source of fiber — and they cost less. Choose them at least once or twice a week. Add drained, canned beans or lentils to make leftovers go further, such as to a macaroni dish, spaghetti sauce or stew.

Here are some other ways to eat beans, peas and lentils:
- For lunch, make the Taco Soup on page 162, enjoy a split pea or black bean soup, or add beans or lentils to a vegetable soup to make a "meal in a bowl."
- Add cooked beans to a pizza (page 166), burrito or wrap.
- Add yellow lentils to a chicken curry (page 188). Then you can cut back on the chicken in your recipe.

More ideas from our *Diabetes Meals for Good Health Cookbook*
- Try Mexican Rice and Beans (pictured at right).
- Three of our dinner meals help you cut back on meat by including beans: Chili con Carne, Tacos, and Beans and Wieners.
- Sun Burgers replace meat with romano beans, cheese and sunflower seeds.
- Santa Fe Salad, made with black beans, is delicious. You can make an easy bean salad with a can of rinsed and drained mixed beans, along with sliced peppers or cucumber and a vinaigrette dressing.
- For a snack, try hummus spread on crackers.

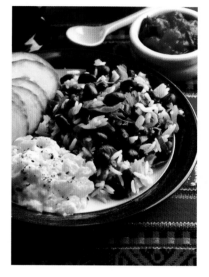

Mexican Rice and Beans

Food Choices	Large Meal	Small Meal
Carbohydrate	5	3½
Protein	3	3
Fat	3	3

Your Dinner Menu	Large Meal (730 calories)	Total Carbs	Net Carbs	Small Meal (550 calories)	Total Carbs	Net Carbs
Vegetable omelet	1 serving	10	8	1 serving	10	8
Baked beans	½ cup (125 mL)	27	22	¼ cup (60 mL)	14	11
Toast, whole-grain	2 slices	27	23	1 slice	14	12
Margarine or butter	2 tsp (10 mL)	0	0	1 tsp (5 mL)	0	0
Honey or jam	1½ tsp (7 mL)	9	9	1½ tsp (7 mL)	9	9
Mandarin oranges	2 small (or 1 medium)	15	13	2 small (or 1 medium)	15	13
		88 g	**75 g**		**62 g**	**53 g**

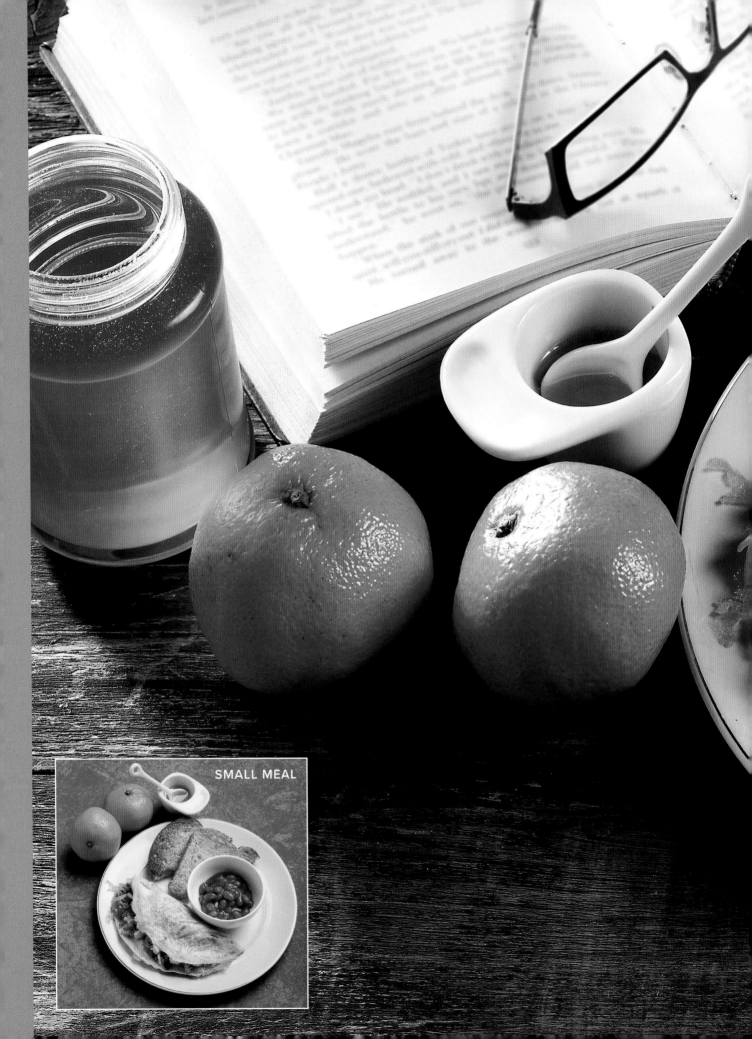

SMALL MEAL

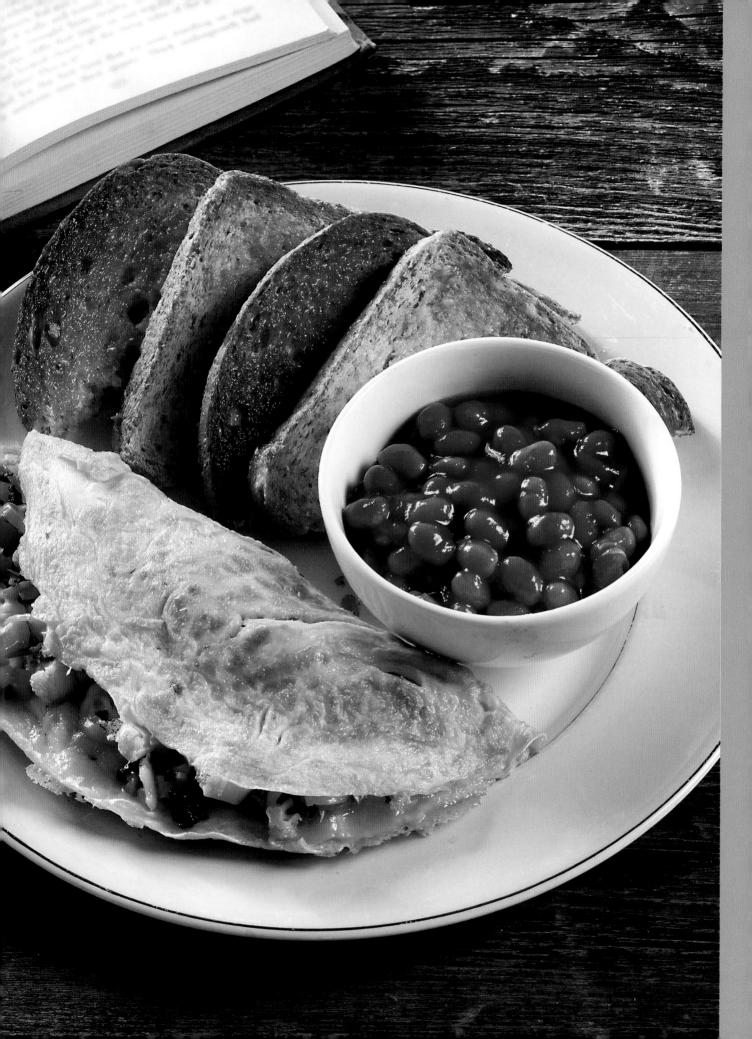

Snacks

Do you want more snack ideas? The *Diabetes Meals for Good Health Cookbook* includes more than 100 additional snack suggestions.

In this section you will find photographs of four groups of snacks. The groups are low-calorie snacks, small snacks, medium snacks and large snacks. The calories for each snack within each group are about the same. The carbs for each snack are listed. The number of snacks you choose will depend on how many calories a day you want. Look at the chart on page 149 that shows the calories of the small and large meals, and different snacks.

Low-calorie: 20 calories or less

Small: 50 calories

Medium: 100 calories

Large: 200 calories

For most of us it's good to choose no more than three of the small, medium or large snacks a day.
Three small snacks add up to 150 calories, three medium snacks add up to 300 calories and three large snacks add up to 600 calories.

Salty snacks

Salty snacks with 300 to 499 mg of salt are shown with one salt shaker. These should be limited to no more than once a day or even a couple of times a week.

Snacks with 500 mg or more are shown with two salt shakers and should be limited to no more than once a week.

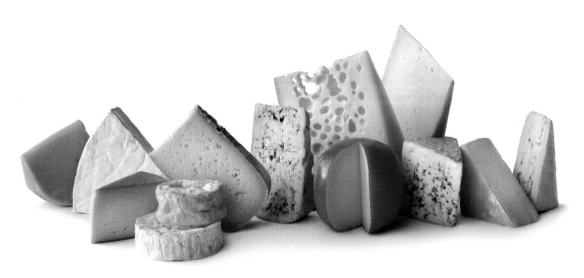

Low-calorie snacks or meal condiments

20 calories or less in each snack

Carbs in grams is marked in red. As portions
are small, total carbs and net carbs are the same.

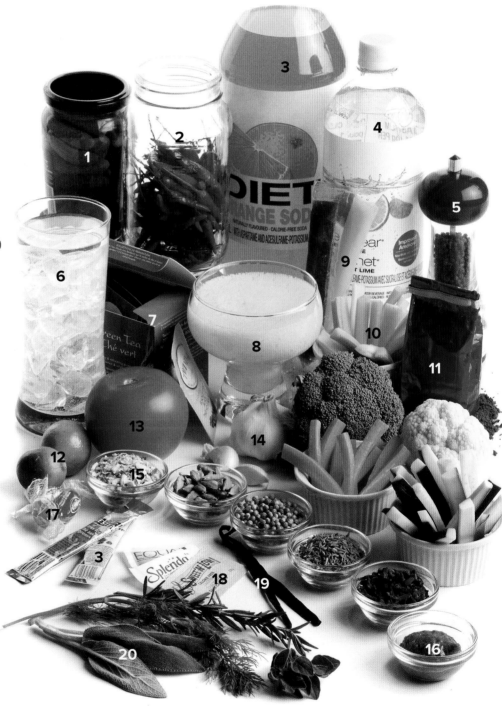

1. 1 to 2 mini pickles **0**
2. Hot peppers **0**
3. Diet soft drinks, diet iced tea and packaged diet drink mixes **0**
4. Flavored waters (no sugar added) **0**
5. Pepper **0**
6. Water **0**
7. Herbal tea or other tea **0**
8. Diet gelatin (whipped Jell-O shown) **0**
9. Sugar-free Freezee 4 tsp (20 mL) **1**
10. Celery sticks, or broccoli or cauliflower bunch, or carrot, cucumber or zucchini sticks **2**
11. Coffee or chicory root coffee substitute **1**
12. 1 to 2 mini limes **2**
13. Tomato **3**
14. Garlic **2**
15. Salt-free spice blends and a variety of other dried spices and herbs **0**
16. 1 tsp herb paste **1**
17. 1 to 2 sugar-free candies or mints **3**
18. Low-calorie sugar substitute **1**
19. Vanilla flavoring **0**
20. Fresh herbs **0**

Small snacks

50 calories

Total carbs are shown in dark blue and net carbs follow in red.
Both are in grams.

1. $\frac{1}{3}$ cup (75 mL) cranberry cocktail (on ice) **12 / 12**

2. 1 cup (250 ml) hot apple cider (half apple juice, half water, plus vanilla or cinnamon stick) **15 / 15**

3. 1 cup (250 mL) V8 juice **11 / 9**

4. $\frac{2}{3}$ cup (150 mL) low-fat milk **8 / 8**

5. 12 oz (355 mL) hot frothed coffee (half coffee, half low-fat milk) **8 / 8**

6. $\frac{1}{2}$ oz (15 g) cheese (slice) **1 / 1**

7. 1 cup (250 mL) low-calorie Vegetable Soup (see Diabetes Essentials) **11 / 9**

8. 1 orange **15 / 13**

9. $\frac{1}{2}$ cup (125 mL) frozen grapes **14 / 13**

10. $\frac{1}{2}$ cup (125 mL) no sugar added pudding **14 / 13**

11. 13 baby carrots **11 / 8**

12. 5 small pineapple spears **13 / 12**

13. 1 small apple **15 / 13**

14. $\frac{1}{2}$ cup (125 mL) unsweetened applesauce **14 / 12**

15. $1\frac{1}{2}$ oz (45 g) slice of luncheon meat **0 / 0**

16. 3 tbsp (45 mL) nuts and bolts **7 / 6**

17. 1 cup (250 mL) raw vegetables with 1 tbsp (15 mL) light dressing **6 / 5**

18. $\frac{1}{2}$ cup (125 mL) pickled beets **13 / 11**

19. 2 tbsp (30 mL) dried cranberries **13 / 12**

20. 5 animal crackers **9 / 9**

21. 2 Graham wafers **11 / 10**

22. 4 whole wheat soda crackers **11 / 8**

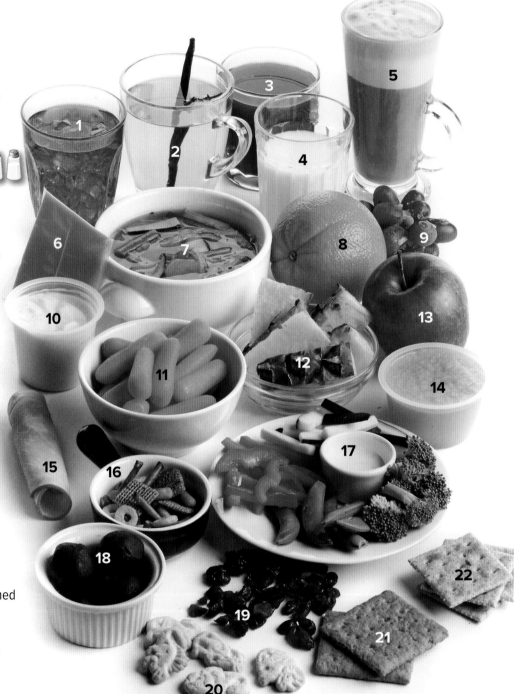

Medium snacks

100 calories

1. 100 calorie mini snack bag **21/18**
2. ½ cup (125 mL) low-fat chocolate milk (with ice!) **13/12**
3. Float (12 oz/355 mL of diet cola plus ½ cup/125 mL frozen yogurt) **12/11**
4. 1 open-face sandwich (unbuttered) **14/12**
5. 3 stone wheat crackers **16/14**
6. ¾ cup (175 mL) low-fat yogurt (no sugar added) with pomegranate seeds **16/16**
7. ¾ cup (175 mL) fat-free pistachio pudding **15/15**
8. 2 donut "bits" **12/12**
9. Ham and cheese slice (rolled) **3/3**
10. 1 hard boiled egg **0/0**
11. 1 medium pear **26/21**
12. 1¼ cups (300 mL) blueberries **26/22**
13. 1 piece of toast with 1 tsp (5 mL) margarine and diet jam **16/14**
14. 1 small banana **23/21**
15. 1 medium apple, sliced, with a sprinkle of sugar and cinnamon **23/20**
16. 14 almonds **4/2**
17. 13 baked rice thins crackers **23/21**
18. 100 calorie ice cream stick **22/18**
19. 1½ cheese string sticks **1/1**
20. 100 calorie granola bar **15/13**
21. 1 to 2 celery sticks with 1 tbsp (15 mL) peanut butter or 3 tbsp (45 mL) light cream cheese **4/3**

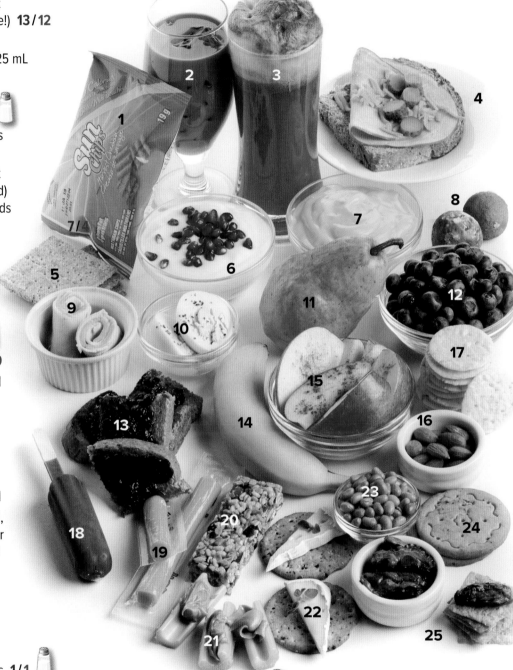

22. Two 3-inch (7.5 cm) crackers with ½ oz (15 g) cheese (try brie or blue cheese) **11/10**
23. 2 tbsp (30 mL) roasted soybeans **7/5**
24. 2 healthy lifestyle cookies **14/14**
25. 7 oysters on 7 mini wheat crackers **11/8**

Large snacks

200 calories

1. 1 cup (250 mL) of cream soup made with milk **15/15**

2. Chef salad made with 2–3 oz (60–90 g) cheese and/or ham and 1 tbsp (15 mL) dressing **6/5**

3. Piece of thin crust cheese pizza **30/28**

4. 1 cup (250 mL) cooked oatmeal with $\frac{1}{2}$ cup (125 mL) low-fat milk **34/30**

5. 5 cups (1.25 L) of popcorn (made with 1 tsp/5 mL of oil) **31/26**

6. $\frac{3}{4}$ cup (175 mL) frozen yogurt in a cone **31/31**

7. Omelette (made with 1 egg plus 1 egg white, 1 oz/30 g of cheese, green onion and 1 tbsp/15 mL bacon bits) **4/3**

8. 1 cup (250 mL) cereal (such as bran flakes) with $\frac{3}{4}$ cup (175 mL) milk **33/28**

9. 1 cup (250 mL) fruit salad with $\frac{3}{4}$ cup (175 mL) no-sugar-added yogurt **39/36**

10. 1 tomato and cheese sandwich (with 2 tsp/10 mL fat-free mayonnaise) **29/25**

11. Half 3-inch (7.5 cm) bagel with 1 tbsp (15 mL) light cream cheese **29/26**

12. 1 chicken drumstick with a slice of bread and 1–2 tbsp (15–30 mL) cranberry sauce **21/18**

13. 6 soda crackers with $\frac{1}{4}$ cup (60 mL) salmon or tuna mixed with 1 tsp (5 mL) fat-free mayonnaise **17/14**

14. $\frac{1}{4}$ cup (60 mL) peanuts or other shelled nuts **7/4**

15. $\frac{2}{3}$ cup (150 mL) sunflower seeds in the shells **6/3**

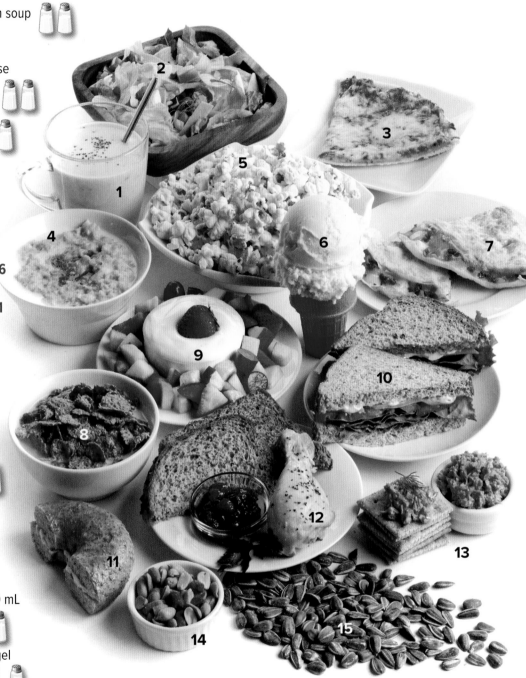

Step 2: Be Active

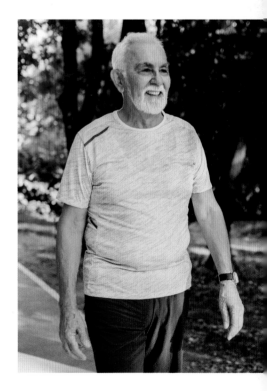

A Prescription for Exercise

You've been really tired the last two months. Your blood sugar is higher than usual. You go to see your doctor and she gives you two possible answers.

Answer one:
Doctor: "Here's a prescription. Take this pill twice a day. It will help with your blood sugar and the tiredness you have told me about."

You: "Yes, thank you, Doctor."

When you say yes:
- You trust your doctor.
- You are willing to try something to feel better.
- It sounds easy.
- You can start right away.

Answer two:
Doctor: "The best prescription for these health issues you have told me about is for you to go for a walk every day."

You: "Well no, I can't walk. I don't have time to walk during the day. Anyway, it's too cold outside, my knees hurt and I just don't have the energy."

When you say no: You still trust your doctor and would like to try something to feel better, but walking is more of a challenge. It requires you to change your daily routine.

- If you answer "yes" to the pills, you are like many others. We all wish that doctors will find a pill that will make us better without too much change on our part.

- Yet when you say "yes" to the pills, it shows you are willing to change. You are thinking of your future. You want to be the healthiest you can and live longer.

- If you answer "yes" to the walk, then you recognize that exercise can be one of the most powerful medicines that we have for good health.

This chapter will help you find ways to include exercise as part of your prescription for good health. You can choose a fitness plan that will be easy and comfortable for you. An exercise plan will give you energy, not take it away.

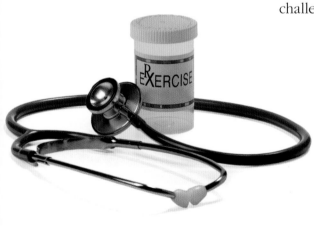

℞ DOCTOR'S ADVICE

Nearly half of North Americans don't exercise. Skipping exercise is as harmful as smoking. Exercise is a powerful medicine for good health.

Getting Started

In this chapter you will read how others have overcome their barriers to exercise and become active. You can, too.

One step at a time

Increase exercise gradually. You should always be able to do the "talk test." This means you can talk comfortably when exercising.

Avoid sore muscles by warming up or cooling down before and after exercise. One easy way to warm up and cool down is to begin and end your exercise session at a slower pace. For example, walk slowly for the first few minutes, then increase your pace to a comfortable level. Walk slowly again for the last few minutes of your walk.

First, move more at home and work

Even small changes in how we live can make a difference. Take walks at home or at work. Use stairs instead of the elevator. Park or get off buses further away from buildings and walk. Little things add up. People who move a little all day long burn more calories than people who sit a lot.

Second, take longer walks or do other aerobic exercise

Replacing just a half hour of television or screen time every day with a walk or other aerobic exercise can help fight against weight gain. There are lots of options for aerobic exercise in this section.

Third, do strengthening and flexibility exercises

Strengthening and flexibility are parts of your walking, biking or swimming. You may also now be ready to do some specific exercises for optimum overall fitness for your age. Read ahead to learn more about flexibility and strength training.

Watching television, texting, using computers or video games and commuting are activities that occupy more and more of our lives. Yet these activities burn virtually no calories. They contribute significantly to the rise of obesity.

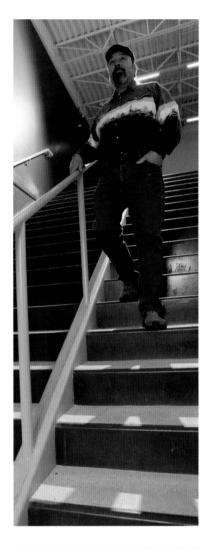

BE ACTIVE

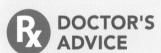

DOCTOR'S ADVICE

It is helpful to exercise about half an hour after you eat a meal. This helps bring down blood sugar.

The best exercise is the one you enjoy and can fit in your life.

Choose a fitness plan

A plan will help you put everything together, manage setbacks and motivate you. There are three different Fitness Plans in this section. Fitness Plan 1 includes exercises while seated and short walks. Fitness Plan 2 starts off with a 15-minute walk and works up to a 45-minute walk after 8 weeks. Fitness Plan 3 includes longer walks or other aerobic exercise. The body is an amazing machine, and almost everyone can gradually increase their fitness level.

If you plan to do exercises more vigorous than brisk walking, talk to your doctor first. Also, please read the *Precautions* section.

Use a pedometer, wearable wristband or watch to count how many steps you take each day

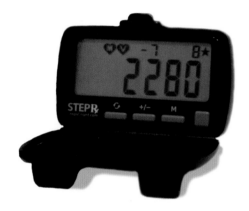

Wearing a pedometer helps you learn how many steps you take each day.

- If you are older or in poor health, you may only be doing a few hundred steps a day. Building up to 1,000 or 2,000 steps would be an achievement.
- Walking 2,000 steps is about equal to walking a mile (1,250 steps equals a kilometer).
- If you already do 2,000 steps a day, then try to add an extra 1,000 steps to your day. Take a month to do this.
- For improved health, it may take several months to build up to 5,000 steps a day.
- Doctors consider 10,000 steps a day an ideal goal.

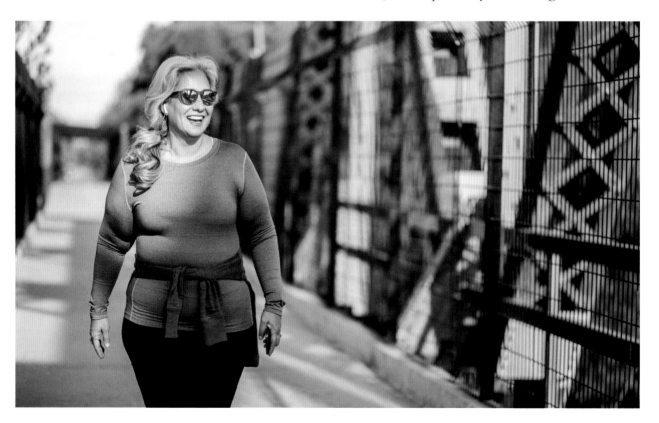

Ten Benefits of Regular Exercise

1. Reduces blood sugar

- Exercise helps insulin work better. If you are overweight, walking can help you lose body fat. Then insulin does a better job of lowering your blood sugar.
- When you exercise, your muscles need fuel (sugar). Insulin goes to work and moves sugar out of your blood and into your muscles.
- When you take a short walk after a meal, this reduces your blood sugar. You get more benefit if you walk farther.

2. Strengthens your blood vessels and heart

Your heart pumps faster when you exercise. This helps move the blood around your body. This improves circulation and reduces swelling in your hands and feet. Regular exercise improves your blood pressure, cholesterol and immunity, and helps prevent heart attacks and strokes. It reduces your risk for dementia. Exercise also prevents or reduces erectile dysfunction in men.

3. Helps you breathe easier

Exercise will improve your breathing. That's because it strengthens the heart's ability to pump oxygen. If you have asthma or emphysema, this is especially important.

4. Reduces your body fat

Exercise boosts your metabolism so you burn more calories. This can help you lose weight or maintain weight loss.

5. Helps digestion and reduces constipation

Your stomach and bowels are muscles. Exercise and increased blood flow helps them work better.

6. Reduces your risk for certain cancers

Studies show that exercise helps reduce cancer, including colon and breast cancer. Exercise reduces constipation, so waste and toxins leave the body more quickly. This reduces the risk of colon cancer. Exercise can help reduce excess weight. This decreases certain hormones like estrogen. This can reduce the risk of breast cancer.

BE ACTIVE

Exercise helps your body's insulin work better for 12 to 24 hours.

You will have fewer diabetes complications if you improve your blood sugar.

Make a list of reasons you choose to exercise. Why? Because you value your health.

Exercise is crucial for everyone, no matter what body size, for a healthy long life.

Recommended amount of exercise

The American Diabetes Association and Diabetes Canada recommend at least 150 minutes of walking or aerobic exercise a week. This is about 20 to 25 minutes a day or 30 minutes a day for five days a week. This is less than 3% of your day while you are awake.

7. Strengthens your muscles and bones

As your muscles get stronger, you'll have more energy. Exercise while you're young builds strong bones. As you get older, exercise helps maintain strong bones and reduces osteoporosis and hip fractures.

8. Reduces lower back pain

Exercise gives you better posture and balance. It keeps your back muscles and joints strong and flexible.

9. Helps you sleep better

Exercise tires you out and calms your body and mind. This happens, in part, because of the release of hormones such as serotonin. These help you fall asleep easier and sleep longer.

10. Reduces stress

Exercise releases "happy hormones" into your blood. This helps you relax. Taking a walk can give you time to think through stressful situations and come up with solutions. A walk gives you time to make positive plans for the future.

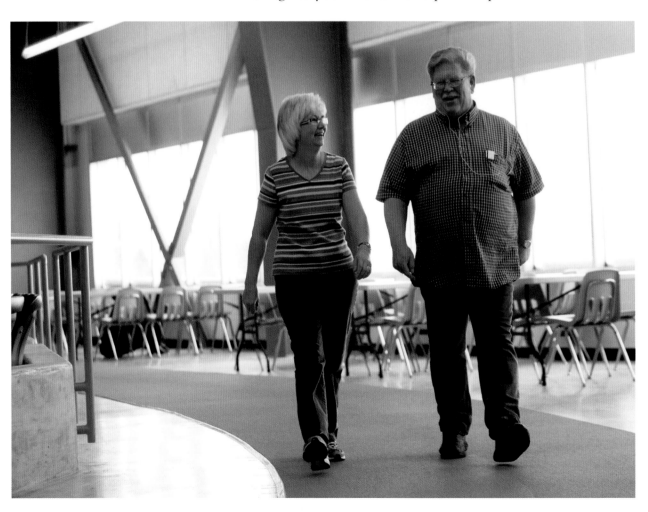

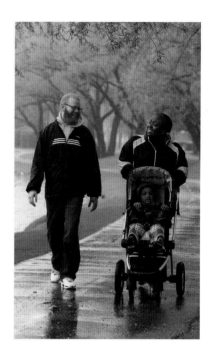

Low-Impact Aerobic Exercise

Aerobic exercise involves continuous movement of your legs and arms, for example, walking or swimming. When you do aerobic exercise, your heart rate rises and stays above your heart's resting level. Oxygen flows through your blood vessels to your organs, muscles and your brain. You'll feel your heart beating faster and your breathing is a bit deeper. You may feel warm and start to sweat. To do productive exercise, you don't need to overwork your heart. You just need a gradual increase.

Low impact means the exercise increases your heart rate (it's aerobic) but doesn't cause sudden jarring that stresses the joints, bones and muscles. Walking is one of the best low-impact exercises. Walking doesn't put excess stress on your joints and feet. There is just enough impact to strengthen your bones. Swimming is very low impact, as the water buoys your body weight. Biking on a smooth surface is also low impact, because the bicycle carries your upper body weight.

Here are some of the most common aerobic exercises that adults with diabetes enjoy:

- Walking (or using a treadmill)
- Biking (or using a stationary bike)
- Swimming and aquafit (water aerobics)
- Aerobic workouts at home or a gym

Other aerobic exercises include:

- Walking up and down stairs
- Raking leaves and heavy gardening (hoeing and digging)
- Wheeling yourself in a manual wheelchair
- Golfing, when walking the course and carrying your clubs
- Rollerblading, ice skating, or road or ice hockey
- Cross-country skiing, snowshoeing or curling
- Rowing, canoeing, hiking or rock climbing

Every time an ad comes on TV, stand up and walk on the spot. You'll get quite a lot of exercise during a one-hour program.

High-intensity "start and stop" exercise
This includes snow shovelling, chopping wood with an axe, heavy carpentry, tennis, pickle ball or badminton. These can be strenuous. Take rests as needed — pace yourself.

If you have advanced retinopathy (diabetes eye damage), take precautions when doing these high-intensity exercises. See page 40–41 and 243.

Studies show that dog owners do almost twice as much walking each week compared to those who don't have a dog.

Make a regular date with a friend to go for a walk. Consider joining a walking or hiking group.

Wear shoes that support and cushion your feet and have good traction. Boots should keep your feet warm in the winter. See pages 276–279 for more information on footwear.

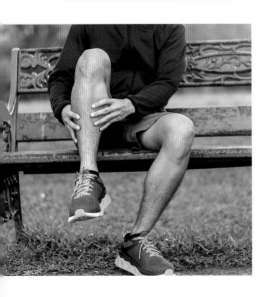

Walking

Walking is the best exercise choice because:

- It is low cost. All you need is your walking shoes.
- You can do it anywhere, indoors or outdoor: in an apartment hallway, indoor track, down a city street, country road, or in a mall.
- You can walk alone, with a friend or family member, or with your dog. Or offer to walk a neighbor's dog.
- You can listen to music as you walk, enjoy the sounds of nature or be part of a bustling city.
- Walking is an activity you can do throughout your life.

Is safety a concern for you when walking?

- Walk in open, well-lit areas, and vary your route. If possible, walk with someone else or a big dog.
- If on your own, tell someone where you're walking and when you'll be back. Carry your cell phone.
- If you walk in the dark, wear a reflective safety vest (available at hardware stores) so vehicles can see you.
- To be more aware of your surroundings, remove your music earbuds or keep the volume low.

If you get pain or cramping in your lower legs:

This is often due to decreased blood flow (poor circulation) in your leg muscles. This means that as you walk, your lower leg muscles are short of oxygen. This is a common sign of peripheral arterial disease (PAD). Talk to your doctor if you have these symptoms.

If you have PAD-related pain, it's still important to exercise daily. Try this:

1. "Stop and go." This means walk for 2 minutes, then slow down, stop or sit down if you can for 1 minute. Then walk 2 minutes and stop for 1 minute, and so on. This allows time for the oxygen to get to your muscles. Do this regularly and you may be able to gradually increase the "go" portion to 3 minutes, then 4 minutes, and so on.

2. Limit or avoid walking up hills or prolonged stair stepping. This can make the pain worse. Try swimming, cycling, walking slowly on a treadmill, using an elliptical trainer, or doing chair exercises instead.

3. Do ankle rotations once or twice a day to help improve blood flow to your lower legs.

📖 PAULETTE'S STORY: I love my walking poles

I'm 71 years old. Exercise is more important to me than ever. Really, it's common sense. "If you don't use it, you lose it."

Before I got my walking poles, I was afraid of walking, in case I fell on uneven ground or a slippery patch. One day I saw a woman using walking poles on a path near my home. She was slim and looked younger than me. I thought to myself, "If she can use walking poles, maybe I can too." So, I bought a pair, but I felt awkward and silly using them the first time.

Well, the second time I used them, I didn't see the crack in the pavement and tripped but the walking poles steadied me, and I kept my balance and stayed standing. Then I knew the walking poles were for me. Now, I use them every time I go for a walk, and I go for walks almost every day. I am getting to know my neighborhood and even walking a bit further on some days. Sometimes I drive to the park and walk in a different area for some variety. I am proud of myself. I have found the poles helped strengthen my arms. My back doesn't seem to ache as much as it used to. I try not to be bossy, but now I tell my friends they have to buy a set of walking poles too!

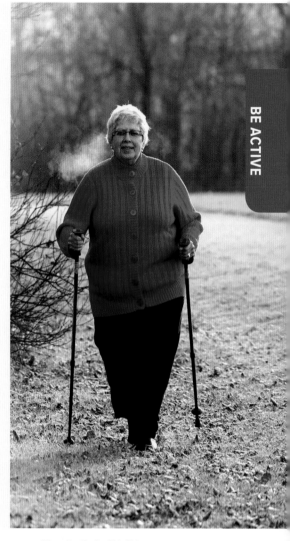

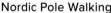

Nordic Pole Walking

BE ACTIVE

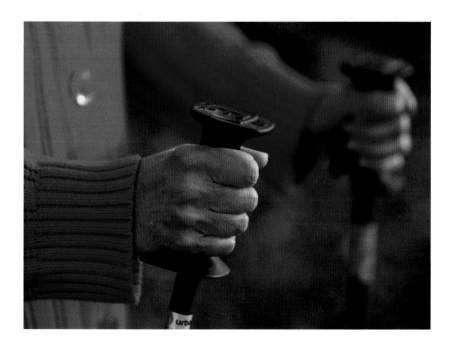

The tips of the poles have a rubber end for summer walking. There's an option with spikes for winter ice and snow.

The poles should be adjusted to your height. Generally, your arms should be bent at your elbows at a 90-degree angle.

📖 JOHN'S STORY: Fitting in exercise around long commutes and a hectic job

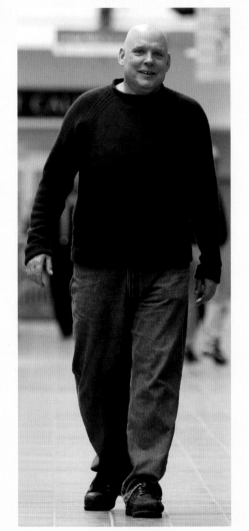

Exercising is difficult for me because I am so busy. I commute to work, and there's never time for a break at work. On weekends, I volunteer, and there's always work to do at home and in the yard. When I finally get some time to myself, watching TV is my way of relaxing.

When I found out I had diabetes, my doctor told me I should walk everyday. I felt angry. I thought that my doctor didn't understand how busy my life was. Exercise was just one more thing to have to cope with. I'm an "all or nothing" kind of guy, and it was either get really active or not at all.

So I kept on doing what I had always done. After a few months, I had a hard time reading because my vision was often blurry. I thought it might be my diabetes, so I went back to see my doctor. Sure enough, my sugars were up. He gave me a diabetes pill this time but said I needed to become more active, or the sugars would go up again. He said if I could fit in even some short walks, it would help.

Let me tell you, I was scared about losing my vision. I thought about what my doctor said and realized I had to make changes.

This is what I did. I tried to take a 15-minute walk on my lunch break. If I had a lunch meeting, then I tried a 15-minute walk in the afternoon. The first few weeks, I missed quite a few walks, but at least I was thinking about it. After several months, I was walking at least three days a week. Now six months have passed. What I found was that on the days I walked, I wasn't as tired. I actually got more done, especially in the late afternoon. I still don't get for my walk some days, but if the weather is nice, I try to walk a little longer. Plus, I try to walk on the weekend.

I now know it's possible to fit exercise into your life, even into a busy life like mine. I'm not having any more blurry vision. I feel better. In the end, that's probably most important.

Other ways to fit walking into a busy schedule

- You don't need hours — only minutes. Walking just 8 minutes after each meal adds up to about 25 minutes a day. This meets the recommendation for 150 minutes of aerobic exercise a week. A walk after a meal helps bring down blood sugar.

- Every hour on the hour, get up and walk the hallway or stairs for 20 seconds.
- Consider cutting out a half hour of television or screen time to take a walk.

Treadmills

If the weather is bad or you'd rather walk indoors, consider using an electrical treadmill. You set the treadmill speed and you can increase it for a challenge. The most useful treadmill features are for setting the speed, length of time and elevation. Then you can get a consistent workout. Start off and end your session at a slower pace. Slowing down your pace for the last 5 minutes helps prevent dizziness when you step off the machine.

Safety strap and pulse rate monitor

Wear a safety strap so the machine will stop if you fall off. If you have a heart condition, use a treadmill with a heart rate monitor. This is an important safety feature. Use the guidelines provided by your doctor, with the treadmill or on page 240.

A manual treadmill usually will cost a lot less and take up less space. It works without electricity. You need to work harder to get the walking belt moving which can put too much strain on your knees. Generally, an electric treadmill is better for protecting your knees.

A treadmill takes up space, so people often put it in a storage room or basement. You may forget to use it there. You are more likely to use it if the treadmill is easy to see and in a nice environment near music or a TV.

Before buying home exercise equipment, try it out for fit and comfort. A more expensive treadmill may have:

- A bigger motor, usually 2 or more horsepower (if you are a heavier person this is a good feature)
- A quieter motor (works at less than 4,000 rpms)
- A walking belt that is long enough for most people to walk a full stride (usually at least 54 inches/135 cm)
- A warranty on the motor of 5 to 10 years
- Special features such as the ability to program walking speeds and times
- Option for moveable handle bars for upper body strengthening

Try not to hang on to the treadmill handles. Swing your arms as you do when you walk. Then you'll burn more calories and improve your balance. Use the handles if you feel unsteady or need to relieve some weight off your knees.

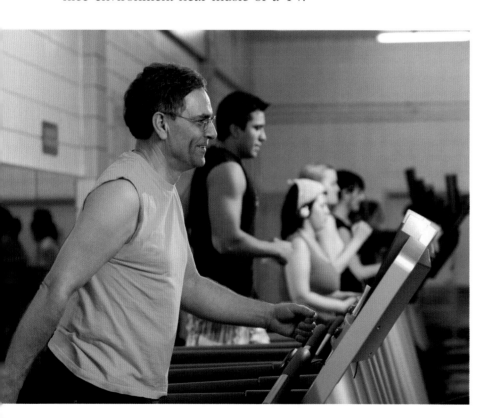

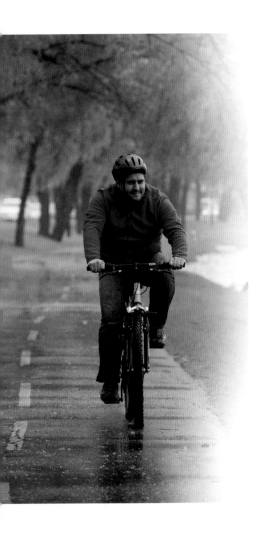

Biking and Exercise Bikes
Outdoor biking

Warm up and cool down. Start off and end your ride at a slow pace.

Increase calorie burning and further reduce your blood sugar. Bike up hills, for longer distances, or at a higher speed or resistance (in a higher gear). Also, combine biking with some walking.

Think safety. Wear a helmet. Ring your bell when you pass walkers. Carry water for longer bike rides. If biking at night, wear a fluorescent vest and have a light at the front and back of your bike. If using a recumbent bike, attach a bright flag so drivers can see you in traffic.

Remember proper positioning. Keep your elbows slightly bent for better shock absorption. Try to shift your hand positions often to prevent strain. Set the height of your bike seat so that when you pedal, you extend your legs almost completely.

Go for comfort. For extra comfort, replace the standard seat with a wide seat. A recumbent bike (with a chair-like seat and back support) may be more comfortable. Recumbent bikes are also easier to climb on and off and are good if your balance is poor.

Stationary exercise bike

- Look for the same features on a stationary bike as on a street bike, such as a wide padded seat or a recumbent position for sitting.

- Put your stationary bike in front of your television as a reminder to get on it! Make it convenient to use.

- Movable handlebars provide upper body exercise while you are pedaling.

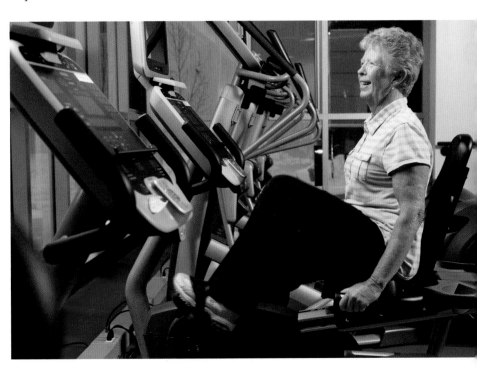

Recumbent bike

MILLY'S STORY: Keep your feet healthy even if you can't walk much

I wasn't really a very well person. I felt my weight limited me from doing a lot. I have a small apartment and I mostly stayed in. A home care nurse came into my home twice a week to help me with my bath. My favorite place was my lazy chair in the living room. My next favorite was my kitchen chair. I liked to look out of the window, watch TV, read my book, and visit with my granddaughter. But then my eyes started getting worse, and I couldn't even see my feet very well.

I developed a problem on one of my toes. It became infected, but I didn't realize it at first. Now the nurse also checks my feet and trims my toenails. She told me I had very little circulation in my feet, and that I needed to do some exercise or next time I might lose my toe.

I bought myself a mini exerciser. I started doing a couple of minutes after breakfast. I find time passes faster if I pedal while watching TV. Now after a month I can do almost 10 minutes at a time. Usually I pedal after supper. My granddaughter put the exerciser up on my table, so I turn the pedals with my arms when she visits.

The funny thing is that since I started doing all this for my feet, it has helped me in many other ways. I never thought I would be an active person again, but I'm finding I can do more about my home, and can get out a bit more. So far, I haven't had any more problems with my toes. I have less swelling in my feet and legs. Mostly I just feel better.

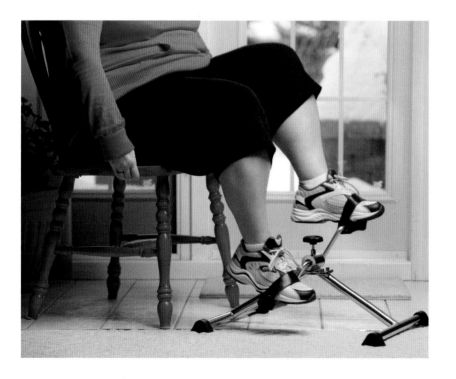

Mini exerciser

A mini exerciser is a cheaper option than an exercise bike and you can buy one at an online store.

It takes up less space. You can pedal it while sitting in your favorite chair.

Do you have smooth flooring rather than carpet? If so, you may want to put your mini exerciser against the wall so it doesn't move as you are cycling.

Swimming and Water Exercise

If you can't swim:

- Take lessons. You are never too old to learn to swim.
- When you feel confident, use a kickboard and kick your way down the pool.
- Find a program that works for you. For example, some pools offer special exercise programs for people in wheelchairs that allow for muscle movement and exercise.
- Walk or jog in shoulder or waist-deep water:
  - Walking in deeper water reduces the weight on sore hips, knees, ankles and feet.
  - Keep your feet flat on the bottom of the pool rather than walking on your toes.
  - Keep your body straight, rather than leaning forward.
  - Swing your arms, keeping them close to your body.
  - Walk forward, backward, or sideways taking side steps.

Join water aerobics. Also called aquafit, it's a class with an instructor who uses resistance training. These are routines done in a shallow pool or in deeper water. In deeper water you can wear a flotation vest. This helps keep your body straight as you walk in the water.

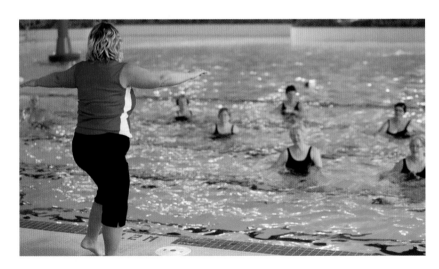

Swim laps. Over time, increase your laps and vary your strokes.

Build strength. Water gives good resistance, which helps build strength and endurance.

Get flexible. Swimming involves long strokes that increase flexibility. When swimming, kick from your hips, not your knees, for greatest benefit. You may find your range of motion is larger in water than on land (for example, you can swing your legs higher).

You weigh less in water!

Water buoys you upward, so in water there is about 50% less weight on your joints. If you have knee, hip, ankle or back pain, you may be able to swim or do the water exercises with less or no pain. This is also a great exercise option for most pregnant women.

Aquafit tips

- Try water shoes (also called "aqua socks") to cushion and protect your feet.
- Exercising in a group with an instructor can help motivate you.
- Have fun!

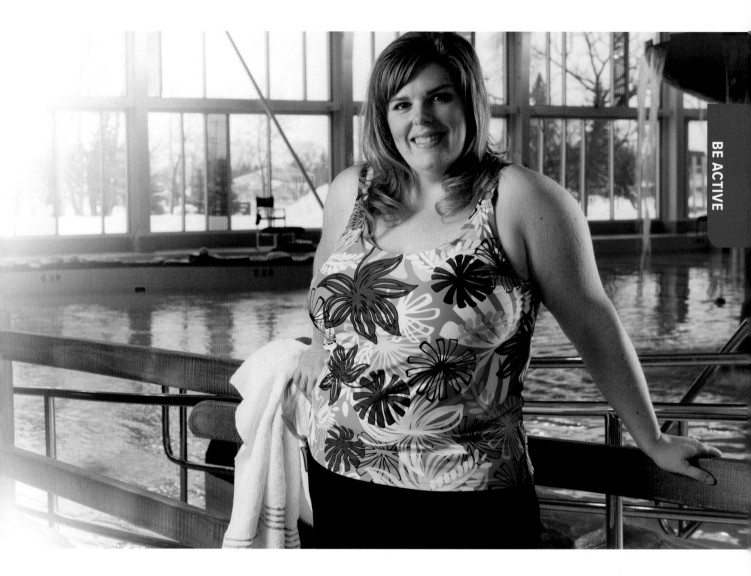

What to wear in the pool? There are many styles of bathing suits for different body sizes. On the internet search "modest swimwear," "plus size swimwear," or "UV protective swimwear" for some great styles with discreet coverage. Look for swimwear that is comfortable for you.

For women, choose:

- Shirt-like tops and skirt-like bottoms or leggings
- Bright color at the chest and a darker color below
- Up-and-down patterns or stripes to make your hips look smaller

For men, choose:

- Dark solid colors with option of vertical stripes on the side
- Bold graphics or funky patterns or colors attract the eye, so there is less focus on your body
- Longer bathing trunks
- A T-shirt or tank top; many pools allow them now

Try a "rash guard." This is a shirt made of swimsuit material that covers you up. They are sold in all sizes. It reduces your risk of sunburn when outdoors.

Prevent injuries

- Give yourself room to exercise so you don't bang into anything.
- A cool home temperature will be more comfortable and safe.
- Start slowly. Don't feel you have to keep up with the program until you're ready.
- Some tiredness and muscle stretching is expected, but if any move really hurts, don't do it.
- To reduce the impact on your ankles, legs and knees, exercise or dance on an exercise mat, carpet or softer floor rather than tile or cement. To protect the bottoms of your feet, wear a pair of shoes with good support.
- Always keep knees slightly bent, avoiding straight leg sit-ups, or raising both legs at once. Avoid deep knee bends.
- Stand tall, as if someone is pulling a string at the top of your head.
- Breathe deeply.

Aerobics and Dancing

Exercise at home

- March on the spot or dance at home to your favorite music. Try chair dancing; see page 232. Take one or several song breaks during the day. This improves circulation to your feet and brain.
- Play a YouTube aerobics or dance clip. Check local TV channels for home exercise programs or cable music channels.
- Equipment for home exercises may include:
  - a set of weights
  - rubber exercise bands for stretching and strengthening
  - a small towel for stretching
  - a yoga mat
  - a small step (to step up on as you exercise)

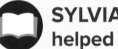 **SYLVIA'S STORY: Here's what helped me lower my blood sugar**

After I developed diabetes, I did two things that helped my blood sugar. First, I kept careful food records. And second, I used my Leslie Sansone walk at home DVD or watched it on YouTube every day. In the privacy of my own home, I did my exercises and still do. No one sees me do this or sees me sweating.

The DVD I bought had three levels to it. I started with the easiest level and I really struggled with this. It wasn't easy. After three months, I was surprised that I could manage the second level. I was a large woman but I lost weight. My doctor is really pleased with my blood sugars.

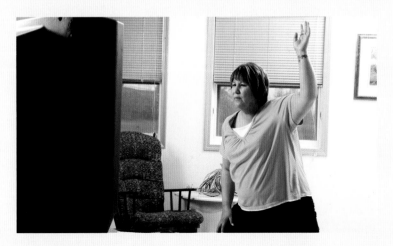

Exercise at a class or gym

- Join an exercise class on your own or with a friend. Most community centers and gyms have different exercise classes such as low-impact, chair exercises, zumba and spin classes (cycling).
- Exercise programs, such as Curves for women or SilverSneakers in the United States for men or women, are popular too. They can be a great option for doing a set of controlled exercises.
- Try square dancing, country line dancing, tap dancing, jazzercise, salsa, hip hop, belly dancing, swing dancing or ballroom dancing. Try an ethnic traditional dance or a seniors' dance night.

Hiring a certified fitness instructor for yourself, for even one or two sessions, is a great investment for getting started right. A trainer coaches and encourages you on a regular basis.

Questions to ask when using an exercise or dance video or attending a class

- Are the instructors certified in their field?
- Is low-impact exercise a priority?
- Is the difficulty level suitable? Some exercise programs go from beginner to moderate to advanced, as well as classes for different ages. You can move up a level as you become stronger.

- Does the instructor encourage you to monitor your heart rate during the class?
- Are the moves easy, with clear instructions and safety precautions? For example, are there tips on how to protect your back or knees?
- Is there a warm-up and cooldown?

 ## WAYNE'S STORY: Being overweight is not easy

If you've never been overweight, you don't understand the physical and mental toll it has on your life. Going to the public gym was not what I wanted to do. I didn't want people to stare at me, but I knew I had to start somewhere. So, I started exercising at home. I got some weights and a mini pedal exerciser. I'd lean on the kitchen counter and stretch my legs, bend my knees a bit and get more comfortable with moving more.

I finally got out to the gym and I was sweating before I even got started. But I kept going back and one day, a really buff, older guy said to me, "Good to see you out again today." Now we know each other's names and I kinda feel like I belong. Believe me, everyone is working toward their own goals at the gym and they all have their own struggles. I learned from experience that you don't succeed until you believe you are worth it.

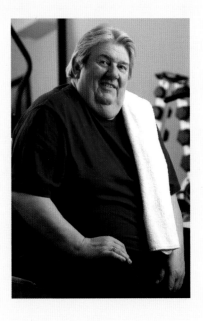

Home or Gym Exercise Equipment

- For your comfort, it's best to try out a piece of equipment before you buy it. Go to a fitness store or consider a one-day pass at a fitness club to try out various machines.
- Read reviews about exercise gear online. YouTube.com is a good place to watch online videos to learn how people use equipment for working out.
- Find good deals on exercise equipment at secondhand stores, in newspaper ads or online. And remember, walking is free!

The exercise equipment mentioned here is safe when in good condition and used properly; note the cautions listed.

Deciding what to buy

- Treadmills and exercise bikes are the most common exercise equipment. These are safe and excellent options. A bike (or mini exerciser) is easier to move into your home, while a treadmill is heavy and takes up space.
- Ellipticals, ski machines, stair steppers, rowing machines and weight machines are also good options for use at home or at a gym.

⚠️ **CAUTION**
Mini trampolines or full-sized trampolines can result in a fall with a serious neck or head injury.

Weight loss with no exercise?
Vibrator belts and chi machines vibrate your body without you doing exercise. They won't help you lose weight, but they may help relax you.

℞ DOCTOR'S ADVICE
Some people find that if they do their exercise at the same time each day or evening, this makes it a habit — a good habit!

Remember, even 5 minutes, three times a day, can add up to 15 minutes a day, and can make a difference. One good time to schedule exercise is half an hour after breakfast, lunch or dinner. Blood sugar goes up after you eat. Exercise brings it back down.

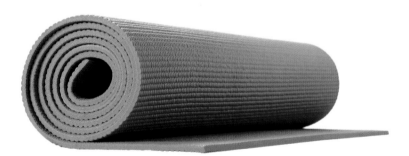

Protect your feet by standing on a mat while exercising.

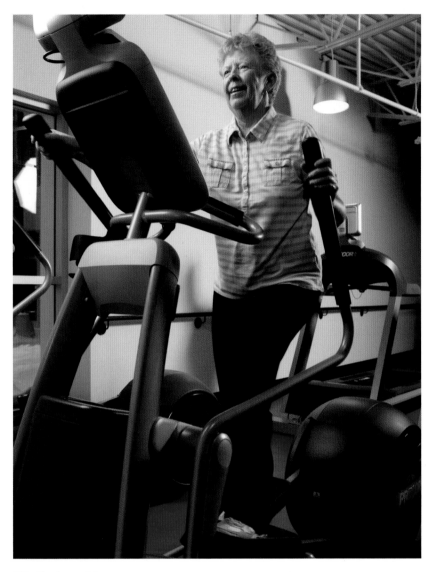

Elliptical machine

The elliptical machine is easy on your joints. It combines upper and lower body muscle work, so you burn more calories. Your feet never leave the pedals. You can pedal forward and backward. It's described as "running in mid-air," making it very low-impact. It's quieter and uses less electricity than a treadmill.

A cross-country ski machine feels like the gliding motion of cross-country skiing. It also combines upper and lower body muscle work. The machine should have adjustable poles for greatest comfort. There should be a smooth leg sliding action and independent arm-lever motion.

⚠️ **CAUTION**
Both the elliptical and ski machine take practice to learn how to use them. If you have a painful disc in your back, this may not be the best choice. Talk to a physiotherapist.

Stair climbing: Want a low-cost workout? Walk up and down stairs at home and in buildings every day.

Stair steppers in gyms exercise your legs, yet are easy on your joints, like ellipticals. They often have movable handles for upper body strengthening.

Home stair steppers without handles are light and easy to store, but can be hard on sore, arthritic knees. Look for a smooth stepping action, a solid frame and an adjustment for your height. The pedals should be parallel to the floor when stepping.

Home steppers with arm handles provide support and balance. Some steppers are available with movable handles.

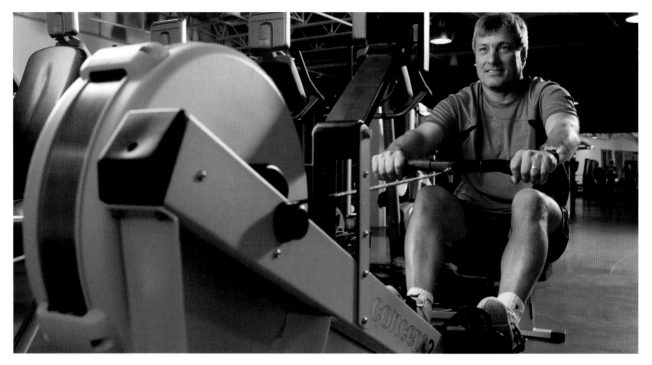

Rowing machine

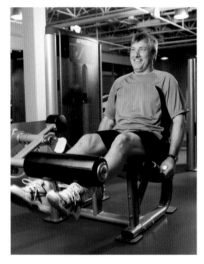

Weight machine

A rowing machine provides a full body low-impact workout. This is a good option if you have foot or balance problems, or lower leg weakness.

Get out in a kayak or canoe. Enjoy exercise in nature! Always take safety precautions, including wearing a life jacket. If you aren't comfortable on water, use the rowing machine.

Weight lifting, either using machines or free weights, burns sugar and calories and builds muscle. With a weight machine, the weights attach to the machine rather than free dumbbells.

⚠ **CAUTION**

Rowing machines: When rowing, keep your back in a straight position. Don't bend so far forward that when you pull back you use your lower back instead of your legs. Doing it the wrong way stresses your back. Remember to breathe deeply while rowing.

Weight lifting: Go to a reputable gym or sports store for training before doing this alone. To avoid injury, use proper technique, increase weights slowly, and breathe properly. Never hold your breath when lifting. Don't use weights you can't comfortably manage. Do not use heavy free weights without supervision. If you have advanced retinopathy or have had blood pressure that has been chronically high for many years, don't lift weights over your head. This increases the pressure at the back of your eyes.

If You Have Arthritis

Good blood sugar levels are important to manage arthritis. High blood sugar over many years causes changes to muscles and bones. These changes make joint pain and stiffness worse. Here are some tips on exercising when you have arthritis in your hips, knees, ankles or shoulders.

1. **Take your pain medications** regularly, as prescribed.

2. **Choose the right time to walk.** Walk when your pain is less and you feel most relaxed.

3. **Limit your walks** to just 5 to 10 minutes but consider walking several times a day.

4. **A good pair of walking shoes** supports your feet and provides cushioning for your knees. You may benefit from a rigid or semirigid orthotic in your shoe. Talk to your foot specialist or doctor. If you have an option to walk on a soft surface such as a rubber track, this will be easier on your knees.

5. **Even a small weight loss helps** to decrease the weight on your hips, knees and ankles, and lessen joint pain.

6. **Use heat before and cold after.** Before you exercise, put a hot cloth on your joint. This will warm it up and make your tissues and joints less stiff. After you exercise, apply a cold cloth (or ice inside a cold cloth) for 5 to 10 minutes. At the same time, elevate your legs. This reduces pain, inflammation, swelling and muscle spasms.

7. **Low-impact exercises** are the best for your joints. They include swimming, biking, using an elliptical trainer, chair exercises, walking, tai chi, yoga or Pilates. On a bike, start with a low resistance so you pedal easily, and build up gradually. A recumbent bike further reduces knee strain. When walking, reduce the weight on your knees by using a shopping cart, walker, cane or walking poles.

8. **Avoid exercises where you squat or do deep knee bends.**

9. **Rest your knees.** When standing for a long time (for example, doing dishes, or standing at a work bench) shift your weight from one side to the other every few minutes to relieve pressure off that knee.

10. **Don't overdo it.** When your knees hurt, rest them; sit or lie down.

BE ACTIVE

Arthritis Association
If there is an arthritis support group in your community, they may be able to provide you with exercise ideas or an online link to exercise videos. Also, ask your doctor for a referral to a physiotherapist or exercise specialist for individualized recommendations.

Being active helps arthritis in two ways:
1. It keeps your muscles and joints as movable and strong as possible.
2. It improves your blood sugar.

After exercise, some mild soreness is normal. If you develop joint pain that lasts two hours or more, cut back. Consult your doctor if the pain is severe and has gotten worse.

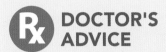

DOCTOR'S ADVICE

Remember, exercise should never be painful. Stretch your muscles slowly and gradually. Stretches should be done smoothly and slowly. Hold each stretch for 5 to 10 seconds.

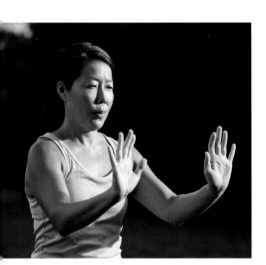

Staying Flexible

Flexibility means the ability of your muscles to stretch. Flexibility gives you a better range of motion. Stretching improves your body's circulation and posture. It also helps to warm up and relax muscles. Do these exercises before your walk or aerobic exercise, or combined with strength training.

What do you do every day that helps you to stay flexible? Do you stretch to tie your shoes or put on your coat, or stretch to reach the top shelf? All of these things help keep you flexible. See the next page for easy exercises you can do at home.

Exercises with good stretching include:

- swinging your arms while you are walking
- bowling
- swimming and dancing
- Tai Chi, yoga and Pilates

Take care when doing flexibility exercises

- Take it slowly and gently. If you push your muscles to be too flexible too soon, you will injure small muscles and have inflammation and pain. This can increase your blood sugar.
- Be safe. The exercises shown in this book are safe for you as a person with diabetes. However not all exercises found in books or on the internet are safe.

 CAUTION
Do not do these unsafe exercises.

- Neck rotation: Turning your head in a complete circle puts too much stress on your neck. A safer neck exercise is to lean your ear into your shoulder or to tuck your chin into your chest.
- Forced or bouncy stretching: Do not overstretch. If you are forcing a joint beyond its normal range of motion, this can tear muscles, ligaments and tendons. For instance, if you are desperately trying to touch your toes, even though you haven't done it in 50 years, you are overstretching!

Flexibility Exercises
Neck stretch

Sit in a chair and relax your arms and shoulders. Start with your head to one side. Slowly lower your head forward and move it across your chest in a smooth semicircle to the other side and then back. Do this three times.

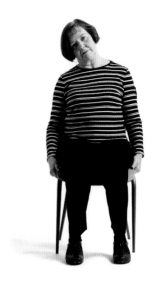

Ankle rotations

Sit in a chair. Extend one leg. Make complete circles from your ankles. Repeat with the other foot. Do 10 rotations.

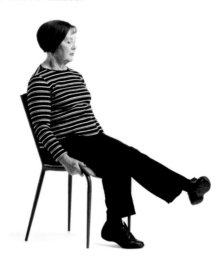

Calf stretch

Stand with your hands resting against a wall. Place one leg forward and the other leg straight back. Point toes straight ahead and keep both heels on the floor. Lean forward, keeping back knee straight. Hold for 5 to 10 seconds. Return to starting position, relax. Repeat five times with alternate legs.

A variation of this exercise can be done sitting with one leg up on a chair, knee slightly bent. Lean forward and hold the stretch.

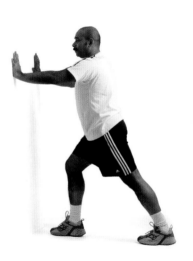

Seated hamstring stretch

Sit up straight on the edge of your chair. Straighten out one leg (but don't lock your knee), with your heel on the floor. Pull your toes back as much as you can. Keep your back straight and lean forward from your hips. You will feel a stretch in the back of your legs; the hamstring is the muscle at the back of your thigh. Hold for 5 to 10 seconds. Return to starting position, relax. Repeat five times with alternate legs.

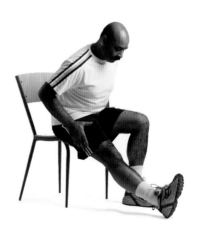

Do you wonder if sex is good exercise?

If you enjoy sex, then the answer is yes! The aerobic benefit is on average about equal to climbing two flights of stairs. But there's more! Regular sex keeps you flexible and strengthens muscles inside and out.

Strengthening Exercises

Making your body stronger and more flexible is a part of walking, biking, swimming and all aerobic exercise. Boosting the strength of your muscles and bones is important. Here are some specific exercises that make you stronger.

Exercises to strengthen muscles include:

- Lifting weights to strengthen arm and shoulder muscles
- Using stretch bands for upper and lower body strengthening. Bands are an alternative to lifting weights, but sometimes take a bit more coordination. The thicker or shorter the band, the more strength you need to stretch it. To learn proper and safe use of stretch bands, consult a physiotherapist or an exercise trainer at a gym, or watch a YouTube video by a qualified instructor (search "resistance band demo").
- Stomach tucks to strengthen and tone the abdomen
- Back exercises to further strengthen your abdominal and back muscles
- Climbing stairs and doing leg lifts with weight machines to strengthen the legs
- A weight lifting and strength training workout at a gym

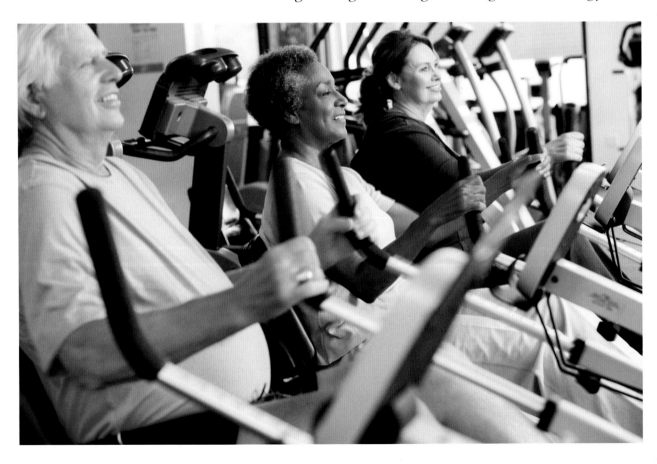

DOCTOR'S ADVICE
Strength training and blood sugar

Exercises that make your muscles stronger are important for people with diabetes. What does increasing muscle tone and muscle mass do for you?

- It improves your metabolism.
- It helps your body's insulin work better.
- It improves your blood sugar in the long term.

If you check your blood sugar right after weight lifting, you may find that it goes up a bit. This is caused by the release of adrenaline that occurs with any intense, intermittent activity. An hour or two later, you'll see your blood sugar come down.

Take care when doing strengthening exercises

- **Keep the exercise smooth and slow.**
- **Don't lift above your head** if you have advanced retinopathy or have had blood pressure that has been chronically high for many years.
- **Remember to breathe** while you are exercising; otherwise your blood pressure could go up. Breathe in through your nose when lifting weights. Breathe out through your mouth when bringing weights down.
- **Do one set at a time and rest in between.** A common set is lifting a weight 5 to 10 times. Follow the Fitness Plans on pages 230–236.
- **In general, to increase your strength, you need to fatigue your muscles.** Therefore, choose a weight that you have a hard time lifting 10 times. Increase your repetitions and, when you are ready, move to a heavier weight.
- **When you start doing strengthening exercises, it's normal to feel mild muscle stiffness lasting one day.** If this stiffness lasts longer, then reduce your length of exercise or the weight you use.
- **If you feel pain or discomfort** stop the exercise. If you have severe pain in a joint, a physiotherapist or trainer needs to adapt the exercise so you can do it safely.

How often should I lift weights to strengthen my muscles?

- To maintain strength, do one or more sets twice a week.
- To build muscles, do one or more sets three times a week.

Doing exercises properly helps prevent injury
If you are unsure how to do an exercise, try to meet with a fitness specialist at a gym.

At all ages, it's possible to become more fit and reverse the natural loss of muscle tone. People in their 80s and 90s can maintain or increase their strength through weight training. Bone and muscle strength helps reduce the risk of falls as you age.

Arm and Upper Body Exercises

These exercises don't take long to do. For example, you can do one or two sets during the television ads of your favorite show. If sitting, sit straight up and have your feet flat on the floor. If standing, place your feet shoulder width apart and slightly bend your knees.

You can do one arm at a time or both together. Do these exercises slowly for the greatest benefit.

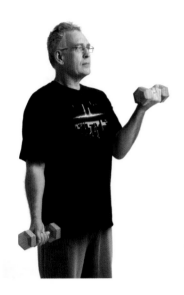

Arm roll

Holding a weight in each hand, extend your arms straight out slightly below your shoulder height. Move your hands in slow, controlled small circles. Moving your hands in larger circles and lifting a heavier weight will increase strengthening. Repeat, alternating your arms or doing both together.

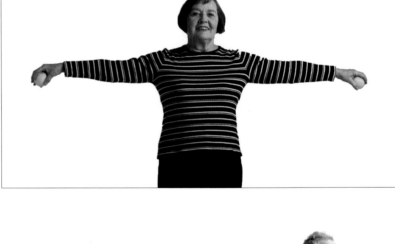

Bicep curl

Hold the weight in your hand with your palm facing up and *slowly* curl your arm up to your shoulder, bending at the elbow. *Slowly* return to extended position and repeat, alternating your arms or doing both arms together.

Armchair pushup

Sit in an office chair or other chair that has arms. Put your hands on the arms and lift your bottom off the chair. Hold this position for for a few seconds. Even lifting slightly will exercise your arms. Over time, work up to lifting for 10 seconds.

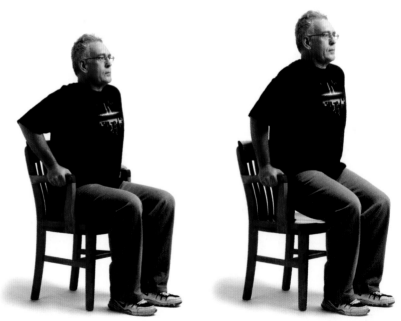

Stomach and Lower Body Exercises

For all three of these exercises, remember to:

- Keep breathing. Do not hold your breath.
- Hold your exercise for 2 to 3 seconds. Over time, work up to a 10-second hold.

> Exercise that strengthens your abdomen also strengthens your lower back.

Option 1

Sit upright against the back of a chair. Draw in your belly button. Hold in your stomach, then relax.

Option 2

Go on your hands and knees. Keep your back straight, parallel to the floor. Don't move your back. Hold in your stomach, then relax.

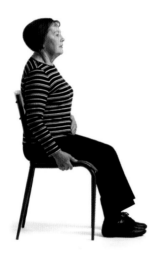

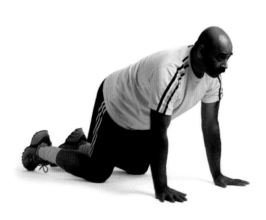

Wall squat

This exercise helps strengthen your back, abdomen, buttocks and thighs. It's a great exercise if you sit a lot. Stand with your back flat against a wall (including the back of your head). Keep your tummy tucked in. Keep your feet flat on the floor and about 2 feet (60 cm) out from the wall. Bend your knees slightly and slide down the wall. Sliding down just a little is a good start. Over time, work up to a deeper squat. Your knees shouldn't extend forward beyond your ankles. Hold. Slowly return to starting position and repeat.

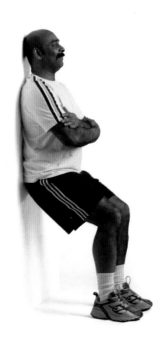

> The best exercise for your legs is walking, biking or swimming. If you don't walk, bike or swim, check out the chair leg exercises shown on page 232.

Talk to your doctor or physiotherapist about back exercises.

If a health professional treats you for a back injury, please follow the exercises that he or she recommends.

Lift carefully

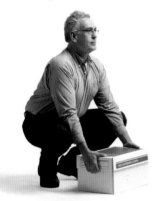

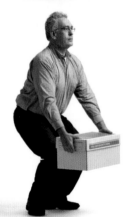

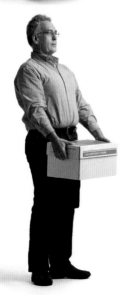

Ten Tips for a Healthy Back

1. **Do back exercises.** Simple back exercises help keep your back strong, allowing you to stay active.

2. **Go for a walk every day.** This helps strengthen the muscles that support your back. If you lose weight around your waist, even 5 to 10 lbs (2.5–4.5 kg), this can relieve pressure from your back.

3. **Stand and sit tall.** When you walk, keep your back straight and chin up, relax your shoulders and tighten your stomach muscles. This helps maintain good posture. Sitting posture is also important. If you work at a computer, look straight ahead at the screen, not up or down. Keep your knees level with or slightly higher than your hips. Your elbows should be at a 45° angle from your body. To relieve back strain, take short breaks. Walk or move around or do the two back exercises.

4. **Use a support, if needed, when walking.** Using a walker, walking stick, cane or Nordic walking poles reduces the weight on your back. Also, lean on a shopping cart while walking in a mall or store. As your back gets stronger, you may no longer need support.

5. **Take the pressure off your back while standing.** Slightly bend your knees or shift your weight from one leg to the other.

6. **Avoid arching backward.** When doing exercises while lying or sitting, always keep the knees bent or slightly bent. Don't raise both legs at one time.

7. **Lift carefully.** Before lifting, especially heavy or bulky things, place your feet at shoulder width. Bend your knees, keep your back straight and hold the object close to your body as you lift it. Don't twist your back. Use a push cart or wheelbarrow to move heavy things. Get help as needed.

8. **Get a lower-back massage.** Ask a friend or family member to gently massage your back, or go to a licensed massage therapist.

9. **Find a good sleeping position.** If you like to sleep on your back, place a pillow under your knees. If you sleep on your side, lie with your knees bent with a pillow between them. This cuts down on pain if you twist your back as you sleep. A good mattress also helps.

10. **Take pain pills only as prescribed.** Use appropriate pain pills. Exercise at the time of day you feel your best.

Back exercises

Pelvic tilt

This exercise stretches your back.

- Lie on your back on the floor or on a hard mattress. Bend your knees.
- Keep your feet flat on the floor and your arms at your sides.
- Tighten your tummy to press your lower back against the floor (or bed). Hold 5 seconds, then relax.
- Repeat five to ten times.

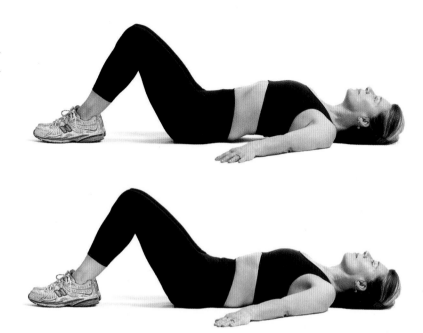

The bridge

This exercise strengthens your back.

- Start in the same position as the pelvic tilt.
- Separate your knees slightly.
- Slowly lift your hips upward so your weight is on your feet and shoulder blades. Even lifting just an inch or two is beneficial.
- Keep your stomach tight and your abdomen in line with your thighs. Hold for five seconds and return to the starting position. Relax.
- Repeat five to ten times.

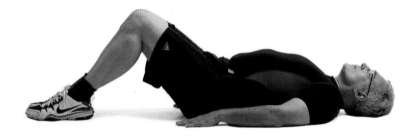

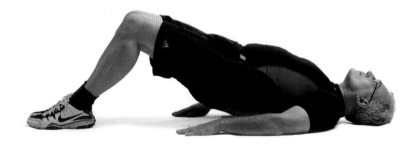

Try doing these exercises daily or several times a week.

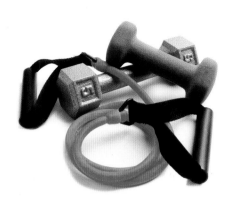

Your Fitness Plan

Right now, how much walking or aerobic exercise do you do? Based on your present amount of exercise, choose one of the three fitness plans below.

Each fitness plan increases in difficulty over an eight week period. At the end of eight weeks, you may be ready to move to the next level. Make daily walking or other aerobic exercise a priority. Add in the strengthening and flexibility exercises as you are able.

Amount of exercise I do right now		My fitness plan
My exercise is limited. On average, I do less than 15 minutes of walking or other aerobic exercise each day. **Other considerations** • I limited my exercise in the past because of arthritis, muscle pain, shortness of breath, or my weight. • I have poor balance. • I have had a stroke or partial leg amputation. • I use a wheelchair or walker sometimes or all the time.	▶	**Fitness Plan 1** **Basic** (pages 231–233)
I am relatively fit. I want to maintain or increase my fitness. On average, I do 15 to 25 minutes of walking or other aerobic exercise every day.	▶	**Fitness Plan 2** **Active** (pages 234–235)
I am fit and I want to stay this way! On average, I do 30 minutes or more of walking or other aerobic exercise every day.	▶	**Fitness Plan 3** **More Active** (pages 236–237)

If you have a different fitness level:

- If you have partial or full paralysis, consult a physiotherapist or exercise specialist.
- If you are a runner, train for marathons, triathlons or competitive sports, consult your doctor, diabetes educator, or sport specialist. A specialist who is knowledgeable about diabetes can advise you. It's important to learn about risks, ways to avoid injury, and your need for fluid, carbohydrates and calories.

Fitness Plan 1 (Basic)

This plan includes short walks and exercises you can do while sitting in a chair. As needed, use a cane or walker, or walk with a companion for support. Even if you are not as mobile as you'd like, you can become stronger, more flexible, move faster and improve your circulation. This decreases your risk of diabetes complications.

Over eight weeks, this plan increases your exercise from 5 minutes to 20 minutes a day.

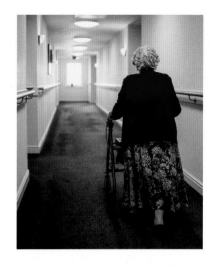

BE ACTIVE

Progress	Minutes a day of walking or chair exercises	Strengthening and flexibility
Week 1 – Week 2	**5 minutes** (as one session or two 2½-minute sessions)	**Twice a week:** • Do 5 bicep curls with each arm, using a 1-lb (0.5 kg) weight.
Week 3 – Week 4	**10 minutes** (as one session or two 5-minute sessions)	**Twice a week:** • Do 10 bicep curls with each arm, using a 1-lb (0.5 kg) weight. • Add in 5 stomach tucks (option 1, seated).
Week 5 – Week 6	**15 minutes** (as one session or two or three shorter sessions)	**Twice a week:** • Do 10 bicep curls with each arm, using a 1 lb (0.5 kg) weight. • Do 10 armchair pushups. • Add 5 stomach tucks. **Once a week:** • Do one set of neck stretch and ankle rotations (see flexibility exercises on page 223).
Week 7 – Week 8	**20 minutes** (as one session or two or three shorter sessions) Consider joining a swimming program, or getting home exercise equipment such as a mini exerciser or recumbent bicycle.	**Two to three times a week:** • Do 10 bicep curls and 10 arm rolls each arm, using a 1-, 2- or 5-lb (0.5, 1 or 2.5 kg) weight. • Also add 5 to 10 stomach tucks. • Fit in one set of the neck and arm flexibility exercises. • Do daily back exercises if needed (see page 229).

Many standing exercises can be adapted to do while sitting. For example, try the bicep curl and arm roll.

Chair Exercises

On this page are a few exercises especially designed for strengthening. For all of these exercises, sit up straight, hold in your tummy and push your bottom to the back of your chair. This helps protect your back.

Leg walk

Place your hands on your hips with your feet flat on the floor. Raise one foot about 6 inches (15 cm) off the floor. Return foot to the floor and repeat with the other foot. Alternate left and right legs in a rhythmic manner. Walk for several minutes, and increase your time as you are able.

Moving chair exercises

Sit in an office chair or wheelchair. With your feet flat on the floor, pull yourself forward or backward.

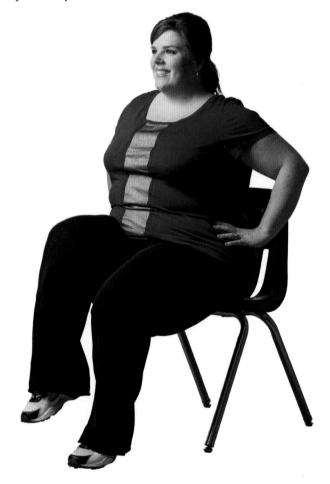

 DONNA'S STORY: You can dance in your chair!

Chair dancing is good for anyone who has an issue with their feet or their legs and can't walk easily outside. It's important to be in a comfortable chair with good back support. Mine is in front of my computer. I play some peppy music, like Mama Mia, because it's got a great beat and I love to sing along. I'll pick four or five songs — that's about 15 minutes, which goes by fast when you're exercising to the music.

Then I start my set of exercises. I lift my left foot 5 times, the right foot 5 times, I move each foot sideways 5 times and back and forth 5 times. Then I lift my right foot and straighten out my leg in front of me 5 times, and do the same with my left leg. That's my set, which I repeat until the tunes are over. Sometimes I put my arms above my head and cross them over, or make circles out to the side, or just move them back and forth like I'm walking. I'm always surprised how much better I feel after the 15 minutes of exercise. Try it — you might like it.

You are never too old or too large to start moving.
The key is to find the right kind and amount of exercise for you. Even a small amount of exercise can make a big difference. People of all ages, including older adults, can become stronger and healthier by becoming more active.

DARREL'S STORY: Always keep moving!

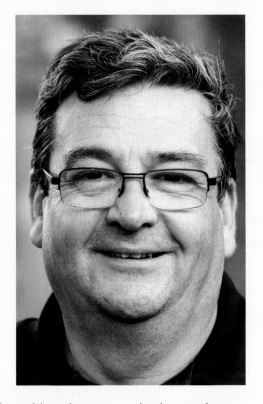

I am 53 years old. I live in Cherry Hill, New Jersey. I had a stroke four years ago. The stroke left me in a wheelchair and affected the left side of my body. I've had diabetes for more than 10 years.

I ended up in long-term care and they told me I would never go home. I was very discouraged at first, but then I didn't believe that I'd have to stay there. I started moving a little bit of my limbs at a time. I believed I could move for 5 minutes, then I knew I could move for 10 minutes. I had a therapist at the beginning, but then I started doing it by myself, because the therapist only had a limited time to work with me. With hard work every day, I got well enough to go home.

At home, I started moving around in my kitchen. My kitchen is what got me well, believe it or not. I started moving. I started bending. I started lifting pots. I started standing, you know, trying to get things out of the cabinet, because nobody was there to get them. So I started doing things like that and then I said, wow, what a workout! And then I tried it again and again. I started to appreciate my kitchen. I started loving my kitchen. I wanted to love the food that I eat. I was able to start cooking with one hand and enjoying the food that I prepared. I didn't want to eat as much food as before, but I wanted to enjoy what I did eat.

Now, I am walking a distance of 50 feet (15 m). I can sit in a regular chair when I have a visitor. I can stand a little bit longer. I use a walker. Now I have a therapist again. I am learning how to walk more without the walker. I don't really like the walker, but I have it for support. The leg and arm on my left side can work now about 80 percent. I am amazed at what my body can do. I think positively and challenge myself and I'm much happier.

Fitness Plan 2 (Active)

Start off slowly and gradually increase the amount and pace of exercise that you do.

Over eight weeks, this plan increases your aerobic exercise from 15 to 45 minutes a day.

Progress	Minutes a day of walking, biking, swimming or other aerobic activities	Strengthening and flexibility
Week 1 – Week 2	**15 minutes** Warm up and cool down by walking slowly for the first and last few minutes of your walk or other aerobic exercise.	Twice a week: • Do 10 bicep curls each arm using a 1-lb (0.5 kg) or 2-lb (1 kg) weight.
Week 3 – Week 4	**25 minutes** of aerobic exercise (as one or two sessions a day)	Twice a week: • Do 10 bicep curls each arm using a 2-lb (1 kg) weight. • Add in 5 stomach tucks (option 1, seated) and wall squats.
Week 5 – Week 6	**35 minutes** (as one or two sessions a day) To burn more calories, increase your pace a bit. If walking, swing or pump your arms.	Twice a week: • Do 10 bicep curls and arm rolls each arm using a 2-lb (1 kg) weight. • Do 10 armchair pushes. • Do 5 stomach tucks and wall squats. **Once a week:** • Add in one set of flexibility exercises (see page 223), including neck stretch and ankle rotations.
Week 7 – Week 8	**45 minutes** (as one session, or break into two or three shorter sessions to total 45 minutes) Try something new, like swimming, biking, tennis, skating, curling, dancing or golf. Find an exercise program online or enroll in an exercise class. Go to a gym and have a complete training program designed for you. Keep it interesting! Challenge yourself if you're ready for it.	Two to three times a week: • Do 10 bicep curls and arm rolls each arm using a 2- or 5-lb (1 or 2.5 kg) weight. • Do 5 to 10 stomach tucks and wall squats. • Add in one set of the neck and ankle exercises. • Do daily back exercises if needed (see page 229).

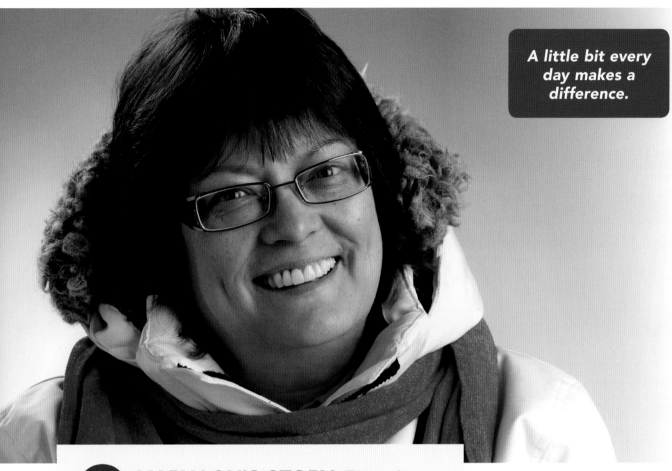

A little bit every day makes a difference.

 MARY-LOU'S STORY: There's no bad weather, only bad clothing!

I find walking is the most convenient for me. Beating the weather was my biggest barrier. It was either too cold or too hot. I decided rather than let the weather beat me, I'd beat it!

When it's cold, I dress in layers, including a big hood on my jacket and warm lined pants. I tend to have cold hands and feet, so I wear a double layer of mitts and lined boots that give me enough room to wiggle my toes and comfortably fit over a pair of wool socks.

In the summer when it's hot out, and I'm walking, I carry a water bottle with me. This way I can walk further without getting so thirsty. I love the sun, but I know too much is not good for me. If it's hot, I cover up with a hat and light clothing, and wear sunscreen. Mostly, I go for my walk early in the morning or in the evening when it's cooler. My whole family is into making me healthier. My daughter gave me an umbrella to keep the sun off me!

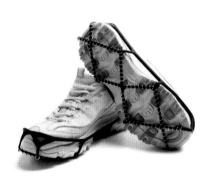

Shoe grips for winter walking

To prevent falling, try shoe grips, a walking stick with a spike on the bottom, or a pair of ski poles or Nordic walking poles.

235

When you do strengthening exercises, remember take a break of 1 or 2 minutes between sets of 10.

Fitness Plan 3 (More Active)

As with Fitness Plan 1 and 2, start off slowly and gradually increase the amount and pace of exercise that you do.

Over eight weeks, this plan increases your aerobic exercise from 30 minutes to 60 minutes a day.

Progress	Minutes a day of walking, biking, swimming or other aerobic activities	Strengthening and flexibility
Week 1 – Week 2	**30 minutes** Warm up and cool down by walking slowly for the first few and last few minutes of your walk or aerobic exercise. To burn more calories, increase your pace. If walking, swing or pump your arms.	**Twice a week:** • Do 10 bicep curls and 10 arm rolls each arm using a 2-lb (1 kg) weight. • Do 10 armchair pushes. • Do 10 stomach tucks (try option 2 if you are able) and wall squats.
Week 3 – Week 4	**40 minutes** (as one session or two 20-minute sessions) Try a different aerobic exercise to add variety to your workout.	**Twice a week:** • Increase weights to 5 lbs (2.5 kg) and continue with upper and lower body exercises. • Add in a set of each of the four flexibility exercises (see page 223).
Week 5 – Week 6	**50 minutes** (as one session, or two 25-minute sessions)	**Twice a week:** • Continue with above exercises.
Week 7 – Week 8	**60 minutes** (as one session, or two 30-minute, or three 20-minute sessions) Go to a gym and ask about high-intensity interval training (HIIT). For example, on a stationary bike, do 30 seconds of high-resistance cycling as fast as you can, followed by several minutes of slower low-resistance cycling. Do 4 to 6 repetitions in one workout.	**Three times a week:** • Continue as in Week 5 and Week 6, but increase to two sets of each. • Consider enrolling at a gym for extra strengthening and stretching, and for a weight program designed for you. • An exercise specialist can recommend more types of exercises and stretches. • Do daily back exercises if needed (see page 229).

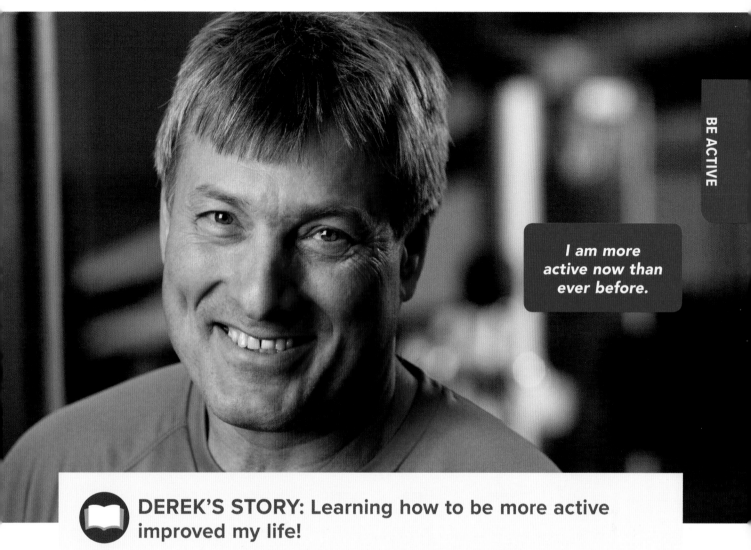

I am more active now than ever before.

📖 DEREK'S STORY: Learning how to be more active improved my life!

I am a lawyer. Even with all that education, I knew very little about nutrition and fitness. I always thought that I ate a balanced diet and kept busy, but over the years I gained weight, bit by bit. I was diagnosed with diabetes five years ago. At that time, I weighed 220 lbs (100 kg).

My wife bought me your cookbook. It consolidated a lot of basic nutrition information that I did not know, especially about calories and portions. I found it very easy to follow. It provided the road map. I lost 30 pounds (14 kg) over a one-year period. I have kept my weight at this level ever since.

At the beginning when I started to lose weight, I deliberately did not do the 30 minutes a day of walking you recommended in your book. I wanted to know for sure that the weight loss happened because I followed the portions in your book. Once I could see I was losing weight from eating less, I started adding in exercise.

First, I started walking. Losing some weight gave me the confidence to join a gym. I started a combination of fast walking on the treadmill, using the elliptical trainer, and doing some weight training for my legs and arms. I am now able to do 40 minutes on the treadmill and rowing machine — and I wasn't even doing that as a young man! I feel a lot more fit. That has led me to take up other kinds of exercise. For example, my wife and I now play pickle ball.

Shorter, more frequent exercise works

Several shorter exercise sessions — for example, two 10-minute sessions — can be as beneficial as one longer one of 20 minutes. Do what you can, when you can. It all adds up.

By following these Fitness Plans, you will be adding small amounts of exercise each week, and you will see benefits. If you go too fast, you may feel overwhelmed and give up.

Here's an easy way to keep a record:

✓ Give yourself one check for 10 minutes of continuous walking or other aerobic exercise.
✓✓ Give yourself two checks for 20 minutes, and so on.

If you are following Fitness Plan 1, you could give yourself a check for each 5 minutes.

At the end of the week or month, look back on your record. At a glance, you'll see how you've done.

Managing Setbacks

Setbacks happen. You may get sick, bored, have an injury or a personal crisis. If you've had a setback and stopped exercising, here are some tips to get back on track.

Don't delay. If you've missed a few days or a week, try to get back to your usual schedule.

Don't double up. Don't do two days of exercise in one day.

Go back to an earlier level if needed. If you missed a few weeks, go back to an easier level in your Fitness Plan. Then work your way back up.

Consider a walking buddy. If you're having a hard time exercising alone, would a walking partner motivate you?

Choose a time to exercise. The best time to exercise is the time you'll do it! Most people do well with a routine, so choosing a regular time, whether it's morning, afternoon or evening is helpful. Half an hour after you've eaten is a good time to exercise. Exercise brings down your blood sugar from the food you've eaten.

Log your exercise. Keeping a log of your exercise can help motivate you. Use an app on your phone with an activity tracker wrist band or put one check on your calendar for 10 minutes of continuous aerobic exercise such as walking. If you skip exercising, use a calendar, journal or app to record why. See if you can find solutions to avoid any future setbacks.

Remind yourself to exercise! Set an alarm on your cell phone. Put notes on your bathroom mirror, TV remote or computer.

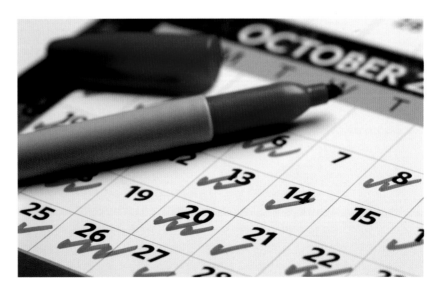

Exercise Precautions

Ten Heart Precautions

Please ask your doctor "Have I been diagnosed with a heart problem?" If yes, read these 10 points.

1. **Avoid or limit high-intensity and high-impact activities.** High-intensity exercise includes strenuous weight lifting or heavy snow shoveling. If shoveling a heavy wet snowfall, do the shoveling for short periods of time over several days. Don't lift the snow above your head. Ask for help from healthy relatives or neighbors, or hire help.

   High-impact exercises include jogging or sprinting. These can damage your feet and joints. They can also cause blood pressure to go up to a dangerous level.

2. **Monitor your heart rate.** Here are three different ways to monitor your heart rate.

   The "talk test"
   If you can't talk in a normal voice during your exercise, you are pushing too hard. Slow down. Listen to your body.

   Take your own pulse
   Use your first two or three fingers (not your thumb) to gently press on your pulse at either your wrist or neck. Count for just 10 seconds and then multiply by 6 to get your number of beats in a minute. See Target Heart Rate chart on the next page. Practice so you can do this quickly, as your heart starts slowing down as soon as you stop exercising.

   Use a monitor
   Use an activity tracker wrist band or an electronic monitor on a piece of exercise equipment, such as a treadmill.

   Use the target heart rate as a guide for what your pulse should be.

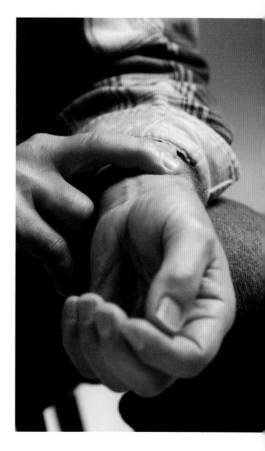

239

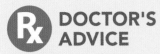

DOCTOR'S ADVICE

Target heart rates are only a guide.

If you feel discomfort, slow down below the lower limit. If you are pregnant, keep slightly below the upper numbers. Some heart conditions and medications (such as beta blockers for high blood pressure) can change your heart rate. Ask your doctor about your safe target heart rate.

Target heart rate during exercise

Depending on your age, there is a target heart rate for you that includes a range of two numbers. It's good to exercise with your heart beating somewhere between the two numbers. At first, you may exercise at a lower pace than your target heart rate. Gradually build up your stamina. After a while, you may be able to comfortably exercise closer to your upper number. Try not to go above your upper number, or you'll be overworking your heart.

Age	Target heart rate	
	Beats per 10 seconds	**Beats per minute**
20 to 30 years	23–28	140–170
31 to 40 years	22–27	130–160
41 to 50 years	20–25	120–150
51 to 60 years	18–23	110–140
61 to 70 years	16–21	100–130
Over 70 years	15–20	90–100

3. **Avoid bending your head lower than your heart,** especially right after exercising. For example, sit down and put your foot up on a stool to take off your shoes rather than bending down.

4. **Don't exercise right after eating a heavy meal or drinking alcohol.** After you eat, your blood diverts to digest food in your stomach. Exercise can then overwork your heart. Alcohol can speed up your heart rate. Alcohol also increases your risk for low blood sugar if you are on insulin or certain diabetes pills.

5. **Don't exercise in hot environments** or sit for long periods in saunas or whirlpools. The heart has to work extra hard to cool you down when you're hot.

6. **Drink water when exercising.** Drink water before and after your walk. When your blood sugar is high and when the weather is hot, water is especially important so you don't get dehydrated. You may need to carry a water bottle too.

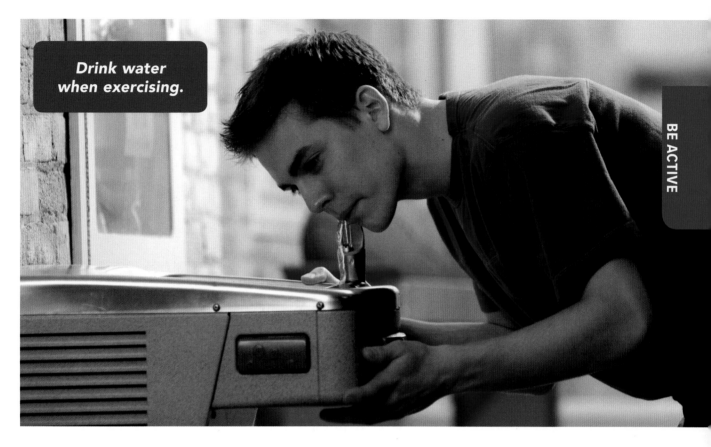

Drink water when exercising.

7. **Breathe deeply** while exercising to increase the amount of oxygen in your blood.

8. **Warm up before vigorous exercise.** Cool down afterward.

9. **Take heart medications** as prescribed by your doctor. Use prescribed drugs, like nitroglycerine, as recommended.

10. **Your doctor may order an electrocardiogram (ECG) stress test.** This is a test that measures your heart's health. An ECG can expose an undiagnosed problem such as a partially blocked blood vessel leading to the heart that could make exercise dangerous. An ECG stress test also measures blood pressure, heart rate and heart rhythm. A medical professional supervises you while you are doing this test. It helps give your doctor answers about what exercise you should or shouldn't do.

Diabetes and overheating

If you have had diabetes for a long time, you may notice that you don't sweat as much as you used to. This is because the sweat glands are stimulated by nerves. Diabetes can damage nerves. Sweating is the body's natural way of cooling down. With less cooling, it's really important to drink water and avoid getting overheated.

Your doctor may order an ECG stress test if you:

- are at high risk for heart disease, and
- were previously inactive, and
- wish to do an exercise program more vigorous than brisk walking.

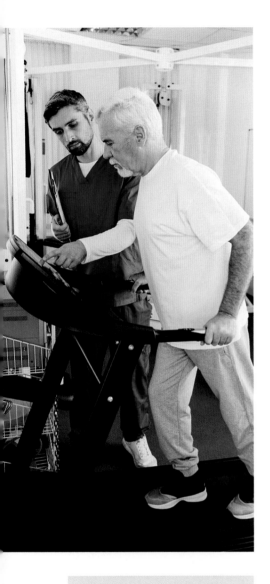

Page 28 outlines warning signs of a heart attack or stroke.

If you've recently had a heart attack

- Doctors recommend an activity program for almost all heart patients. Talk to your doctor.
- The goal is to help heal your heart through a very structured exercise program that gradually increases how much you do. It often includes walking and use of a treadmill or bicycle.
- In your community, there may be an exercise facility for people who have had a heart attack. Their programs usually include a physician or other health professional nearby and safety precautions in place.

Regular exercise should never cause serious pain or distress. Increase your exercise slowly to help avoid or decrease soreness and fatigue. Also avoid exercising right after you eat. If you do get a sore muscle or cramp, massage and stretch it gently.

 WARNING SIGNS: Stop Exercising
Immediately seek medical help if you have:

- Chest pain or tightness in your chest, if it is severe or persists more than two minutes
- Pain in arm or jaw
- Difficulty breathing or you can't talk
- Profuse sweating
- Severe joint or muscle pain
- Pain at the back of your calf that suddenly worsens or becomes severe
- An irregular heartbeat
- A feeling of faintness, dizziness or nausea
- A very pale or "off" color
- Extreme fatigue

Keeping Your Eyes Healthy When Exercising

Exercise helps improve the circulation of oxygen and nutrients to your eyes. However, if you have diabetes retinopathy (damage to the back of the eye), there are certain exercises that you should avoid. Talk to your eye doctor. Ask if you need to limit any exercises.

If you have early non-proliferative retinopathy (see pages 40–41), you may not need to restrict any exercises.

With more severe retinopathy damage, you will have to avoid high-impact exercises or strenuous activities that increase your blood pressure. These exercises could worsen the damage to your eyes (retinopathy) or lead to severe eye complications, such as a detached retina.

Exercises to avoid when you have severe diabetes retinopathy

- Running, jumping or jogging
- Boxing, karate or hockey
- Tennis, squash or pickle ball
- Sky diving, scuba diving or bungee jumping
- Strenuous exercise at altitudes higher than 5,000 feet (1,500 m)
- Lifting heavy weights
- Lifting any weights above your head
- Strenuous shovelling, for example, of heavy, wet snow where you lift the shovel above your waist or are pushing hard
- Dropping your head below your waist (unless recommended to do this by your eye doctor following eye surgery)
- Strenuous blowing into a trumpet or other musical instrument

For advice on exercises you should avoid, please talk to your eye doctor.

Have you had laser eye treatments or eye surgery?
If so, carefully follow your doctor's exercise restrictions before and after surgery.

BE ACTIVE

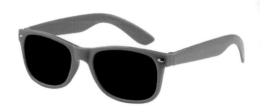

Wear sunglasses to protect your eyes from ultraviolet light when walking outdoors in the sunshine.

Keeping Your Feet Healthy When Exercising

For more information on footcare, see pages 268–281.

- Avoid activities that cause damage or injury to your feet. Don't run or jump.
- Wear shoes that protect your feet.
- Check your feet every day. Take care of your feet.
- After exercise, check your feet for any red or warm spots. This might be a sign of an infection underneath your skin.
- Follow your doctor's recommendations if you have an open sore or ulcer on your foot. In some cases, you may need to stay off your feet until it heals. Chair exercises or biking (if you use a part of your foot that isn't hurt) may be an option. If you have an open sore, you should not go swimming.

Walking is a low-impact exercise

When you walk, the force on each foot is about one and a half times your weight.

When you walk, one foot is always on the ground. Each foot lands with a force one and a half times your weight. For a 200-lb (90 kg) person, the force on each foot would be 300 lbs (135 kg).

Low-impact exercise reduces your chance of injury.

Jogging is a high-impact exercise

When you jog, the force on each foot is about three times your weight.

When you jog, both feet are off the ground together. Therefore, each foot lands with a force of three or more times the weight of your body. For a 200-lb (90 kg) person, the force would be at least 600 lbs (270 kg).

That's a lot of weight on the bottom of your feet, or on a worn or older joint.

Talk to your doctor or exercise specialist if you want to run for exercise. You must speak to a doctor if considering a marathon. This high-impact exercise will increase your risks for injury, especially if you:

- are older
- are overweight
- have any diabetes complications such as foot problems or retinopathy, or
- have other health conditions such as high blood pressure

ELSIE'S STORY: Choose the right shoes to take care of your feet

Nearly one in every four people has what we call "sugar diabetes" in my community. I have seen many people suffer because of the sugar. Now so many young people have this disease. When my doctor told me that I had diabetes, I knew I wanted to do something right away. I am an Indigeneous elder and people look up to me. I talked to the dietitian who comes to our community twice a month. She helped me learn what I should and shouldn't be eating. I drank a lot of soft drinks, so this is the first thing I got rid of and replaced with diet drinks. I made other changes too. One thing I did was I started walking. I walked a lot. Over a period of six months, I had got myself up to walking almost one hour every day. My blood sugars were a lot better and I felt better too. That is the good news.

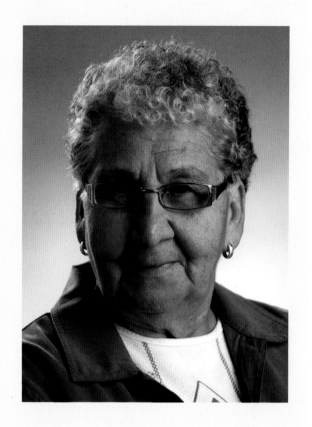

The bad news is something else. I didn't know about proper foot care. I wasn't checking my feet at all. I wasn't wearing a proper pair of shoes. I walked so much that my right foot shoe got a small hole in the bottom. I didn't know this because I had lost the feeling on the bottom of my foot. No one told me that this could happen with diabetes. There are so many things I didn't know about diabetes.

That hole in the bottom of my shoe caused a bad sore on my foot. By the time I got to the clinic, the sore was worse and went all the way to my bone. It got infected. To make a long story short, I lost my right foot and then my leg to below my knee. Now I wear an artificial leg. Looking after my diabetes is more difficult because I can't walk as much.

I am telling my story so you don't make the same mistake I did. Exercise is so important to fight diabetes. I still believe it, but please do the exercise safely. I could have prevented all of my foot problems if I had just known about checking my feet and the importance of wearing the right kind of shoes.

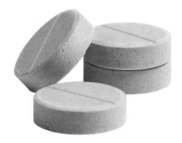

Glucose tablets

Low and High Blood Sugar When Exercising

Low blood sugar

A low blood sugar is when your blood sugar goes below 70 mg/dL (4 mmol/L). You may feel shaky and dizzy. Treat this by eating three to five glucose tablets or 1 tbsp (15 mL) of sugar (which equals 15 grams of carbohydrate). Low blood sugar can happen when you exercise if you are on insulin or certain diabetes pills. Low blood sugar can happen even a few hours after exercise. For more information about low blood sugar signs, symptoms, causes, prevention, treatment and safety guidelines, see pages 329–336.

High blood sugar

You may be surprised to learn that exercise can cause either low blood sugar or high blood sugar.

In type 2 diabetes, there are two main reasons exercise can cause blood sugar to go up.

1. Your body is warm and you may be thirsty or a bit dehydrated right after you finish exercising. This causes your blood sugar to go up. After you drink some water and rest, it usually will come down in about half an hour or less. Unless you think your blood sugar is low, wait at least half an hour after exercise before testing your blood sugar.

2. You have high blood sugar staying at about 300 mg/dL (16 mmol/L) or higher for days, weeks or months. This means that you are short of insulin or your insulin is not working properly. If you do strenuous or prolonged exercise such as long walks or heavy weight lifting, your blood sugar may actually get worse rather than go down.

    Why can it get worse? Even though you have lots of sugar in your blood, it can't get to your exercising muscles, because of a shortage of insulin. Your muscles send a message to your brain that they need sugar. Then your body sends more sugar to your blood from your liver stores. This extra sugar still can't move into your muscles because of the shortage of insulin. The sugar builds up in your blood, and your blood sugar goes up.

Step 3: Become a Nonsmoker

QUIT SMOKING

I quit because I want to see my grandson grow up.

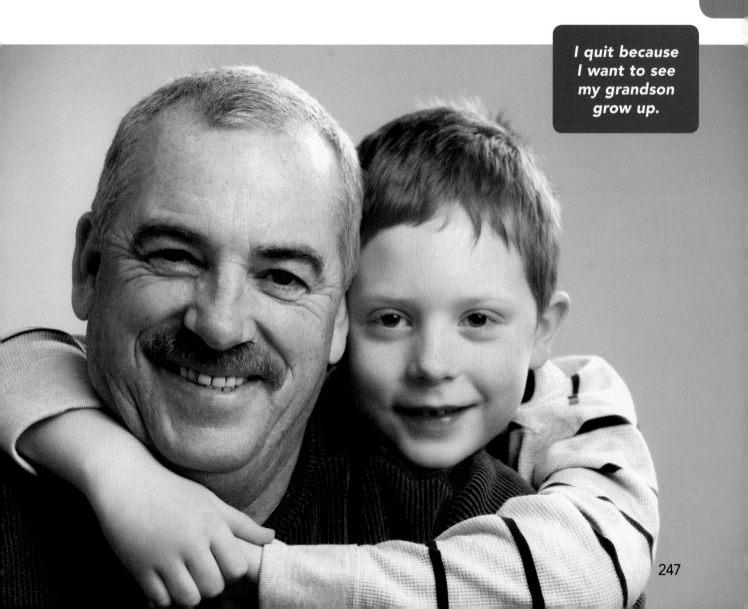

247

Who needs to quit?

Anyone who uses:

- cigarettes
- e-cigarettes
- cigars or pipe
- chewing tobacco or smokeless tobacco (snuff)

These all have nicotine and toxins and cause health problems. These addictions require similar steps in order to quit.

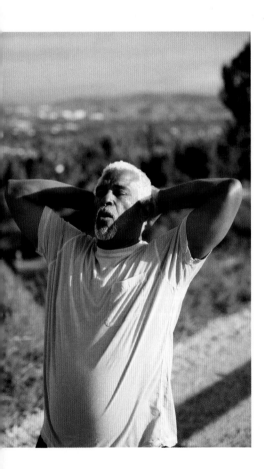

Reasons to Quit

Most smokers would like to be nonsmokers. You may have quit many times and then returned to smoking.

Here's why quitting smoking is so important for a person with diabetes.

You want to feel better

You will have less shortness of breath and have more energy. You'll have fewer colds and lung infections. You'll feel clean and fresh. Food will taste better as your sense of smell and taste improves.

You want to stay as healthy as possible

Smoking has three major health effects on your body:

1. **Cancer.** Smoking is the main cause of lung cancer. Smoking also contributes to cancers that affect the mouth, throat, pancreas, colon, rectum, kidney, bladder and cervix.
2. **Breathing difficulties.** Smoking can cause a variety of breathing problems such as bronchitis or emphysema.
3. **Heart attack and stroke.** Smoking damages and narrows blood vessels throughout your body. It can increase blood pressure.

If you quit, benefits start right away

No matter how long you have been smoking, you'll benefit within the first hour of quitting.

- Right away, your blood pressure and pulse will improve.
- After the first day, the carbon monoxide clears out of your body.
- In just a couple of days, you'll have more energy and feel less breathless.
- In a few weeks, your body has better circulation.
- In a few months, your lung function improves by about 10%.
- One year later, your heart attack risk will be half of that of a smoker with diabetes. Your risk for a foot amputation will be one-third less.

This is amazing!

Smoking and diabetes together are a bad combination

When you have diabetes and you smoke, you are more likely to have diabetes complications. This is because both nicotine and high blood sugar narrow and damage blood vessels and decrease the flow of oxygen in your body. They also both decrease your body's ability to use insulin properly.

People who smoke and have diabetes have more of these health complications:

- Heart attack and stroke
- Gangrene and amputations to a lower leg or foot
- Kidney problems
- Vision loss (retinopathy)
- Nerve damage
- Gum disease
- Hip fractures
- For men, erectile dysfunction

Save money
Smoking costs a lot of money. If you're on a limited budget, you could use that money on healthy food, medicine and fitness opportunities.

Be a good example for your family
- You can reduce your family's risk of smoking. Studies show that children are less likely to smoke if their parents are nonsmokers.
- If you are pregnant, you want to have a healthy baby.
- You can eliminate the danger of secondhand smoke by not smoking in the home, workplace and vehicles. This keeps the air clean.
- You want to get rid of the thirdhand smoke. This is the smoke that adheres to your clothes, hair and skin, even when you smoke outside. You want to be fresh smelling and clean.
- Make your home a safe one! Smoking is the major cause of home fires.

You can do this. There are lots of ex-smokers out there — join them!

It's never too late to quit smoking.

QUIT SMOKING

249

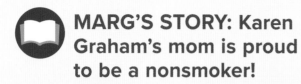

MARG'S STORY: Karen Graham's mom is proud to be a nonsmoker!

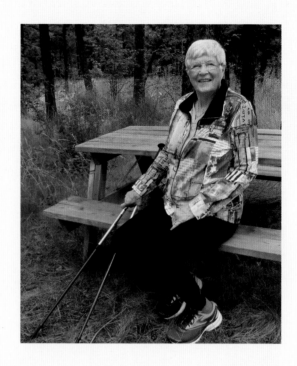

I am 90 years old. My best friend and I started smoking at the age of 15. We all did it — secretly. We smoked while on the school grounds, and we'd go downtown to the bus depot and sit in the ladies restroom and have our lunch and smoke. It was grungy, but we had a private place to smoke.

Of course, my mother eventually caught me. She was very disappointed and she told me how bad it was for my health and she hoped that I would quit. I was about 18 by this time.

I continued to smoke after I got married and until I became pregnant with my first child. For the reason that I did not want to harm my baby, it seemed easy to quit. Nevertheless, I did start again when my child was about 9 months old. My husband continued to smoke during this time.

My next quitting time was pregnancy again. I am not sure when I started smoking again. In my defense, I did not smoke while breastfeeding or holding babies. However, there was secondhand smoke all around. We were not aware of the dangers of secondhand smoke in those days.

With my third pregnancy, I also quit smoking and again started months later, after the baby's birth. I do not remember that it was difficult to quit when I had such an important reason.

Later, to quit just for myself with no real impending reason — that was not easy. Over 30 or so years, I tried at least seven times to quit. I tried nicotine gum, I tried cold turkey, I joined the Seventh Day Adventists' no-smoking program, I tried total relaxation and I tried overkill (smoking cigarette after cigarette one after the other till you felt sick — it was supposed to turn you off smoking). I would quit for a while and then start again. My husband smoked all this time.

One fine day, we both decided to quit smoking. We finished off the cigarettes that we had (a dozen or so) and then quit cold turkey. We had each other and there was no smoking or cigarettes in the house. Doing it together was what I needed and also what my husband needed. We quit because we knew and had known for years that it was a very stupid thing to do.

I guess the story here is that one has to be honestly motivated to quit. You do it for your own health or the health of loved ones or finally recognizing how very ignorant and wasteful it is. Also, it is a very expensive habit, and for my husband and I, we smoked over two packs a day. Quitting allowed us to save money and then do things in our retirement that we would not have been able to afford.

I don't remember that it was extremely difficult, but then it is a long time ago — 45 years now. We have never, not for one second, regretted giving up that filthy habit.

As a 90-year-old nonsmoker, I am healthy and fit. For me, quitting smoking paid off.

Ten Steps to Stop Smoking

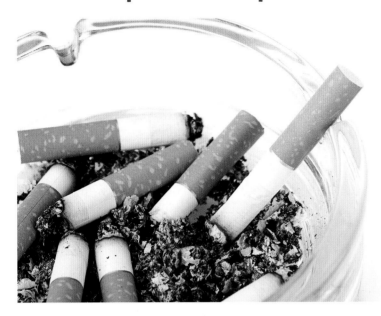

1. Prepare

If you are like most smokers, you began smoking as a teenager. Most of us tried it and some never became smokers. But others kept trying and became addicted. Today, many people, especially young people, are becoming addicted to nicotine through e-cigarettes. Whether you smoke cigarettes or e-cigarettes, the process of quitting nicotine requires determination, planning and support.

The 10 steps in this chapter give you important information and ways to prepare you to quit, and to help you stop smoking for life.

Here's a few questions for you so you can start thinking about quitting:

What are your reasons to quit?
Your reasons are the best ones. Make a list.

What are your smoking triggers?
Triggers are times or things that make you want to smoke. Examples of triggers are drinking coffee or alcohol, finishing a meal, watching TV, playing cards or bingo, driving or coping with a crisis.

How will you manage your smoking triggers?
One way is to develop healthier habits. Relieve stress by going for a walk, drinking water, deep breathing and a hobby that keeps you busy.

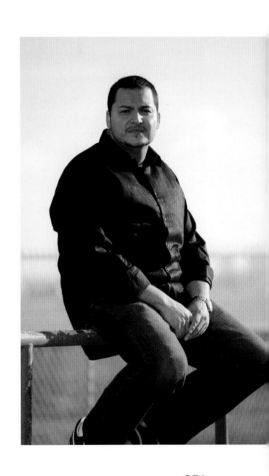

**Support Groups
and Phone Support**

- American Cancer Society
- Canadian Cancer Society
- American Lung Association
- National Cancer Institute
- Addiction support organizations

Available services

- Toll-free telephone counseling
- Online counselling
- Web-based message boards
- Handouts and booklets
- Support groups

Set up support

You will have more success with at least one person to listen to you and support you. This could be a friend, family or professional. You may want to:

- Talk to family or friends that have quit.
- Talk to your family and coworkers about your intention to quit. Seek their support.
- Talk to your doctor about methods of quitting and quitting aids. Your pharmacist (or diabetes educator) can also be a great help.
- Ask about quit smoking programs and support groups available online and in your community. See sidebar.
- Ask your health educator for the number of your local toll-free quit line or on-line quit-smoking service.
- Ask if your health plan covers the cost of quit-smoking aids (for example, nicotine patches) or medications.

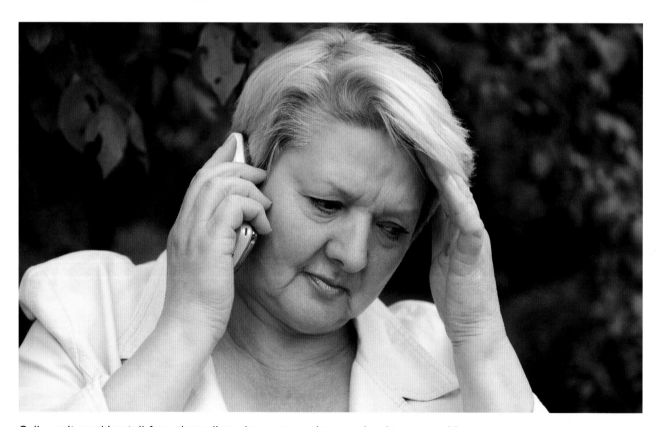

Call a quit smoking toll-free phone line whenever cravings are hard to cope with. It helps to speak to a smoking cessation counsellor.

2. Set a Quit Date

It's natural to keep putting off quitting. This is a very hard but important change. You might find it easier if you set a quit date. Then you can work toward a goal. Don't set the goal too far away, or it will feel unreachable. Consider setting a quit date within the next month. Choose a time without a lot of stressful events planned. You need to be prepared mentally and physically for quitting.

It's easy to find excuses for not quitting. Put your quit date on your calendar.

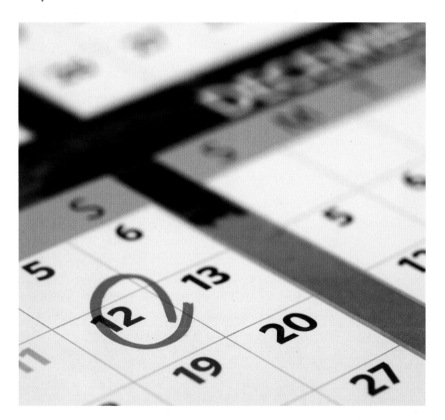

**Imagine yourself as a nonsmoker.
If you can imagine it, you can do it!**

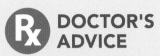

DOCTOR'S ADVICE

After an emergency such as a heart attack or stroke, some people quit cold turkey with great success. Please don't wait that long to make your change.

Take it one day at a time. Every cigarette you don't smoke gets you closer to your goal.

Talk to your doctor or pharmacist

You can buy almost all of these NRT treatments over the counter. Some sprays and the inhaler need a doctor's prescription in the United States.

Ask for information about how to use these, especially if you have other health issues or are pregnant or breastfeeding. Use the products correctly, so that you don't get too much nicotine.

3. Go Cold Turkey or Reduce Slowly

Cold turkey

This means when you reach your quit date, you quit all at once, without any quit-smoking aids. Most people who quit cold turkey have had many previous attempts to quit. Research shows that people who use supports like quit-smoking aids or toll-free quit phone lines can quit with fewer attempts. If you tried to quit cold turkey in the past, and then returned to smoking, next time consider using quit-smoking aids.

Cut back slowly

This means you cut back on smoking gradually over several weeks until you reach your quit date. Some people find it helpful to smoke the cigarettes that they feel are the hardest to give up, like first thing in the morning, or after a meal. Instead, decrease smoking at other times of day. Then gradually cut out cigarettes during the harder times. Set a reasonable goal for yourself. Cut a certain number of cigarettes per day. Gradually reduce the number.

4. Quit-Smoking Aids Help

Quit-smoking aids help many people quit. They include nicotine replacement therapy (also called NRT), medications and alternative therapies. All NRT contain nicotine. They come as gums and lozenges, an oral inhaler, a mouth spray and a nasal spray, and as skin patches. The medications don't contain nicotine but can help you quit. Examples of alternative therapies include talk therapy, hypnosis, acupuncture and laser therapy.

If you tried to quit with one method and it didn't help, consider trying it again, or trying something else. Find out about quit-smoking aids from your doctor, nurse or pharmacist. Also contact a support group or addictions organization.

Nicotine replacement therapy

NRT helps you with cravings. It provides an exact amount of nicotine, but without the carbon monoxide and toxins that come from burning tobacco leaves and inhaling cigarette smoke. NRTs help decrease your physical withdrawal symptoms so it's easier to skip having a cigarette in your hand.

No matter which NRT you choose — gum, lozenges, inhaler, spray or nicotine patch — over time, you will use a lower and lower dose until you can totally quit.

The NRT you choose depends in part on how many cigarettes you smoked a day. Some people don't like the taste of the gum or lozenges and prefer the patch. Some people's throats get irritated with the inhaler or mouth spray; others get irritation in their nose with the nasal spray. With your doctor's advice, you may want to use more than one product. This may increase your chance of success.

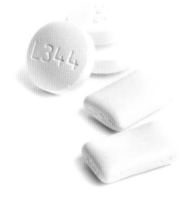

Nicotine lozenges and gum

How much should I take?

- See a doctor, pharmacist or smoking cessation specialist for the right NRT dosage.
- If you are a heavier smoker, you'll start with a higher dose than a light smoker.
- Do not take more than the maximum dose.
- It's important to follow the prescription. You don't want too much nicotine. You want just enough so that it works for you.
- If you don't use NRTs correctly, they can make you feel sick.

How long should I use them?

Some people will only use NRT for a short time, while others may use them for four to six months, or longer.

Nicotine gum or lozenges

After you quit, if you have an urge to smoke, take a piece of gum or a lozenge. They will help with your craving. Also use gum or lozenges when you're not yet quite ready to quit but as a first important step to cut out smoking in your home and car, and during work hours.

How to use nicotine gum or lozenges

- **Gum:** Bite it twice then "park" the gum inside your mouth against your cheek for 1 minute. Then repeat. It will last about 30 minutes. Don't chew it like regular gum, and don't swallow.

- **Lozenges:** Don't chew or swallow. Tuck it into your cheek and let it dissolve slowly.

Don't eat within 15 minutes of using gum or lozenges.

Nicotine inhalers, mouth spray and nasal spray

These sprays and inhalers work so quickly that you can become addicted to them. For this reason, doctors recommend gum or lozenges as the first option. In the United States, sprays and inhalers are still prescription-only. These need to be used with caution. Follow all the directions carefully. Use the right dosage and for the correct length of time.

Nicotine oral inhaler

This is a small tube that looks like a cigarette. When you inhale, you get a smaller dose of nicotine than if you smoke a cigarette. You might use 6 to 12 cartridges each day. You would slowly decrease the daily amount. When you are down to 1 to 2 a day, you can quit. The inhaler shouldn't be used for more than six months.

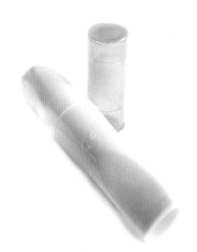

Nicotine oral inhaler

Nicotine mouth spray

This spray or mist works within a minute. When you spray it in your mouth, your body absorbs the nicotine right away through the inside of your mouth. Do not use more than recommended.

Nicotine nasal spray

This comes in a small spray container that you spray into each nostril. You might use it 8 to 40 times a day. Use it for the length of time listed on the package. This may not be a good choice if you get hay fever or sinus infections.

Nicotine patch

Doctors recommend the nicotine patch in two cases:
- If you smoke more than ten cigarettes a day.
- If you have a strong craving for a cigarette as soon as you get up in the morning.

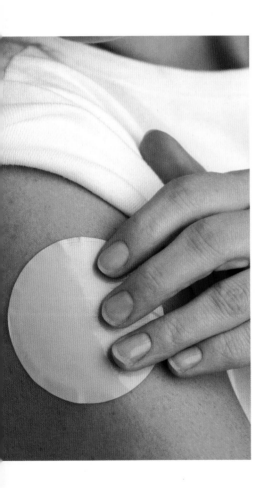

You attach the nicotine patch to your skin. The patch releases nicotine into your blood. You wear it for 16 or 24 hours, and then replace it with a new patch the next day. You start with a stronger patch and decrease to a lower dose. Over 6 to 12 weeks, you decrease the nicotine levels with patches containing less nicotine. The patch is easy to use.

Some people find that the nicotine patch plus an occasional nicotine gum or lozenge work well together. The patch provides a steady supply of nicotine. The gum or lozenge provides a boost for an extra craving.

Facts about e-cigarettes, or vaping

- There are many different names and brands, and they all deliver nicotine. They may be called e-cigarettes or vape pens. The brand name JUUL is an e-cigarette that is smaller, and does not produce the vapor but still contains nicotine.
- The nicotine in e-cigarettes is just as addictive as the nicotine in regular cigarettes.
- There is not enough government regulation on the amount of nicotine in e-cigarettes. Some e-cigarette cartridges have as much nicotine as an entire pack of cigarettes.
- E-cigarettes still have cancer-causing chemicals, but less than cigarettes.
- There is not enough research to fully understand the harm of breathing in nicotine, artificial flavorings and other toxins in an aerosol form. A recent jump in vaping-related lung injury and even sudden deaths has raised concern.

 CAUTION
E-cigarettes are not an NRT.
The amount of nicotine in e-cigarette cartridges is not listed. When you vape, you don't know how much nicotine you get. You can actually become more addicted to nicotine if you switch to e-cigarettes.

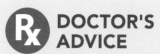 **DOCTOR'S ADVICE**

E-cigarettes are not a good way to quit smoking

When you quit smoking using NRT, you start with a higher dose of nicotine at the beginning and then reduce the dose over time. The nicotine patch or gum allows you to do this, as the exact amount of nicotine is listed. E-cigarettes do not list the amount of nicotine.

QUIT SMOKING

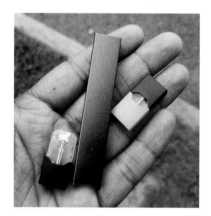

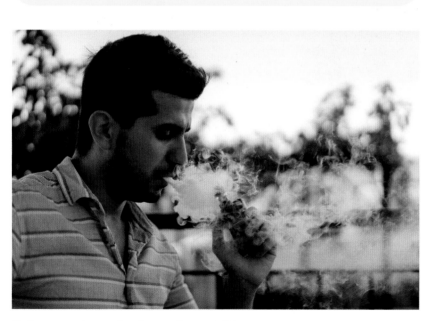

E-cigarettes have nicotine and are addictive just like regular cigarettes. Don't buy them.

Medications that help you quit

There are several prescription pills that help you quit smoking. These include bupropion (Zyban) and varenicline (Champix or Chantix). These don't contain nicotine but they do reduce withdrawal symptoms and your urge to smoke. You can take these pills along with quit-smoking aids. Ask your doctor or pharmacist if one of these pills would be safe for you. Learn about any possible side effects before you take one.

Talk therapy, hypnosis, acupuncture and laser therapy

These treatments help some people stop smoking, especially when combined with NRT, such as the nicotine patch. Also, these treatments often include counseling, support and education about quitting smoking. They also help you to learn to relax.

Talk therapy is also called psychotherapy. A psychologist or other expert will work with you to help you change your behaviors. You will need to attend group or individual counselling sessions. You will be encouraged to think about your smoking habits and especially what prompts you to smoke. You'll be asked to record this. You are then trained to break smoking habits and create new healthy patterns.

Hypnosis involves putting a person into a hypnotic trance. *Only a medical doctor or psychiatrist is qualified to do this.* In this relaxed state, the hypnotist will teach you behavior skills for coping with withdrawal and the urge to smoke. Treatment is typically for three months or longer. Not everyone can be hypnotized.

Acupuncture is a type of traditional Chinese medicine. It involves the insertion of very fine needles into specific points of the body, called acupuncture points. The aim of acupuncture is to help the body achieve its natural balance. There is some research that shows this approach may help smokers cut back or quit.

Laser therapy uses fine beams of pulsating light. These beams shine on specific spots on the body (often, the acupuncture points). This may help release endorphins, which help to relax you.

Studies show you are more likely to benefit from alternative quit-smoking therapy if you have many treatments with a skilled health worker. Ask for a referral from your pharmacist, doctor or local quit-smoking organization.

5. *Time to Quit*

Today is your quit date. Take some deep breaths.

This is the first day of your new life as a nonsmoker. It will be challenging — but this is something you have wanted to do for a long time. It will be worth it! Remember, quit-smoking aids and the toll-free quit phone lines and online supports are there for you. It's helpful to know that the first one to three days are the most difficult. It gets a little easier as time passes.

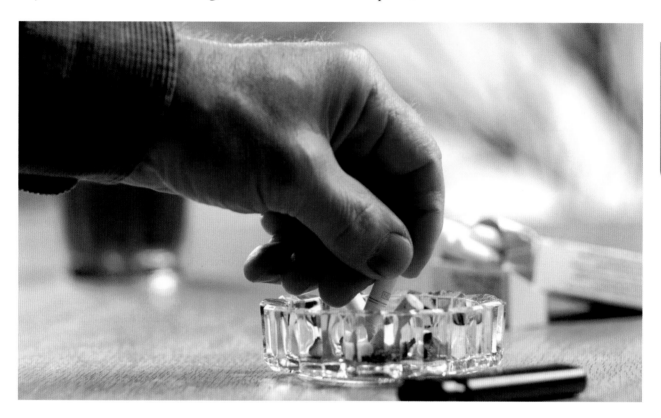

Tips for family and friends of someone who has just quit smoking

- It's likely that the person who has just quit will be grouchy. They are fighting a very difficult addiction withdrawal. Quitting smoking isn't easy and isn't fun for them. Please be sensitive to their moods. Let them vent. Give them space but be a wall of support for them. They will get easier to live with and they will be smoke free.

- If you are a smoker, don't smoke in their company.

- If they slip or relapse, don't make them feel guilty. Be supportive. This is a long process and they will need you to be there for them every step of the way.

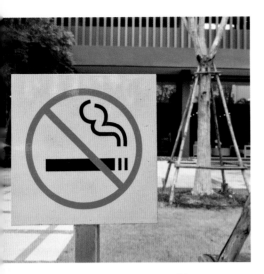

Get out to a nonsmoking location.

Put into action the Four Ds of dealing with cravings:

Delay

Deep breaths

Drink water

Distract yourself

6. *Control Cravings*

Each craving for a cigarette is like a wave. It is the strongest at the beginning, then it lessens. These tend to last a couple of minutes. Get through them one craving at a time. Eventually, your "nic fits" will taper off.

Change your smoking routines

- Reduce time spent in your favorite smoking places. For example, if you have a "smoking chair" at home, try sitting on a different chair. If you are at home a lot, go to a nonsmoking location such as a library or mall. Go for regular short walks.

- If you smoked in front of the TV, then limit your TV watching at first. Maybe listen to the radio, a podcast or music instead of smoking. You will quickly save enough money to buy yourself a new phone or tablet to download all your favorite songs. Each time you want to smoke, put on your earphones and focus on a special piece of music.

- During the first critical days and weeks after quitting, avoid smokers who want you to smoke with them. Reduce activities where you associate with other smokers. Avoid the homes of friends or family who smoke, bars, bingo halls and smoker coffee breaks. Look for nonsmoking facilities.

- Is smoking a cigarette part of your bedtime routine? If so, before you quit, it's a good idea to think about a different bedtime routine. See pages 358–359 for bedtime and sleep tips.

Fill up the space and time without cigarettes

If you were a pack-a-day smoker, you puffed on a cigarette up to 300 times a day (12 puffs per smoke). Each time you think of reaching for a cigarette, take several long deep breaths.

You already know the benefits of drinking lots of water. Learn more about deep breathing on page 359. And distracting yourself is part of delaying — finding something to do other than smoking. So how do you distract yourself?

Distract yourself

- Walk around for a few minutes.
- Do a few stretches.
- Chew a stick of sugarless gum.
- Do your nails.
- Some people find it helpful to sniff a strong scent like lavender oil, peppermint oil or black pepper oil. Others find that chewing on a small piece of fresh mint or parsley helps. These can help break the association with smoking.
- Drink peppermint or strong-flavored herbal tea.
- Suck on a sugar-free peppermint, small wintergreen mint, or cinnamon stick.
- Play a hand of solitaire (with cards or on the computer).
- Play a game on your mobile phone.

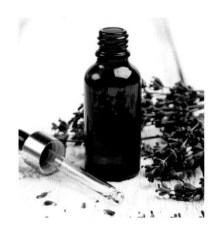

Keep your hands busy

- Roll a pencil or coin in your hands.
- Play with a rubber band.
- Doodle.
- Twiddle a key holder with an interesting ornament.
- Do a puzzle, some needlework or knit.
- Count the beads on a necklace. Prayer beads or meditation beads work well.
- Using a moisturizer, massage your fingers and hands.
- Read or write down how you are feeling in a journal.
- Wash dishes or clean your home. This is a great chance to wash walls, curtains and furniture to get rid of the stale smoke smells and stains.
- Squeeze a stress ball (a soft spongy ball) or some play dough.
- If you are musical, play an instrument or sing.
- Text a friend. Tell them you're texting them instead of smoking.

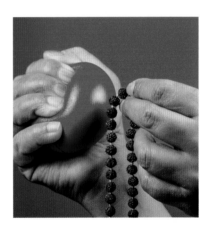

Remember your reasons for quitting.

QUIT SMOKING

Weight gain in people who quit smoking is not just related to metabolism. After quitting, many people substitute food (especially sweets) for cigarettes. This is why it's so important to make a plan and get support before you quit, both for healthy eating and for exercise.

Go for a walk. Exercise is one of the best ways to control cravings and prevent weight gain.

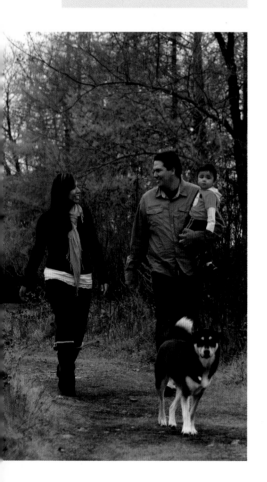

7. Avoid Gaining Weight

If you gain a little weight when quitting, it's less of a health concern than a lifetime of smoking. However, if you exercise and eat properly, you may not gain weight. Nicotine increases metabolism, and so does exercise. So after you quit, exercise helps keep your metabolism and weight in balance. Here are some tips to lessen or prevent weight gain after quitting smoking.

Visit a dietitian before you quit smoking

Talk to a dietitian about healthy meal choices. You can make a plan of what foods you should and shouldn't have in your home when you quit. It is also good to have regular follow-up to monitor your weight. If you don't have access to a dietitian, read the beginning of this book and make meals like the ones shown.

Things to do before you quit

- List tasks and chores you want to get done.
- List fun activities you want to get involved in.
- Stock your cupboards and fridge with lots of low-calorie snack foods: veggie sticks, ingredients to make homemade vegetable soup, sunflower seeds with the shells on, sugar-free popsicles and sugar-free gum. See the low-calorie, small and medium snacks on pages 197–199.
- Avoid buying snack foods that are high in fat, salt and sugar.

Put into action healthy alternatives to smoking

Take a walk. Even a short walk removes you from that familiar place where you used to smoke. It's also invigorating. Exercise will help you deal with the anguish and tension you will feel because of nicotine withdrawal.

Keep busy. Smoking takes up a lot of time. It's a social activity as you chat with other smokers. After you quit, you may eat because you're bored. Work through your lists of things to do.

Slow down your eating. Drink water, both with your meal and at the end of your meal. Put your knife and fork down between bites. Drink water along with snacks too.

Delay your snack. When you crave a snack, try to wait a few minutes. Have a drink of water. Progressively increase the time before each snack.

Sometimes you just have to eat something! Remember the low-calorie and small snack choices. Try a few sunflower seeds. The salty taste of the seeds, and the activity of cracking the seed and spitting out the shells can help with a craving. A quarter cup of sunflower seeds with the shells on is equal to a small snack. (See other small snacks on page 198.)

Plan healthy snacks, at regular times. Keep track of your meal size and snack allowance on page 151.

Watch your portions. Follow the meal plans listed in this book. Look for more plans and many tasty recipes in the two companion books in this series (see page 416).

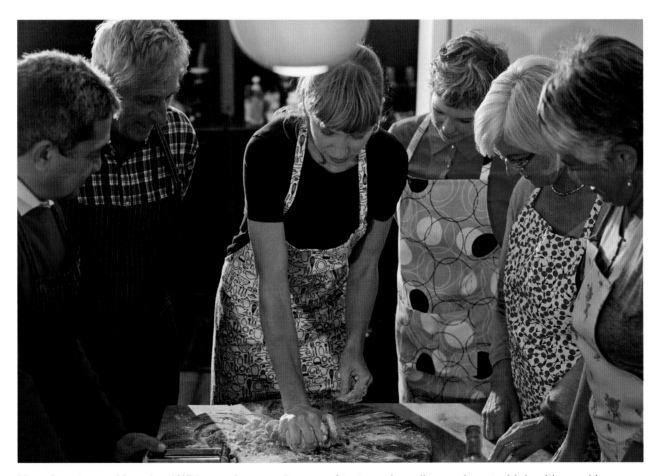

Have fun at a cooking class! With your improved sense of taste and smell, experiment with healthy cooking. Try different recipes with new herbs and spices.

QUIT SMOKING

Resist second helpings. As soon as you finish your meal, get up from the table and help with the dishes. Do something different than when you were a smoker.

Be careful with desserts. It's hard to break the habit of having an after-meal cigarette, and many people replace cigarettes with desserts. Choose a fruit, mini pudding, or one of the light dessert recipes in this book.

After meals, brush your teeth or rinse out your mouth. This becomes a new habit rather than the after-meal cigarette.

Get through social events and "smoke breaks" without smoking

- In the first few weeks after you quit smoking, avoid these social events if possible. You may find that as you cut back on smoking, you also cut back on social drinking, which would also be a positive change.
- Go for a short walk instead of a smoke break at work. Also, see page 78 for tips on managing overeating at work. Have a drink of water or a diet beverage. Fresh fruit is always a good choice.

Instead of smoking when drinking coffee, change your routine

- Drink your coffee out of a different type of mug, or in a different location in your home or workplace.
- Change your drink. Cut back on drinking coffee. Replace some of your coffee with tea, water, flavored soda water or a diet beverage.

Here's a trick to help with a sugar craving: eat one or two Tic Tacs, a cinnamon heart or sugar-free candy.

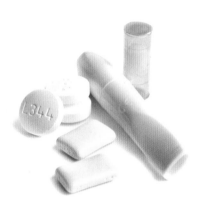

When you have a craving, try one of these:

- a nicotine lozenge
- a piece of nicotine gum
- a puff from a nicotine oral inhaler

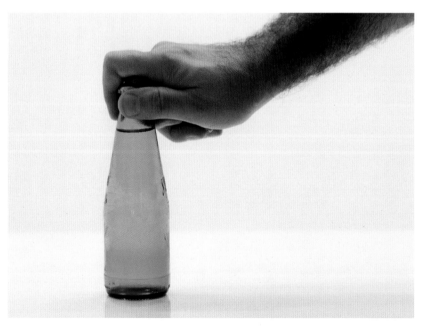

Reach for a bottle of sparkling mineral water.

8. Tips for Other Changes

Irritability or anxiety

It is common to feel irritable when quitting smoking. Warn those around you! Going for a walk perks up your happy hormones and helps you burn off steam. You may find it helpful to call a smoker's support phone line when you are feeling anxious; these phone lines are open 24/7. Try deep breathing or easy meditation (see pages 359–360). Also see other stress management tips in *Coping with Stress* (pages 350–358).

Sore throat or coughs

You may experience this at first. Your lungs are cleaning out the tar leftover from smoking. It's good to get this out by coughing. Drinking lots of water or herbal tea can speed this up. If your throat is sore, sip on water or suck on a sugar-free cough drop. Usually this goes away in a week or two.

Dizziness

This usually only lasts for a few days. It's because your body is getting more oxygen now. Sit down and have a drink of water. Take it slowly. The dizzy feelings should pass.

Headaches

Quitting smoking is stressful. Together, stress and nicotine withdrawal can cause headaches. Lie down in a quiet dark room and rest. Do relaxation exercises. Treat a headache with your usual over-the-counter medication.

Constipation

Nicotine stimulates bowel movements. Some people have difficulty going to the bathroom after they quit smoking. Eat lots of vegetables, fruits and whole grains to get the right boost of fiber. Drinking water and exercise also help.

Difficulty falling asleep

You may feel more nervous and restless at night as you go through your initial withdrawal. In the early evening, do something that will tire you out so you sleep better. Try a short walk or 5 to 10 minutes on your exercise bike or treadmill. Cutting back on caffeine at night might help. Try switching to water, decaffeinated coffee or tea, herbal tea or other caffeine-free diet beverages. Take a short bath or shower to relax.

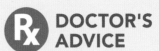

DOCTOR'S ADVICE

After you quit smoking, your nicotine levels go down. Then, caffeine is more potent for your body. You can actually get jitters from this enhanced caffeine effect. Try switching to a decaf later in the day.

Without nicotine in your body, some diabetes and blood pressure medications work better. This means you may need a lower dosage. Plan your doctor's appointment for a month after you quit.

QUIT SMOKING

Sleeping and the 24-hour nicotine patch

As a smoker, did you get up at night to smoke, or did you sleep through the night? If you didn't get up to smoke, then the nicotine released at night from the 24-hour patch might keep you awake or make you restless. Try removing the patch before bed, or switch to a 16-hour patch.

Remind yourself of your goal.

Revisit your reasons for quitting.

Re-enlist help. Smoker help lines are there at any stage — even months down the road. Contact them again.

9. Manage Setbacks

We make mistakes. That's part of being human.

Slipups could be minor — an occasional cigarette here or there. This might involve a day or two where you go back to smoking. The important thing is to get right back to your nonsmoking pattern as soon as you can.

Don't be hard on yourself. Keep focused and stick to your quit plan. Ask yourself, "What triggered this?" "How can I prevent it next time?" Learn from your mistake. Call the toll-free smokers help line. Reconnect with a support group if you need it.

Keep your "reasons to quit list" handy. Read it regularly.

Mistakes can also mean a full-blown return to smoking. You will still be able to quit smoking. For most people, there will be several tries before you become a permanent nonsmoker. When you are ready, get back to your nonsmoking routine. Don't wait too long. Good luck!

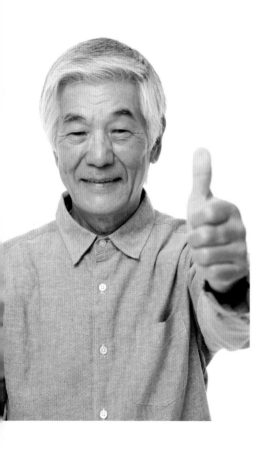

10. Enjoy Being a Nonsmoker

Once you're a nonsmoker, you have achieved an incredible life goal. You reversed something that you likely began as a teenager or young adult. You will now begin to reap the benefits. Enjoy deep breaths, fresh air and better health!

Enjoy a whiter smile

Visit a dental hygienist. Get a teeth cleaning to remove that cigarette tar build-up.

Reward yourself

Watch your savings grow! Use a jar to deposit your daily or weekly cigarette money. Consider rewarding yourself along the way or save your money for something larger. Whatever you decide, you earned it!

Celebrate your success

After 30 days, celebrate a smoke-free month. Then, look forward to celebrating your first year anniversary of being a nonsmoker.

Congratulations!

Step 4: Prevent Infections

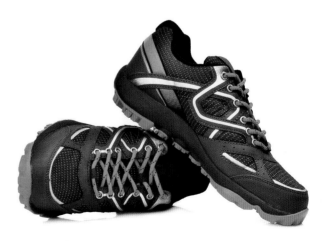

Keep Your Feet Healthy

People with diabetes can have foot problems.
Learn why you are at risk on pages 29–32.

Learn why you are at risk on pages 29–32.

⚠ WARNING
Signs of Infection

- Redness, which can spread, moving from the toe up the foot or from the foot up the leg
- Any unusual swelling or warmth
- Oozing pus
- Unusual pain (although there may be no pain)
- Fever, chills or fatigue
- Any part of your foot or leg turning a darker color or changing color
- Sudden unexplained increase in your blood sugar

1. See a Doctor Right Away if Your Toe or Foot Is Infected

An infection can spread quickly. If you can't get an appointment with your doctor within a day or two, go to a clinic or your hospital's emergency room.

Note the two images below. The picture of the foot on the left shows an infection of the skin called cellulitis. In this case, the skin is warm, red, and swollen. The infection probably began when a bacteria called staphylococcus (commonly referred to as staph) entered the foot through small cracks in the skin. Often this bacteria is resistant to several antibiotics. Treatment must be given right away. Often the medical team uses antibiotics given in the hospital through an intravenous (IV).

The picture of the foot on the right shows redness just around the big toe. Blood around the toenail is a sign that the infection started with an injury. Even though the pain and redness appears localized (limited to the toe), there could be a more serious infection deep beneath the skin that must be drained.

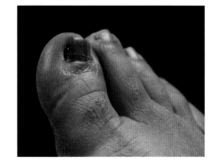

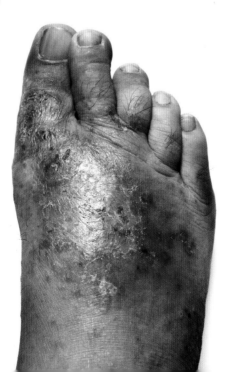

2. Maintain Good Blood Sugar, Blood Pressure and Blood Cholesterol

If you maintain good blood sugar, good blood pressure and good blood cholesterol, you are less likely to get a foot infection. Here are three things you can do to help you reach those goals:

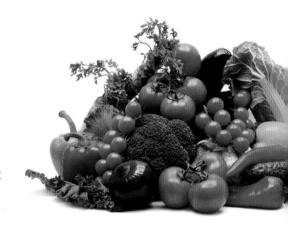

Eat well

The foods you eat make a big difference to your blood sugar and circulation. Drinking alcohol can increase your blood pressure, so be careful. If you need to lose weight, try cutting back gradually on portions. Weight loss will reduce the weight on the soles of your feet. It also improves blood sugar, blood pressure and blood cholesterol.

Become more physically active

Here are specific tips to improve circulation to your feet.

- If you've been sitting for an hour, get up and walk around.
- Pedal an exercise bike.
- Wiggle your toes.
- Do ankle rotations (page 223). Also, move your feet, up and down and side to side.
- Do chair exercises (page 232).
- If your feet swell, raise your feet when you sit or lie down.
- Don't sit with your legs or feet crossed. This reduces circulation and compresses nerves.
- Gently massage your feet if they are cold.

Become a nonsmoker

Smoking significantly narrows blood vessels and decreases blood flow to the feet. It also reduces healing. As a smoker, having diabetes means you are at higher risk for foot problems and amputations.

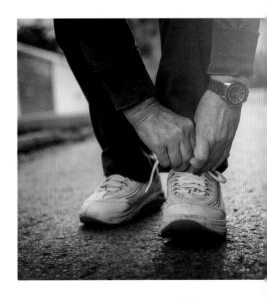

STOP INFECTIONS

⚠️ **CAUTION**
Look for redness, blisters or sores, swelling, dryness, cracks or a change in shape. Be aware of anything that wasn't there yesterday. Check the top and bottom of each foot and between your toes.

3. Check Your Feet Every Day

You may have lost feeling in your feet, so look and touch your feet with your hands daily. Catch infections early.

Check your feet at the same time every day. For example, check after your bath or shower, or before bed. Checking your feet will become a good habit!

If it's difficult for you to look at the bottom of each foot, try one of these options:

- Hold a mirror or put a mirror on the floor. You can buy a special mirror with a long handle to look at the bottom of your feet.
- Sit on a chair in front of a full-length mirror. Put your foot on a stool and look in the mirror.
- Extend your leg backward with the top of your foot flat on the floor. Look back at the sole of your foot.
- Get help from a family member, friend or home care support person.

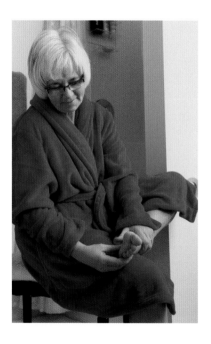

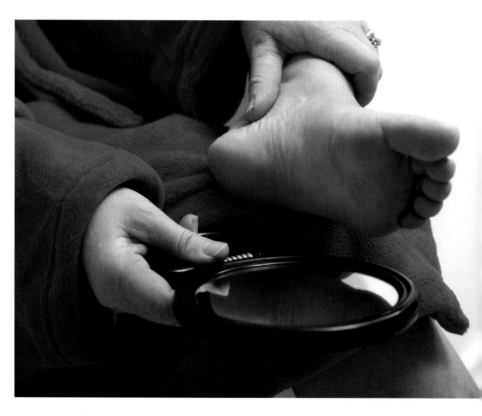

Is it difficult for you to see your feet?

Many people who are visually impaired learn to check their feet by carefully feeling them. However, you could still miss a problem area. It's best if you have someone help you.

What to look for when checking your feet

Redness or color change

- Bruising, or areas that are white, darkened or red
- Red streaks
- Skin that lightens for a few seconds after being pressed and released. This could mean decreased circulation.

Swelling

This is a sign of poor circulation or infection.

Cold or hot spots

- A cold spot can mean an area is not getting enough circulation.
- A hot spot could mean an infection underneath your skin. This could turn into a blister or sore.
- Is one foot warmer or cooler than the other?

Sensation changes

You might feel "pins and needles," a numbness or burning in your feet that can mean decreased nerve function. Your feet may feel like "blocks of wood."

See pages 29–32 for more information on what these changes can look like.

Cracks, bleeding, sores or ulcers, or blisters

- Dry skin can cause cracks in your skin, typically on your heel.
- Tight shoes, irritation or dry skin can cause a blister, cut or sore.
- Look between your toes for cracks, cuts or athlete's foot (flaky, red or white areas with itching and cracking).
- Pus or bad odor is a sign of an infection.

An ulcer is an open wound or sore with severe skin breakdown.

Changes to toenails

- Ingrown toenails will look red and bleeding at the edge of the nail. Tight shoes or bad nail trimming can cause this.
- Toenails that are thick, brittle and yellowish-green may have a fungus infection under the nails. It usually starts in the corner or end of the nail.
- If the whole toenail is discolored, this may be due to poor circulation, which means a lack of oxygen to the toe.

Corns

A corn is a small, round hard spot on the top of your toe, or it could be a thickened but softer spot between your toes.

Most corns occur because of friction from a tight, poorly fitting shoe.

STOP INFECTIONS

271

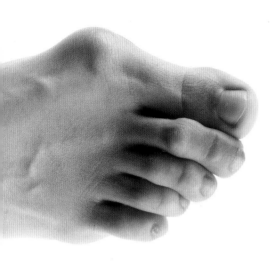

Bunion

Calluses

A callus is thickened skin on the side or bottom of your foot. A callus is usually larger and flatter than a corn. Like corns, friction causes calluses. Pressure on the bottom of your foot also causes this. An infection can develop underneath a callus or corn.

Changes to the shape of your foot

Bone changes happen more gradually. You may develop a bunion, or a change in the arch of your foot. Arches allow your foot to absorb pressure as you walk. When the arch is lost, pressure points develop on your foot. Hammertoes (toes that rise up at the knuckle) are another foot change that might happen.

Loss of hair

If you have less hair growth, or hair stops growing on your feet or lower legs, it could mean reduced oxygen flow and nerve damage.

4. Ask Your Doctor or Nurse to Check Your Feet

Your health care provider should check your feet once a year. Get checked more often if you have foot problems.

Whenever you have an appointment for medical concerns, take off your socks and shoes while waiting for your doctor or nurse. That way, you won't forget to get your feet checked too.

What will my doctor or nurse check?

A doctor or nurse will check the same things that you look for, such as cracks, sores, color changes and swelling, and how your feet look and feel.

- They may check your nerve sensation on top of your big toe or on the bottom of your feet, using either a monofilament or a tuning fork. These tests don't hurt at all.
- They may test circulation, by measuring the pulses in your feet or legs.
- They may check your blood pressure in your legs or feet. If it is lower than the blood pressure in your arms, that means there is reduced blood flow to the legs or feet.

Checking for nerve sensation using a monofilament

5. Wash, Dry and Moisturize Your Feet

Gently wash your feet every day

- Wash your feet with mild soap every day. Use warm but not hot water.
- When taking a shower or bath, check with your elbow or wrist that the water isn't too hot. This is important! If you have nerve damage on your feet, you may not realize the water is too hot.
- When cleaning your tub, use soap or baking soda, and rinse well. Do not use bleach or harsh cleaners.
- If you have an open sore, check with your nurse or doctor about whether you should put your foot in water.

Dry your feet with care

- After a shower or bath, dry both your feet — top and bottom and between the toes. This prevents fungus and germs, which need moisture to grow.

Moisturize dry feet

- Put moisturizing lotion or cream, such as a hand moisturizer, on dry or cracked areas. Gently work it in. Avoid putting lotion between your toes, or on cuts or open sores. Common moisturizer brands are Nivea, Vaseline Intensive Care, Aveeno and lanolin-based creams. Vaseline is also an option. Strongly perfumed creams aren't a good idea. They often have an alcohol base, which dries the skin.
- Apply cream every day, or twice a day, to get rid of or reduce dryness. If after several weeks, the lotion hasn't helped, your doctor or nurse may recommend a diabetic lotion with urea, which occurs naturally in your body. When added to lotions, urea helps to smooth out and soften dry scaly skin.
- Try using a lotion at night after your bath or shower and after you have dried your feet. Then put on a pair of loose-fitting socks. The moisturizer will continue to work as you sleep.
- Chlorine in swimming pools can dry your skin. Also, you can get athlete's foot (fungus) and plantar's warts from public showers and swimming pools. Wear water shoes (aqua socks) at the pool to protect your feet. After swimming, wash, dry and then moisturize your feet and skin.

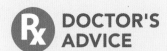

DOCTOR'S ADVICE

If you have dry feet, don't soak your feet, or limit to no more than 10 minutes. Soaking removes natural oils and dries out your feet. Dry, scaly skin is more likely to get cracks and sores.

STOP INFECTIONS

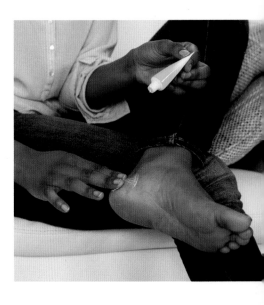

6. Trim Your Toenails Properly

Carefully cut or file your toenails straight across the top of your toe, and not too short.

- Use nail clippers or a nail file rather than scissors. You may be more likely to cut your toe with scissors.
- Cut or file your toenails straight across. Gently file any sharp edges with a nail file or emery board. This will help avoid ingrown toenails. Properly fitting shoes also help prevent ingrown toenails.
- Do not cut your nails too short.
- It's easier to cut toenails after washing or a bath, as your nails are softer. If you have thick toenails, this is especially helpful.
- You should cut your toenails regularly, at least every four to six weeks.

Get help with nail cutting if you need it.

See a foot care nurse or podiatrist (foot doctor) for regular toenail trimming if:

- You've lost feeling in your feet
- You can't see or reach your feet.
- Your nails are thick and difficult to cut.
- Your hands are shaky.
- You have ingrown toenails.

Many senior centers employ foot nurses who are experienced in cutting toenails. You may have to pay for this, but it's worth it to save your feet.

Ask your doctor or diabetes educator to recommend a nurse with training in diabetes foot care.

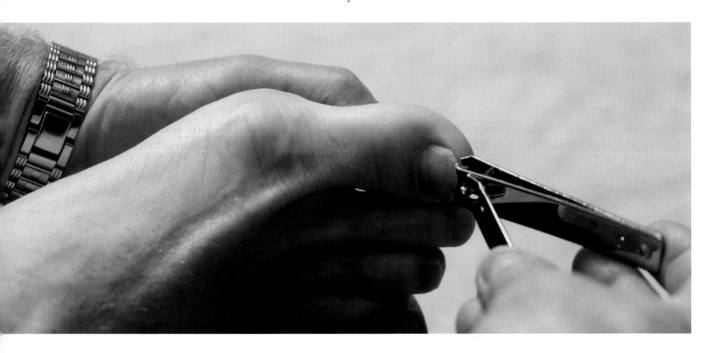

7. Do Not Use Heaters, Razors or Chemicals

If you lack feeling in your feet, you can't tell if something is too hot. You also may do damage to your feet with pedicure tools and chemicals.

Heat

- Avoid using heating pads and electric blankets on your feet, as they might overheat.
- Don't put your feet close to a fireplace or radiator.

Razors, knives or chemicals

Never use sharp razors, knives, corn plasters or wart removal chemicals on your feet to remove calluses, corns or warts.

- Some people are tempted to use a metal grater on their feet, or to shave or cut off calluses, corns or warts using a razor or knife. This can be dangerous. One little slip and you can cut yourself and get an open sore. Also, sometimes there can actually be a sore or infection underneath a hard callus. This makes cutting or filing very risky.
- Corn plasters can rip your skin. Wart removal products can cause open sores that might get infected.
- See your doctor, foot care nurse or podiatrist about how to treat calluses, corns or warts that won't go away. See page 280 about home treatment for minor concerns.

Nail polish

If you have discolored toenails, you may be tempted to hide them under dark nail polish. However, dark nail polish left on for many days could hide a growing infection, so remove the polish after a day or two. Wash your toes with soapy water to remove all traces of the nail polish remover.

Take care to avoid nicks and cuts if shaving

If shaving with a razor, moisten and lather your skin with unscented soap or shaving cream. Be careful. Don't shave an area with any blisters or boils. You could break the skin and cause an infection.

Instead of shaving, some people remove hair in other ways such as threading or leg waxing. For threading, go to a reputable salon. If you easily get infections, it is best to avoid chemical hair removal products, waxing, sugaring and laser hair removal. These processes may cause tiny cuts or burns to your skin. Cuts are slower to heal when you have diabetes, which means you are more likely to get a skin infection.

Never fill a hot water bottle with boiling water and put it directly next to your skin. Check the water with your wrist to make sure it isn't too hot. Wearing socks is a safe way to keep your feet warm.

Both diabetes and getting older can result in some damage to the nerves that go to your hair follicles. This reduces hair growth, for example, on your legs and toes. Women who've had diabetes for a while often say they no longer need to shave their legs.

STOP INFECTIONS

Most foot injuries happen in your house! Protect your feet. Wear shoes and socks both in the house and outside.

8. Wear Comfortable Socks and Shoes that Fit Well

Shoes and socks play an important role in protecting your toes and feet from an infection. A shoe that is tight and squeezes the side of your foot can create an injury point that can later become infected. A worn sock with a hole or no padding won't protect the bottom of your foot or your toe, which then can rub and a sore can develop. The cost of shoes and socks is a lot less than the cost of having a foot amputated.

Socks

Clean and comfortable

- Wear clean socks that fit. These protect your feet from rubbing. This is important when walking.
- If you like, wear pantyhose but avoid elasticized knee highs.
- If your legs swell, you may need socks that are wide at the top or have loose elastic ribbing so that your circulation isn't restricted.

Cotton, wool or cotton-acrylic blends

- Cotton or wool socks are good, as they are natural fibers and absorb moisture.
- Good quality athletic socks, often a blend of cotton and acrylic, are good for walking or sports.

Limit lumps and bumps

- Get rid of any old or mended socks with lumps or bumps that might cause irritation.
- Wear the correct size socks. If socks are too small, they will squeeze seams into your foot. If they're too large, the extra fabric will rub against your feet.
- If your skin is thin and fragile, buy socks with no seams to keep them from rubbing. If your socks have seams, try wearing them inside out so the seams are on the outside.

Padded socks

- These pads cushion the soles of your feet.

Dry and warm

- If your feet sweat a lot, change into a dry pair of socks when necessary.
- Wear warm socks to bed (and during the day) if your feet get cold.
- During cold weather, wear warm socks in your boots.

White socks

If you have a bleeding hangnail or sore, the blood will show on a white sock. This will alert you to take care of it.

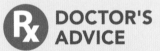 **DOCTOR'S ADVICE**

In certain situations your doctor may recommend you wear support hose for varicose veins, or compression stockings for swelling in legs or feet. In some cases these are recommended to reduce a risk of a blood clot in your leg.

Start with a less tight hose or stocking. These can be difficult to put on and take off. Ask a nurse to show you how.

Shoes

- Look in your shoes, feel inside, and quickly shake them out before you put them on. Make sure there are no cracks, rough seams, pebbles or grit inside.
- On hot days, don't walk barefoot on cement or on a deck. You may not feel the heat on the soles of your feet. You could get a burn or splinter.
- At the beach, wear rubber-soled shoes. These protect your feet from hot sand, sharp shells and sunburn. Apply sunscreen to any parts of your feet and body exposed to sun. Check to see that sand doesn't rub against your feet and between your toes.
- In cold weather, wear warm dry socks and waterproof boots to prevent frostbite.
- Buy a good quality athletic or walking shoe. If your foot changes shape, you may need a specialty or prescription shoe.
- It's good to have more than one pair of shoes, so you don't wear the same pair every day.

At the shoe store, make sure your shoes fit well.

- Shop for shoes in the afternoon or evening. This is when your feet are generally the most swollen, so you'll choose shoes that aren't too tight.
- Try on both shoes. Stand up and walk around. Shoes should be comfortable the first time you try them on. They shouldn't rub or pinch. There should be enough room at the toe.
- Follow the same steps above if you buy shoes online.
- Wear new shoes for less than two hours at first. Check your feet afterward to make sure there are no red areas if the shoes are rubbing.
- When you try on shoes at the shoe store, it's sometimes hard to feel if your foot or toes are being forced into the shoe. One good solution is to stand on the removable insoles and see if your feet fit inside. Some shoes don't have a removable insole, so it's a good idea to bring along an outline of your foot (see sidebar).

Three tips so you don't stub your toe at home:

1. Wear a pair of hard-toed slippers or house shoes.
2. Leave a night-light on in case you need to go to the bathroom.
3. Pick up any odds and ends lying on the floor.

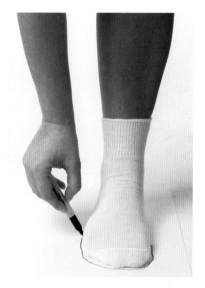

You may want to measure your feet before you go to the shoe store.

At the end of the day, stand on a piece of paper or card stock and draw around your foot. Cut this out and take it with you with you to the shoe store. Place the paper or cardboard inside the shoe, or on top of a removable insole, to see if it fits.

277

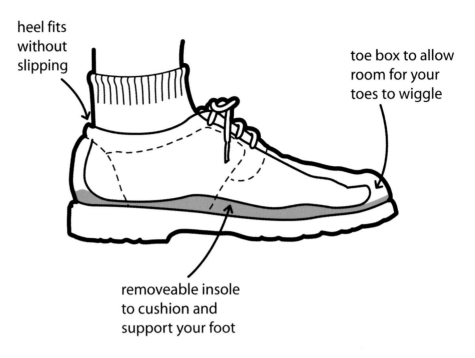

heel fits without slipping

toe box to allow room for your toes to wiggle

removeable insole to cushion and support your foot

- Shoes shouldn't feel too tight. Allow room to wiggle your toes with a deep and wide toe box. Your longest toe should be a finger-width away from the top of the shoe. You will need the shoes to be wide enough to fit bunions or angular bones.
- Leather or canvas upper material is breathable and is a good choice.
- A good insole cushions the bottom of your feet and absorbs the jolts of walking.
- Choose shoes with removable insoles. You can replace them when they wear out. You can also remove the insoles that came with your shoe, and insert a more cushioned insole or an orthotic. Make sure there is still wiggle room for your toes.
- Avoid heels higher than 2 inches (5 cm). High heels increase the pressure on your toes and the ball of your foot.
- Avoid shoes with bare seams or bulges on the inside which may rub your feet.
- Laces, Velcro or buckles are better choices than slip-on shoes. They help to keep your feet firmly in the shoes because you can adjust the fit. Tighten or loosen them if your shoes or feet change shape.

Orthotics or specialty shoes

Orthotics

Orthotics are insoles made from foam or hard plastic that you put in your shoes to provide support. You can buy orthotics over the counter. There are also custom-made ones, which are more expensive but specially designed for your feet problems. Properly sized orthotics help with pain in your feet, and support fallen arches, bunions or curled toes. Orthotics can also relieve a skin irritation, an ulcer or callus.

Modified shoes

A specialty shoe shop can sometimes modify your existing shoes to relieve a pressure point. This is usually less expensive than buying custom shoes. For example, they could cut open your shoe at a pressure point and attach Velcro straps.

Custom shoes

If you have a foot that is difficult to fit, you may need to order custom shoes. A specialist will make the shoe specifically for you.

Go to a foot doctor (podiatrist or chiropodist) or a specialty shoe store for orthotics, shoe modifications or custom shoes. Ask your doctor for a referral. Some health plans covers this.

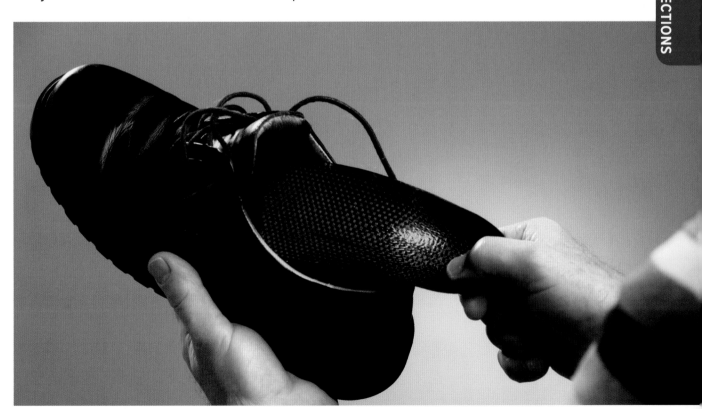

An orthotic is only as good as the shoe that it is in.

STOP INFECTIONS

> ⚠️ **CAUTION**
> A minor injury can become an emergency for a person with diabetes. Go see a doctor right away if you think you have an infection — example, a cut with a red area around it.
>
> If a piece of glass or a nail is stuck in your foot, see a doctor right away.
>
> Avoid or limit walking on an injured foot; give it time to heal.

> If your skin is fragile, a bandage could rip your skin when removed. In this case, hold the dressing in place by wrapping it with gauze, or attach the bandage or tape to the gauze and not your skin. Or use paper tape (sold in drugstores), which is less sticky.

> Keep your cut or blister clean and dry.

9. Take Care of Small Concerns at Home

Corns or calluses

- It's important to remove the source of the pressure that causes you to develop the corn or callus in the first place. This may require you to change shoes, or alter or put an insole or orthotic in your shoe.
- To soften a callus, apply moisturizer first, but not between your toes. If needed, *gently* rub the callus with a moistened pumice stone. Do this once or twice a week.
- Talk to your doctor or diabetes nurse about corns or calluses that won't go away or are getting worse.

Cracks in the skin of dry feet

- Wash your feet and gently dry them.
- Then put on a moisturizer every day, twice a day if needed.
- If the cracks are deep, see your doctor or nurse. They may recommend an antiseptic or antibiotic cream. They may also recommend you temporarily avoid walking on the injured foot.

Small cut or sore

- Wash with mild soap in warm water. Avoid rubbing alcohol, salt, vinegar, iodine or other ointments or antiseptics unless recommended by your doctor. These harsh antiseptics are drying and can slow the healing of a cut. The best treatment is soap and water.
- Cover with a dry sterile dressing or bandage.
- Wash and cover twice daily. Each time, look to see if it's healing or if there are signs of infection.

Moist, pale or crinkly skin between or under your toes

- After washing, gently dry between your toes with a towel or clean tissue.

Blister

- Don't burst the blister. Wash it with soap and water, pat it dry gently, and cover with a sterile dressing.
- If it bursts on its own, gently squeeze out the fluid, then wash, dry, and cover.

10. Get Medical Care for an Open Foot Wound

Get your foot doctor or foot care nurse to treat any open foot wound, commonly called an ulcer. What might they do?

- **Advise you to take weight off the wound.** This may be as simple as wearing a different pair of shoes, or using insoles or orthotics in your shoes. If the wound or infection is on the bottom of your foot, your doctor may ask you to use a pair of crutches or temporarily use a wheelchair. With more serious wounds, the doctor may have you rest in bed or put a cast on your foot to remove all pressure on the ulcer.
- **Give you an antibiotic,** if it's infected. Take the full dose prescribed, even if the sore looks healed.
- **Clean the wound** to examine what's underneath and to allow it to heal from the inside out.
- **Apply sterile dressings, medicated ointments, antiseptics or tissue healing products.**
- **Prescribe pain medication,** if needed.
- **Change your insulin or diabetes pills.** If your blood sugar is up, it's very difficult to get rid of an infection because germs grow on the extra sugar. The doctor may increase your dosage of insulin or diabetes meds. If you aren't on insulin, you may temporarily need some.
- **Change your heart or blood pressure medications** to improve blood flow to the wound.
- **Tell you that you may need surgery** to improve blood flow. Your doctor may refer you to a vascular surgeon or foot doctor.

Once healed, you can prevent another infection or wound with:

- Ongoing diabetes management to improve blood sugar
- Daily foot checks and proper foot care
- New shoes, insoles or orthotics, if the wound was due to your shoes being too tight or worn out
- Surgery to correct the shape of your foot
- Surgery on the blood vessels that go to your feet, to increase the blood flow and healing

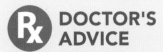

DOCTOR'S ADVICE

Some wounds (ulcers) take time to heal
Foot wounds may take a long time to heal, sometimes six months, a year or more. Closely follow your doctor's advice to ensure complete treatment and healing.

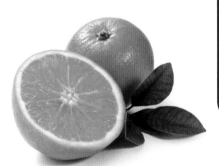

Nutrition for healing
Good nutrition helps improve immunity and aid healing of infections. Include protein at every meal, drink lots of water and eat foods rich in vitamin C, vitamin A and zinc, (see pages 132–133). If you have an infection, your doctor might recommend you take a vitamin and mineral supplement.

STOP INFECTIONS

281

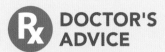

DOCTOR'S ADVICE

As with foot problems, you can prevent skin problems with good blood sugar levels, exercise, washing and skin care. Some skin problems are rare and hard to diagnose. If you have a skin problem that doesn't improve, talk to your doctor, or see a dermatologist (a doctor who specializes in diagnosis and skin care). Your doctor may prescribe medications or treatment.

What kind of soap should I use?

Some people find that soaps with added oils (such as Dove) are less drying to skin. Strongly perfumed soaps or deodorant soaps can dry or irritate your skin.

Corticosteroid creams

Your doctor may prescribe a corticosteroid cream or pill. This may be given for just a short time, as they can increase your blood sugar.

Good Skin Care

Learn why you are at risk for skin problems on page 42.

Here are some tips for good skin care.

Limit showers or baths to 10 minutes

Have a daily shower or bath. Don't use bath salts or Epsom salt, as as they make your skin dry. Check the shower or bath water to make sure it's not too hot.

Dry your skin well

Prevent fungus and yeast infections by avoiding excess moisture on your skin. If your home is hot and humid, an air conditioner helps. After bathing, dry your skin, especially in moist areas where skin touches skin. For example, the groin, in the armpits, under breasts or at your waist, and your feet. Some people find it helpful to dust these areas with cornstarch-based powders or creams. (Cornstarch-based products may be safer than talk, which may contain asbestos.) If this doesn't help, you can use non-perfumed antiperspirants in skin folds. For women, if the rash is under the breasts, wear a clean supportive bra to hold up your breasts.

Apply moisturizers to dry skin

This includes your heels, elbows and hands. Wear rubber gloves when using harsh cleaning agents, solvents, bleach or hot water. Remember to drink lots of water which keeps your whole body, including your skin, hydrated. Use a humidifier in your home in the cold dry months if your house is dry.

Your doctor may recommend skin ointments

The type of ointment will depend on the cause of your specific condition, such as fungus or bacteria.

Avoid excess sun exposure and tanning

Some sun exposure, for example, 15 to 30 minutes a day while walking, helps your body make vitamin D and can be healthy for your skin. However, too much sun in the middle of the day (generally between 10 am and 2 pm) is unhealthy.

Treat cuts right away

Clean minor cuts right away, just as with foot infections. See your doctor if you have a skin problem that isn't healing on its own.

Ten Tips for Mouth Care

Learn why you are at risk for
gum disease on pages 43–45.

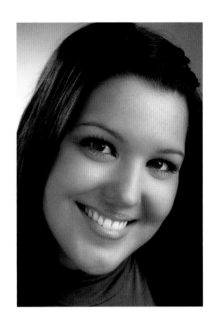

1. Know your ABCs

Take steps to achieve a good A1C (good blood sugar), good
Blood pressure and blood Cholesterol. (Read about these lab
tests on pages 302–303.) These things help your blood vessels
and nerves stay healthy and reduce your risk for infection.
When your blood sugar is high, bacterial and yeast infections
in your mouth cannot heal.

2. If you smoke, quit

If you've struggled with smoking in the past, please give
it another try. See Chapter 3 to learn more about quitting
smoking. It can take several tries before you manage to stop
smoking for good.

If you smoke, you are more at risk for cancer on your lips, the
sides of your tongue and the floor of your mouth. Check your
mouth once a week to make sure there are no lumps, bumps,
red spots or sores. Report any changes to your doctor.

3. Walk and move daily

Exercise helps improve blood sugar. It also keeps the mouth's
blood vessels and nerves healthy.

4. Eat well

Eat less sugary foods. Drink less or stop drinking soft drinks
and juice. Eating smaller portions helps reduce your blood
sugar. Good nutrition helps infections heal.

There are foods especially good for your gums and teeth:

- Milk and milk products have calcium, vitamin D and
  phosphorus. These nutrients build strong teeth and a
  strong jaw bone to support your teeth. They reduce
  the acid in your mouth that comes from other foods.
- Vitamin C, found in fruits and vegetables, is important
  for healing gums.

Fruits and vegetables
have another important
role. As you chew these
foods, the roughness of
the food fiber acts like a
toothbrush to break up
particles of food
between your teeth.
These foods also
stimulate your mouth
glands to make more
saliva. This helps to wash
away bits of food,
helping to clean
your teeth.

STOP INFECTIONS

Sugar-free candies or sugar-free gum

For a product to be sugar-free and safe for your teeth, it should have no dextrose, sucrose, maltose, fructose or any word ending in "ose." These are all forms of sugar.

5. Drink water

Rinse your mouth well with water after brushing and flossing. Also, rinse your mouth or brush your teeth after eating these sticky, sweet or acidic foods:

- Candies, toffees or fruit roll-ups
- Any foods that can get stuck in your back teeth (molars) like potato chips or stuck between teeth like strands of meat or chicken
- Fresh and dried fruits, fruit and vegetable juices, tomato sauces, ketchup and vinegar are acidic
- Carbonated soft drinks (regular and diet) and sports drinks

At the end of a meal or snack, a small piece of cheese, a small glass of milk or a piece of sugarless gum made with xylitol can help reduce acid in your mouth. However, this is not a substitute for rinsing your mouth or brushing your teeth.

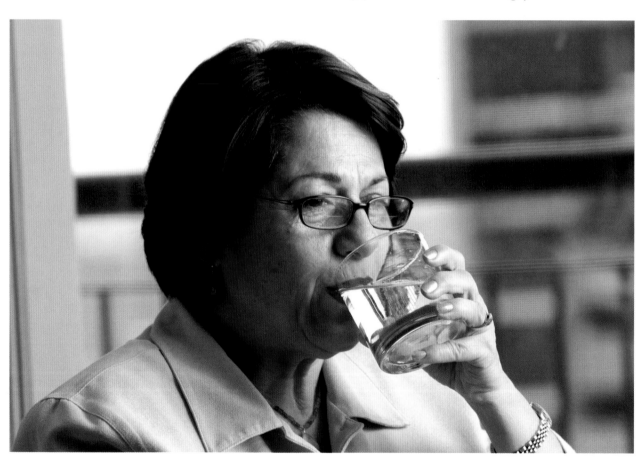

Fluoride is important for hardening tooth enamel and keeping your teeth healthy.

If your tap water does not have fluoride added, ask your dentist about options.

6. Brush

- Brush two to three times each day.
- Use a toothbrush marked "extra soft" or "soft." Overbrushing is a significant cause of gum damage.
- Buy a new toothbrush at least three times a year.
- Put your toothbrush bristles where your gums and teeth meet, at your gum line. Gently massage or vibrate and move the bristles up, away from your gums. Brushing gently and properly is important — if you brush too hard, or up and down, this will damage your gums.
- Brush the inside, outside and chewing surfaces of your teeth. Make sure you brush all your teeth, including your back teeth. Don't forget to brush your tongue.
- The most important time to brush is before going to bed.
- An electric toothbrush is a great option!

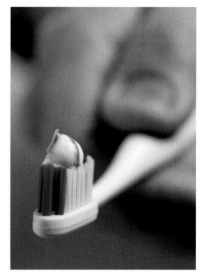

Use a pea-size drop of fluoride toothpaste. After use, keep your toothbrush standing up and not touching another toothbrush. Don't share toothbrushes!

7. Floss

- Floss once a day.
- Floss cleans between the teeth where your toothbrush bristles don't reach, and helps remove plaque.
- The best time to floss is at bedtime before you brush.
- Use a piece of floss that is about 18 inches (45 cm) long.
- Wrap the floss around your middle fingers. Curve the floss around one tooth at a time and move the floss up and down, gently cleaning just under the gumline.

8. Care for your dentures

If you have any of these concerns:

- Rinse your mouth and dentures after every meal if possible.
- If you wear a partial denture, remember to brush and floss your natural teeth.
- Always take your dentures out at night or sometime during the day for four to six hours. This rests your gums. When you've taken out your dentures, do the following:
  1. Brush them with a denture brush and rinse with cool water. Toothpaste is too abrasive.
  2. Soak them in a commercial cleaner or in a solution of 1 tsp (5 mL) of vinegar and 1 cup (250 mL) of water. Rinse them well with water before you put them back in your mouth.
- If your dentures don't fit properly or cause sores, talk to your denturist or dentist.

If your dentures have metal parts, ask your dentist or denturist what soaking solution to use.

STOP INFECTIONS

Is the cost of dental care too expensive? Find out if there is a dental hygiene training school nearby, or perhaps a public dental clinic where care may be more affordable.

9. Visit your dental hygienist every six months

Go even if you think your mouth is healthy. She will examine your mouth and clean your teeth to remove plaque. Fluoride may also be applied to your teeth. She will tell you when you need to see the dentist. Sometimes the dentist will recommend x-rays to look for problems that otherwise can't be seen. This helps the dentist know whether you have gum disease, tooth decay or another mouth problem.

If you have gum disease, your dental hygienist or dentist may give you an anaesthetic to numb your gums, and then and do deep cleaning around your gums. In some cases, gum surgery might be recommended to improve receding gums.

Check your blood sugar when at the dentist office

Do this before you have gum treatment or a tooth pulled. If your blood sugar is too high, your dentist or dental hygienist may rebook your appointment for a day when your blood sugar is better. Having dental treatments when your blood sugar is high may increase your risk of getting an infection. If your blood is low, then treat it before settling into the chair.

Rx DOCTOR'S ADVICE

If you have a gum infection, your doctor may temporarily adjust your insulin or meds to reduce your blood sugar. Take the full dose of antibiotics prescribed for you when you have an infection.

10. See your dentist or doctor if you have any of these concerns:

- Your gums are swollen and red, and bleed regularly.
- Your gums or teeth ache.
- Your gums are pulling away from your teeth.
- When you press your gums, puss comes out.
- You see white patches on your gums or tongue: this could mean you have "thrush," which is a type of fungus infection.
- You have loose teeth.
- You develop sores on your gums from dentures.
- You have bad breath, regardless of what you eat.

Avoid Urinary Tract Infections

Symptoms of UTIs are listed on page 46.
Learn why you are at risk for a UTI on pages 46–48.

If you have an untreated urinary tract infection (UTI), it can increase your blood sugar and become a serious problem.

Treatment

Go to the doctor

Go see your doctor if you have UTI symptoms that won't go away. For women, this includes symptoms of a vaginal infection. Your doctor may diagnose your UTI based on your symptoms, or may order urine or blood tests. You may have either a bacterial or yeast infection. Especially for recurrent UTIs, women may need a pelvic exam to rule out any underlying causes of UTIs. Men may need a rectal exam so the doctor can feel the size of the prostate.

Take medication to treat the infection

For a UTI, your doctor will usually prescribe an antibiotic. If your symptoms don't clear up after you finish the medication, see your doctor again. You may need a different medication, or additional tests.

Unfortunately, antibiotics kill off "good bacteria" as well as "bad bacteria." Taking antibiotics may lead to a vaginal yeast infection. If you have a yeast infection, your doctor will suggest an over-the-counter or prescription medication. While taking the medicine to treat a yeast infection, avoid having sex. This helps healing and may prevent your partner from getting the infection.

Improve your blood sugar

For people with diabetes, infections are more common because of high blood sugar. Although medication treats the UTI, the benefit may only be temporary. If your blood sugar remains high, the infection can return once you finish the medication. To improve your blood sugar, you may need a change in your diabetes medication, or a temporary addition of insulin. You may also need to improve your diet and exercise. Eating healthy foods in the right amounts and being active are important. Doing this improves your blood sugar a well as your ability to fight infection.

Why people with diabetes might get a UTI

With high blood sugar, extra sugar spills into your urine.

▼

Germs feed on sugar in the urine.

▼

Infection develops.

▼

Blood sugars get even higher.

STOP INFECTIONS

To treat UTIs in older women, a doctor may prescribe a low-dose estrogen cream to apply to the vagina.

Follow your doctor or pharmacist's instructions.
Take the medicine for the amount of time recommended, even if the symptoms go away. If it's an over-the-counter drug, follow the package instructions.

DOCTOR'S ADVICE

Take time to look after yourself! You reduce your immunity to infection when you're feeling worn down, stressed, eating poorly or not exercising. This makes you more likely to get sick. That includes UTIs.

UTI prevention tips for women

Maintain good blood sugar levels.

Drink lots of water, so that your urine is a pale color. Try six to eight 8-oz/250 mL glasses a day.

Pee regularly. Don't wait until your bladder feels full. Try peeing at least every two hours during the day. Try to fully empty your bladder each time. Combined with drinking water, this helps flush germs out of your bladder. Always pee after intercourse.

Wipe front-to-back. After you go to the toilet, wipe yourself front-to-back. This will help reduce the spread of bacteria from your back end. Wash your hands afterward. If experiencing diarrhea or incontinence, take extra care to keep clean.

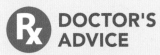

CARMEN'S STORY: UTIs no longer control my life!

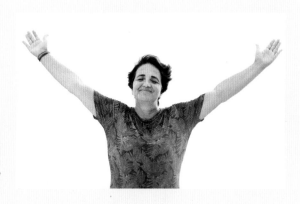

I am in my mid-40s and I've had a kidney and bladder condition since I was young, and now I have type 2 diabetes.

Pee isn't a pleasant topic, but here goes. Most of what I learned may seem like common sense, but it took time to work out a daily routine of care and then stick to it.

People like me with diabetes, we have a higher sugar content than normal in our urine. This is why we have a higher risk of UTIs, because bacteria thrive and grow on the sugar. So, the most important message I can share is that you have to stay clean and dry. Every day, before I go to work and before I go to bed, I use unscented wipes with no added moisturizer or antibiotics. Because my bladder leaks occasionally, I wear a fresh panty liner every time I use the toilet to stay dry.

Also, it's really important to empty your bladder completely, so the extra sugar doesn't stay in your bladder. Before bed, I give myself a little extra time to just relax while sitting on the toilet and then lean forward to help squeeze out one more drop.

I always look at my pee. If it's dark yellow and strong smelling, it's a reminder that I'm not drinking enough water. But if it's cloudy, even bubbly, and it smells really bad, then I know an infection has begun. I take a sample to the lab (I have containers at home), and once I get the results, then my doctor can prescribe the antibiotics I need. You too can prevent UTIs by taking special care of your body.

Healthy sex means a healthy you. Everything that touches your vagina should be clean so that you don't introduce germs. For example, this includes you and your partner's hands, a diaphragm or a vibrator. Consider showering with your partner before sex. If your partner is uncircumcised, ask him to wash under his foreskin where germs can hide. Be sure to pee after sexual activity. Peeing will flush out your urethra. If you have vaginal dryness, this can cause itchiness and friction. Consider using a sterile lubricant (see page 395), which you can buy at any pharmacy.

Using a diaphragm or a spermicide may increase your risk of a UTI. If you use these and are having recurrent UTIs, you may want to consider another birth control method. Talk to your doctor.

Keep genitals dry, clean and perfume free. If you have heavy upper legs, make sure all skin folds are dry. Shower daily, then dry well. If you prefer baths, keep it short, avoid bubble baths, and rinse off after. Be gentle. Extra washing, rubbing and the overuse of soap can lead to irritation and itchiness.

- If you're itchy, apply a cold clean cloth. Try not to scratch your genital area. It needs a chance to heal.
- If you have heavy periods, gently wipe the area with a damp tissue or damp clean cloth or commercial perfume-free wipes, then dry with a tissue. Change your sanitary pads or tampons regularly. If you use a menstrual cup, make sure the cup and your hands are clean before inserting the cup.
- If you have incontinence, change your pads regularly. Keep the area as clean and dry as possible.
- Wear clothes that breathe! Don't wear nylons or tight pants for extended periods. These don't allow air to get to your genital area. Loose clothing is a better choice. Wear cotton, or cotton-lined underwear. Try double rinsing your underwear to remove all soap. Avoid using fabric softeners.
- Avoid vaginal deodorants, scented towelettes and "feminine douches." These kill off the healthy bacteria in your vagina.

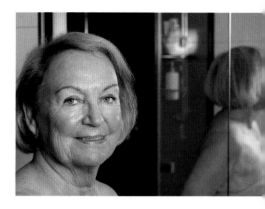

Condoms protect you from germs that cause UTIs

If your partner hasn't washed before having sex, consider using a condom. If you are sensitive to latex, look for ones made from polyurethane or polyisoprene.

STOP INFECTIONS

Other causes of vaginal itch

- Anemia: Ask your doctor to check your iron to make sure your levels aren't low. This can be caused by heavy periods.
- An allergic reaction
- A sexually transmitted infection

See your doctor if symptoms worsen.

Kegel exercises for women with leakage

After childbirth and as you get older, the pelvic floor muscles which support the uterus, bladder and bowel weaken. You may get some bladder or bowel leakage. Kegel exercises can help.

First, try this (once only) to identify the two muscle areas you need to tighten: Sit on the toilet and start to pee, then stop midstream and hold your muscles tight. Next tighten the muscles that keep you from passing gas. Breathe naturally. Hold for 5 seconds. Now relax, and finish peeing.

Now do your Kegels in proper position:

- Sit, stand or lie down; you can do them anywhere without others knowing!

- Hold your muscles for 5 seconds; do ten repetitions, three times a day.

- **Don't do more; more is not better.** Go easy; don't squeeze too hard or do Kegels more often than recommended, as this can actually strain your pelvic floor muscles.

- If you are an older woman and want to do Kegels as prevention, only do several repetitions a couple of times a week, not more.

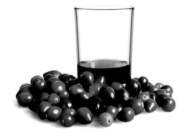

Pure cranberry juice ingredients: Cranberry juice

Cranberry compound may help reduce the growth of bacteria in the bladder. Do not drink regular cranberry juice cocktail, as it is sweetened. Instead, take one of the following daily for six months:

- $\frac{1}{4}$ cup (60 mL) pure cranberry juice (see label in sidebar), available at bulk stores or health food stores. It will be very sour, so may want to add a low-calorie sweetener.

- 1 cup (250 mL) of low-calorie cranberry juice with no added sugar. (This equals 40 calories.)

- 1,000 mg cranberry in pill form, made from powdered whole cranberries, not extract

Nutrition Facts

Per 1 cup (250 mL)

Amount	% Daily Value
Calories 75	
Fat 0 g	0 %
Saturated 0 g	0 %
Trans 0 g	
Cholesterol 0 mg	0 %
Sodium 5 mg	0 %
Carbohydrate 12 g	6 %
Fiber 1 g	4 %
Sugars 9 g	
Protein 1 g	
Vitamin A	2 %
Vitamin C	35 %
Calcium	2 %
Iron	6 %

 DOCTOR'S ADVICE

Interaction with medications

If you are taking an antibiotic, or a blood thinner such as warfarin, cranberry in large amounts may affect your medication. Talk to your doctor or pharmacist.

 CAUTION

Cranberry is not a treatment for an existing UTI.

UTI prevention tips for men

Maintain good blood sugar levels.

Drink lots of water, so that your urine is a pale color. Try six to eight 8-oz (250 mL) glasses a day.

Pee regularly. Don't wait until your bladder feels full. Try peeing at least every two hours during the day. Try to fully empty your bladder each time. This, combined with drinking water, helps flush germs out of your bladder.

Pee after sex or masturbation to flush out bacteria from the urethra.

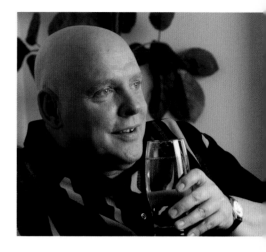

Empty your bladder fully. If you find it hard to fully empty your bladder, try sitting down when you pee, rather than standing. If you feel you cannot empty your bladder fully, tell your doctor. Ask him about options to treat it.

Shower daily. A daily shower or bath is important to keep clean, especially if you have diarrhea or incontinence.

Consider cranberry juice or pills. *Possible* benefits are listed on the previous page.

STOP INFECTIONS

Kegel exercises for men with leakage or after prostate surgery

Kegel exercises are not just for women. As men get older, their pelvic floor muscles supporting the bladder and bowel weaken. You may get some bladder or bowel leakage, or dribble after you pee. Kegel exercises done regularly can help.

First, try this (once only) to identify the two muscle areas you need to tighten. Stand (or sit) to pee. Start to pee, then stop midstream and hold your muscles tight. Next tighten the muscles that keep you from passing gas. Breathe naturally. Hold for 5 seconds. Now relax, and finish peeing.

Now do your Kegels in proper position:

- Sit, stand or lie down; you can do them anywhere without others knowing!

- Hold your muscles for 5 seconds; do ten repetitions, three times a day.

- **Don't do more; more is not better.** Go easy; don't squeeze too hard or do Kegels more often than recommended, as this can actually strain your pelvic floor muscles.

- If you are an older man and want to do Kegels as prevention, only do several repetitions a couple of times a week, not more.

Reduce Risk for Infectious Illnesses

If you do get sick, see pages 138–142 for tips on taking care of yourself when you are ill.

When you have diabetes, you can get more severe colds or flu, which are caused by viruses. Pneumonia is a more serious infection of the lungs that can be caused by viruses or bacteria.

COVID-19 is caused by a new virus called SARS-CoV-2. During the pandemic, we learned that people with diabetes were more likely to get severe COVID-19 symptoms. The COVID-19 illness was more severe in those who were older, had high blood sugar levels, and were significantly overweight.

Once you get sick, your blood sugar may rise and become more difficult to manage, so you may get sicker than someone who doesn't have diabetes. See pages 138–142 for general tips on taking care of yourself when you are ill.

Get up-to-date information from your local or national health authorities on the following: flu strains; how to reduce your exposure to viruses; how to respond if you do become exposed; and available vaccines.

Prevention

Flu and COVID-19 vaccines. These vaccines are important to help protect you from getting serious illness. All people with diabetes should get vaccinated.

Pneumonia vaccine. People with diabetes should also get the pneumococcal vaccine. You are only given this vaccine once or twice in your lifetime, depending on your age.

Social distancing, hand washing and wearing masks

To remove the germs from your hands, wash them for 15 seconds with soap and water. Give a good wash between your fingers, palms and tops, then rinse well.

The evidence from the COVID-19 pandemic has proven that social distancing, hand washing or using sanitizers, and wearing masks can help reduce the spread of airborne viruses. It is likely that certain preventive practices put in place during COVID will be maintained in the future in hospitals and long-term care and other health settings. Also some consumers may choose to continue to practice prevention, for example, eating out less in restaurants and coffee shops, avoiding large gatherings or wearing masks when traveling by airplane.

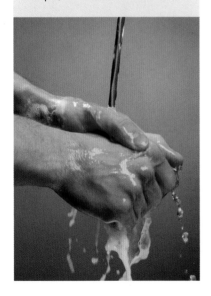

Tips to improve your immunity

Maintain good blood sugar levels. This helps your immunity.

Exercise every day to boost your immunity. Exercise helps white blood cells — the special cells that fight infection — flow throughout your body.

Drink lots of water, about 6 to 8 cups (1.5–2L). This helps flush germs out of your body. This also helps prevent dehydration, which can happen if your blood sugar is high. When you're dehydrated, tiny cracks can form inside your nose. Viruses now have an easy way of getting in your body.

Eat a healthy diet to help keep your immune system strong. For example, choose foods rich in vitamin C and A and antioxidants (like oranges, sweet peppers and broccoli). Vitamin D may also have a role in a healthy immune system. Good dietary sources of vitamin D are milk, fish and margarine. Sunlight is our best source! Taking a vitamin D supplement, at least during the winter, and especially if you have darker skin, is a good idea.

Try to get a good night's sleep. This reduces stress hormones and improves your immune system. See page 358–359 to learn more about sleep.

Limit or avoid alcohol and smoking. These make you more susceptible to illness. Also, when you are smoking or drinking, you recover more slowly.

If you feel worn down, have high blood sugar and don't look after yourself, your immunity will be low. You are more susceptible to getting sick.

STOP INFECTIONS

Tuberculosis and diabetes

Tuberculosis (TB) is a contagious bacterial lung infection. It is spread by coughing and sneezing. Research shows that people with diabetes are a lot more likely to get TB. This may be in part because of reduced immunity. Once you have TB, then blood sugar can worsen.

TB has declined across North America in the past 30 years, but it still exists. The rate of TB is higher for those with diabetes who live in overcrowded homes with poor ventilation and smoking in the home.

Signs and symptoms of TB include coughing for three or more weeks, coughing up blood, chest pain and fatigue. If you think you might have TB, see your doctor. Treatment takes six to nine months. You must take the full prescription of antibiotics and medications, even if symptoms go away.

Prevent Food Poisoning

Food poisoning comes from bacteria and germs and the toxins they release into food. Food that is not handled properly, not cooked properly, or not stored properly can quickly build up high numbers of bacteria that can make you very sick.

If you think you have indigestion or "stomach flu," you might actually have mild food poisoning. If you experience vomiting, diarrhea and fever, again, possible symptoms of a cold or flu, it might actually be severe food poisoning. It helps to think back to what you ate and where you ate in the previous 24 hours.

A complication of diabetes is a lower immune system. Your body is not able to fight off bacterial infections as quickly or efficiently as it used to. Also, if you have some reduced kidney function, your kidneys can't clear toxins as easily. To prevent food poisoning, follow the 10 safe food handling rules below, and eat out less at restaurants.

Ten safe food handling rules

1. **Wash your hands with soap,** especially after touching raw foods or touching your mouth or nose, or after going to the toilet.

2. **Keep your kitchen clean and dry,** especially countertops, dishes and utensils. Change dish cloths at least once a week and allow them to dry between uses.

3. Thaw frozen food in the fridge.

4. **Do not cross-contaminate.** Don't let raw meat or raw eggs touch cooked food. Never place cooked food on an unwashed counter, plate or cutting board.

5. **Cook meat thoroughly.** There should be no pink showing in hamburger meat or chicken.

6. **Keep hot food hot.** Germs grow when you leave foods at a warm temperature. Refrigerate or freeze hot food as quickly as possible.

7. **Keep cold food cold** at refrigerator temperature. Do not leave food sitting out on the counter.

8. **Use up leftovers quickly,** within two or four days, depending on the food.

9. **Do not eat raw eggs,** unpasteurized milk or unpasteurized cheese.

10. **Throw out bad foods.** That means, throw it out if it smells "off," doesn't look good, or you don't know how old it is or how long it has sat on the counter unrefrigerated. If in doubt, throw it out!

Why are people with diabetes more likely to get food poisoning?

- Your immunity is lower when your blood sugar is high.

- If you have had diabetes for many years, your gut may digest food more slowly, and bacteria in contaminated food can stay and grow more in your gut.

- If you have some kidney damage, your kidneys can't remove toxins as easily.

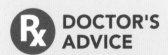 **DOCTOR'S ADVICE**

When you have diarrhea and vomiting, it's important to rest and drink lots of fluids. See your doctor if you have a high fever, or your symptoms last more than 24 hours.

Gastroparesis

This is a condition caused by diabetes where digestion in your stomach and bowel is slowed down. If you get food poisoning, the bad bacteria and toxins have a longer time to grow in your body. You can become very ill because of this.

Step 5: Take Medications and Tests

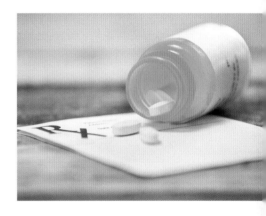

MEDS & TESTS

Appointments with Health Care Providers

When you are ill or in the hospital, the doctors and nurses are your most important health care providers. When you feel well and live with diabetes, you are the most important health care provider. Others will help you, but only you can make lifestyle changes, take your medication and seek advice from your doctor and health workers. At diagnosis, you will need to see your doctor, and ideally a dietitian, diabetes nurse, pharmacist, and optometrist. If you are not used to medical visits, this will be a lot of appointments. This is the time to learn about your diabetes. After you've had diabetes for a while, you may develop early diabetes complications. Then you may need to see other health specialists. The goal is to stay as well as possible.

Appointments at Diagnosis

Your doctor

Your doctor may want to see you regularly until your blood sugar is at a good level. Most people with type 2 diabetes continue seeing their usual doctor. However, if your diabetes is difficult to manage, your doctor may suggest you see a diabetes specialist, called an **endocrinologist**.

What's an endocrinologist?

Endocrinologists are specialists in diabetes and other hormone disorders such as thyroid conditions. Endocrinologists like author Dr. Shomali first earn a medical degree and licence to practice as a medical doctor (MD). Next they complete a three-year residency in internal medicine. And finally they complete several years of training in endocrinology.

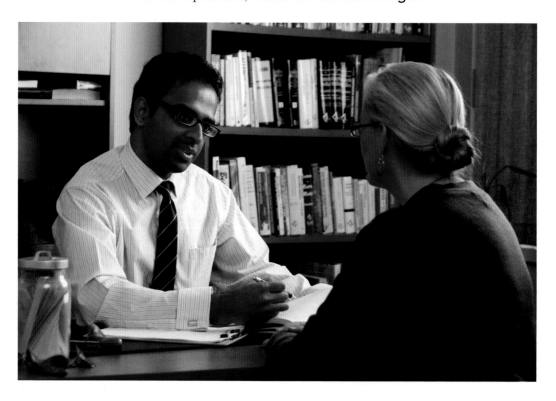

Q & A WITH DR. SHOMALI: Best use of time with your doctor

KEVIN: When I go to see my doctor, he is so busy. He doesn't seem to have enough time for me. I really like my doctor but I feel so rushed. How do I get him to answer my questions?

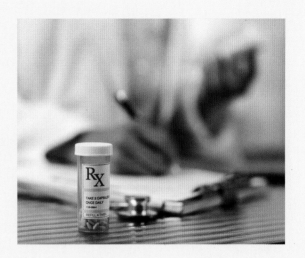

DR. SHOMALI: Kevin, feeling rushed at your doctor's visit is true for many people. Your doctor has dozens of patients to see in a day. Here are three suggestions to help you plan ahead and get the most out of your visit:

1. **Identify key concerns.** Ask yourself what are the one or two diabetes issues that are causing you the most trouble?

2. **Discuss medications.** Bring your current list of all of your prescription and over-the-counter medications as well as vitamins and other supplements that you are taking. If you are having trouble with insulin, bring the pen injection device or vials and syringes with you. I have patients whose high blood sugar is just because they take their insulin or medication the wrong way. Ask if any of your medications should be changed or discontinued. Tell your doctor about any side effects.

3. **Discuss blood sugar.** Bring your blood glucose monitor, diabetes tracking app or blood sugar log book. This is the time to talk about your readings that are unusually high or low. It is most important to note when you have good numbers and what you did right. If you are not checking your blood sugar at home, please be honest with your doctor. If you are experiencing stress at work or home, this may be affecting your blood sugar highs and lows. Your doctor can help support and encourage you to get back on track.

MEDS & TESTS

Patient "to do"
- Write your questions in your note book.
- Write the doctor's answers beside your questions.
- If you don't understand the doctor's answers, ask again.

Dr. "to do"
- Congratulate their efforts to create a list.
- Allow time for your patient to ask all questions.
- Sometimes new questions come from your answers.
- Thank them for their questions.

Dietitian and nurse

Ask your doctor to refer you to a diabetes education center or clinic. Here you will be able to see a dietitian or a nurse. They will teach you about diabetes and what you need to do to improve your blood sugar.

Dentist

See a dentist within the first six months of your diagnosis or sooner if you have concerns. Diabetes can affect your gums and teeth. A dental hygienist will clean your teeth at each visit. Regular visits are a good idea.

Pharmacist

Your pharmacist can help you learn about diabetes medications and blood sugar testing.

What is a Registered Dietitian? Is that the same as a Certified Diabetes Educator?

Author Karen Graham is both a Registered Dietitian and a Certified Diabetes Educator.

Dietitians earn a four-year science or nutrition degree, followed by a one-year dietitian training program to become a Registered Dietitian (RD).

To become a Certified Diabetes Educator (CDE), you need to have worked for at least two years in diabetes and complete an exam or certification process every five years. A variety of health care professionals can become a CDE, including nurses, dietitians and pharmacists.

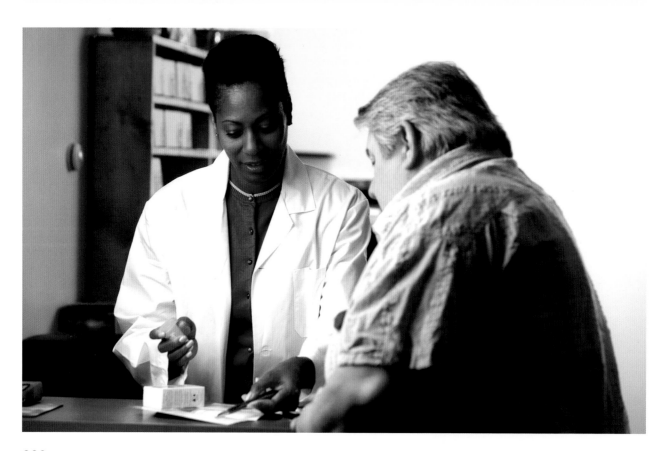

Optometrist or ophthalmologist

Make an appointment to see an optometrist for a diabetes eye check. This is called a dilated eye exam; see page 304 to learn about this exam. If your eyes are healthy, your optometrist will probably suggest you come back for another checkup in one or two years. If you get pregnant, you should also have your eyes checked during the first three months of pregnancy. Doctors need to catch eye problems *early*.

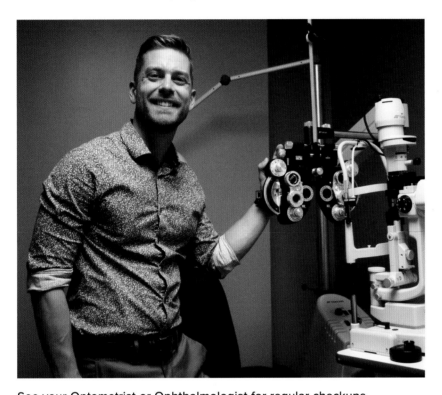

See your Optometrist or Ophthalmologist for regular checkups.

Optometrist or optician?

An optician can fit you for glasses. An optician isn't qualified to do a diabetes eye check or to check your eyes for cataracts or glaucoma. See your optometrist or ophthalmologist for this.

What's an ophthalmologist?

An ophthalmologist is a medical doctor who has special training as an eye specialist. An ophthalmologist will do laser eye surgery or other eye surgeries. You might also see an ophthalmologist for your regular diabetes eye check.

 RUTH'S STORY: High blood sugar affects your vision

About two months ago, my long-distance vision became blurry. I made an appointment to see my optometrist and I saw him later that week. He asked me if my blood sugar was running high or going up and down. I said, "Yes, my blood sugar has been high." The optometrist did an exam and found a change in my prescription. He said he was not going to give me a new prescription for my glasses ... not until my blood sugar stabilized. He suggested that I go back to see my doctor for a checkup and a review of my medications. Then I could come back to see him again in one month if my vision hadn't improved. He also said that sometimes blurry vision can have more serious causes, such as macular edema, which may require treatment by an ophthalmologist. I learned something new that day about how diabetes can affect my sight. I also had an incentive to go back to my doctor, and my dietitian. With changes and improvement in my blood sugar, sure enough, the blurriness went away. Thankfully, I didn't need to get new glasses, but I did need to pay attention to what I was eating and get out for my daily walk.

MEDS & TESTS

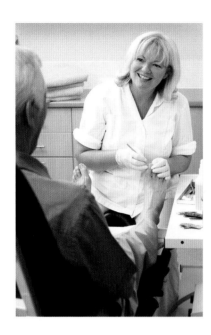

Appointments Down the Road

You may be referred to other specialists:

- A **pedorthist** specializes in fitting you for custom shoes or shoe inserts.
- A **foot care nurse** can trim your toenails.
- A **podiatrist** (or chiropodist) is a doctor who provides foot care and does some foot surgery.
- A **vascular surgeon** specialized in vascular surgery (surgery of your blood vessels) or more extensive diabetes foot surgery
- If you are feeling depressed or require emotional support, a **mental health worker**
- If you need help to develop an individualized exercise program, especially if you have challenges such as arthritis, a **sports medicine clinic** or **physiotherapist**
- If you are pregnant, an **obstetrician**
- If you have concerns with your bladder or with sex, a **urologist**, **gynecologist** or **sex therapist**
- If you have pain related to diabetes nerve damage, a **neurologist** or **pain clinic**
- If you have stomach or bowel problems, a **gastroenterologist**
- If you have skin issues, a **dermatologist**
- If you need further heart assessment, a **cardiologist**
- If your kidneys are not working properly, a **nephrologist** as well as a **renal dietitian**

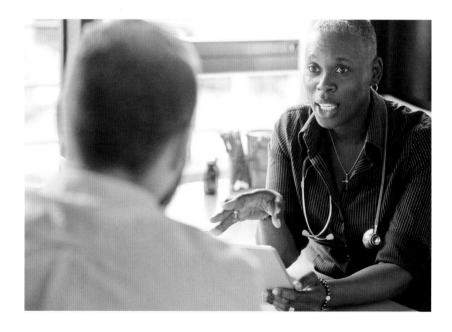

Lab Tests, Foot Exam and Eye Exam

Why are lab tests important?

You may not feel any difference when blood sugar, blood pressure or cholesterol is high. Yet damage is happening. Laboratory tests (lab tests) and exams will tell you and your doctor how healthy you are. These also explain what medications you need and how your positive lifestyle changes help you be healthier.

Which lab tests are important for you?

Pages 302–304 describe the lab tests (blood and urine) that are important for you as a person with diabetes. The chart on pages 305–306 lists these tests and how often you should have them done. It also shows what healthy levels for each test are. The name for those healthy levels is the target. Americans should use the chart on page 305. Information for Canadians is on page 306. If you'd like to photocopy the chart, go ahead. Put your name at the top and fill in any lab information that you have. When you see your doctor or diabetes educator, ask them to help you fill in the blanks from your records. This chart is a reminder of the important tests you need to have done on a regular basis. Your doctor is busy. It is often up to you to request lab work be done.

Other tests

This section covers the most important diabetes-related tests. However, there are many other tests that your doctor might order, such as thyroid and complete blood count (CBC) tests, which measure the health of hormones and blood cells.

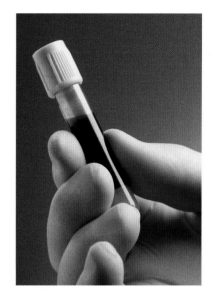

℞ DOCTOR'S ADVICE

Your doctor may set slightly different targets for you than what is on the chart on page 305 and 306, especially if you are older. Also, you may need to take some tests more or less often.

MEDS & TESTS

Tip: Ask your doctor for a lab requisition for three to six months down the road. Then you can get your lab work done two weeks before your next doctor visit. When you see your doctor, the clinic should have your lab information.

What is an A1C?

An A1C is a measure of how much sugar sticks to your red blood cells. Your blood cells live for about three months, and the more sugar that has been in your blood during that time, the more will be stuck on the cells.

Certain health issues, such as anemia, can affect whether an A1C is accurate.

A fasting or random blood sugar test

Unlike an A1C, a fasting or random blood sugar test measures your blood sugar at that moment.

Waist Measurement

- A few times a year, you may want to measure your waist. Measure your waist just above your hip bone.
- Dropping this number by even a small amount helps your health.

Blood sugar tests

A1C ("A-one-C")

This is an important test for you as a person with diabetes. **The lower your A1C, the lower your risk for complications.** This is an average of all your blood sugar ups and downs over a three-month period of time. This test will give you the big picture of how you are doing and adds to any home blood sugar testing results. If your A1C is high, your doctor may want you to have it taken every three months. In between, try to make changes to improve it. When your A1C level is good, the doctor may suggest taking it just once or twice a year.

At-home A1C tests

If you are seeing your doctor at least every three to six months, there is really no need for additional home A1C testing. Your doctor can order the A1C for you.

Fasting blood sugar

This is a blood test done in the morning before eating. It's done either at home or at a lab. See pages 337–345 to learn about checking your blood sugar at home.

Random blood sugar

This test can be done at any time of the day. Record the time you did the test and if you ate beforehand.

Blood pressure

It is very important to have good blood pressure. This protects your blood vessels, eyes and kidneys from diabetes complications. See page 317 for information about blood pressure pills. See page 346 for blood pressure numbers and how to check your blood pressure at home. If you aren't able to check your blood pressure at home, then have your blood pressure checked at your doctor's office at each visit.

Weight

Extra body weight makes extra work for your heart and body organs, including your pancreas. When you weigh more, your pancreas needs to make more insulin. Keeping track of your weight is therefore an important tool to monitor your health. A small weight loss or preventing weight gain are great successes.

Cholesterol panel

Your doctor has various ways of checking your cholesterol levels:

- **LDL cholesterol** ("Lousy" or bad cholesterol): This cholesterol builds up and clogs your blood vessels.
- **HDL cholesterol** ("Healthy" or good cholesterol): This cholesterol helps clear unwanted deposits from the insides of your blood vessels.

Two other ways to measure your LDL cholesterol:

- *ApoB* measures a protein that is associated with LDL cholesterol.
- *Non-HDL cholesterol* takes your total cholesterol and subtracts your good cholesterol.

Triglycerides

This is a type of blood fat that clogs your blood vessels. It goes up when your blood sugar is high or you are drinking alcohol regularly.

Kidney tests

Albumin creatinine ratio

The albumin creatinine ratio (ACR) is a urine test that measures the amount of albumin (a type of protein). Albumin usually stays in your blood, but when kidney damage begins, it leaks into your urine. The ACR is an important test because it can pick up kidney problems early. It also indicates if you are at risk for a heart attack. This will alert you and your doctor to take steps to protect your kidneys and heart, including improving blood sugar and blood pressure. You may need some new medication.

Estimated glomerular filtration rate

The estimated glomerular filtration rate (eGFR) measures the rate that fluid flows through your kidney filters. A lower number means the kidneys aren't working as well.

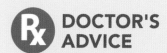

DOCTOR'S ADVICE

Your Diabetes ABCs
The **A1C, Blood Pressure** and **Cholesterol** tests are three important tests. Together, they measure your blood vessels' health.

If you have had a recent kidney or bladder infection, you may have extra protein in your urine. This returns to normal after the infection is gone.

MEDS & TESTS

Foot exam

To gently remind a busy doctor or nurse to check your feet, you might want to remove your shoes and socks before he or she comes into the examining room. You will be all ready for a quick 5-minute foot exam!

It is important to check your feet daily. See your doctor right away for urgent foot problems. In addition, there are certain things that your doctor or diabetes nurse can pick up when they check your feet. A monofilament or tuning fork can determine how much nerve sensation you have on the bottom of each foot. If you have damaged nerves, you are more at risk for foot problems. When the doctor feels your pulses, he learns how much blood flow goes to your lower leg, feet and toes.

Dilated eye exam

Your eyes are like a window into the health of all blood vessels in your body.

When an optometrist (or ophthalmologist) looks into the back of your eye, he can see inside your blood vessels. The only other way to see inside blood vessels is for a doctor to do surgery. If your eye blood vessels seem damaged, there is likely damage in your kidneys and other parts of your body. On a routine eye check, an optometrist may be the first one to see signs of diabetes. He would advise you to go right away to your doctor.

Regular eye checks help to catch eye problems early. This way, you have time to make changes to make it better. If you need laser eye surgery, you can do this early to keep your eyes as healthy as possible. Once your optometrist has seen you for your first diabetes visit, he will tell you how often you need to come back, usually once a year.

How does a dilated eye exam work?

The optometrist or opthalmologist puts medicated drops into your eyes to make your pupils go large. When they are large, he looks through your pupils and can completely see the back of your eye. After a dilated exam, your eyes can be blurry and sensitive to light for a few hours. Someone else should take you home. Wear a pair of sunglasses if you are outside or in bright lights, until your pupils go back to normal size.

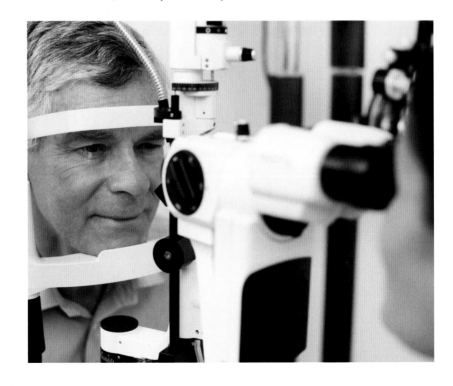

Important Diabetes Tests

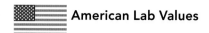 **American Lab Values**

The American Diabetes Association updates their diabetes guidelines (Standards of Medical Care in Diabetes) based on the latest evidence for treating diabetes. The chart below lists the tests used to assess diabetes and the usual targets. The right targets for you will depend on questions such as:

- How long have you had diabetes?
- Is your A1C high?
- Do you often have low blood sugar?
- Are you pregnant?
- Are you elderly or frail?
- Have you had a heart attack or other health issues?

If you are elderly and likely to get a low blood sugar, your doctor may instead recommend a higher target. Or, if you have had heart problems, your doctor may recommend a lower target LDL cholesterol than shown.

Show this page to your doctor and ask, "What targets are right for me?"

Tests and targets	Record results and dates below			
Usually tested at diagnosis and every three months				
BLOOD SUGAR TESTS, BLOOD PRESSURE AND WEIGHT				
A1C (average blood sugar over the past three months) Target: less than 7%				
Fasting Blood Sugar (in the morning before eating) Target: 80–130 mg/dL				
Random Blood Sugar (any time during the day) Target: less than 180 mg/dL after eating				
BLOOD PRESSURE Target: less than 140/90				
WEIGHT Your target: _____				
Usually tested at diagnosis and once a year, more often if abnormal				
CHOLESTEROL TESTS				
LDL Cholesterol (L for "Lousy") Target: less than 100 mg/dL				
HDL Cholesterol (H for "Healthy") Target: more than 40 mg/dL (men) more than 50 mg/dL (women)				
KIDNEY TESTS				
Albumin Creatinine Ratio (ACR) urine test Target: 30 mcg/mg or less				
Estimated Glomerular Filtration Rate (eGFR) Target: more than 60 ml/minute				
FOOT EXAM				
Includes monofilament or vibration test, pulses and general foot exam. Do daily foot checks at home. **Target: Sensation present and pulses felt**				
DILATED EYE EXAM				
Eye drops will be given. **Target: no retinopathy**				

MEDS & TESTS

Important Diabetes Tests

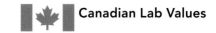 **Canadian Lab Values**

Diabetes Canada updates their diabetes guidelines (Clinical Practice Guidelines) based on the latest evidence for treating diabetes. The chart below lists the tests used to assess diabetes and the usual targets. The right targets for you will depend on questions such as:

- How long have you had diabetes?
- Is your A1C high?
- Do you often have low blood sugar?
- Are you pregnant?
- Are you elderly or frail?
- Have you had a heart attack or other health issues?

If you are elderly and likely to get a low blood sugar, your doctor may instead recommend a higher target. Or, if you have had heart problems, your doctor may recommend a lower target LDL cholesterol than shown.

Show this page to your doctor and ask, "What targets are right for me?"

Tests and targets	Record results and dates below			
Usually tested at diagnosis and every three months				
BLOOD SUGAR TESTS, BLOOD PRESSURE AND WEIGHT				
A1C (average blood sugar over the past three months) Target: 7% or less				
Fasting Blood Sugar (in the morning before eating) Target: 4–7 mmol/L				
Random Blood Sugar (any time during the day) Target: 5–10 mmol/L after eating				
BLOOD PRESSURE Target: less than 130/80				
WEIGHT Your target: _____				
Usually tested at diagnosis and once a year, more often if abnormal				
CHOLESTEROL TESTS				
Either LDL Cholesterol (8-hour fast) Target: 2 mmol/L or less				
OR apoB (no fast needed) Target: 0.8 g/L or less				
Non-HDL Cholesterol Target: 2.6 mmol/L or less				
KIDNEY TESTS				
Albumin Creatinine Ratio (ACR) urine test Target: less than 2 mg/mmol				
Estimated Glomerular Filtration Rate (eGFR) Target: more than 60 ml/minute				
FOOT EXAM				
Includes monofilament or vibration test, pulses and general foot exam. Do daily foot checks at home. **Target: Sensation present and pulses felt**				
DILATED EYE EXAM				
Eye drops will be given. **Target: no retinopathy**				

Diabetes Medications

Managing without Medication

You may wish to avoid the side effects and bother of taking medications. If you can manage your blood sugar through diet and exercise changes, this is a healthy option. It's usually easier to manage without medicine when you have had diabetes for a short period, perhaps less than five years.

Medications Can Help You Manage

Over time, your pancreas may naturally make less insulin. The insulin may become less effective due to insulin resistance. Even if you do all the "right things," such as making good food choices and exercising regularly, you may still need medications. Diabetes is a progressive disease. Needing medicine doesn't mean you failed. Keeping your blood sugar at a good level and preventing complications is most important. Today's medications are better than ever in preventing diabetes complications.

There are many insulins and diabetes medications

The first drug treatment of diabetes was insulin, discovered in 1921, 100 years ago. Today a lot has changed! There are many types of insulins and many ways to give insulin. This includes very tiny needles that you hardly can feel and computerized insulin delivery pumps. The first diabetes pill to help lower the blood sugar was discovered by accident in the 1950's, as a side effect of another medication. Since then, there has been continuous research into medications for managing diabetes and preventing diabetes complications. See page 319.

Seven groups of medications and four groups of insulin

There are seven major groups of diabetes medications that come as pills or as liquids that you inject. These liquid medications are not insulin. The first part of this section gives information about these medications. The four groups of insulin are covered later.

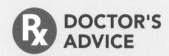

DOCTOR'S ADVICE

Take your medications as prescribed by your doctor.

Medications work best when you take them regularly. Yet it can be easy to forget whether you have taken your meds. Try a pill container. Some pharmacies will organize your pills into blister packs. You can use an alarm on your phone. There are even pill reminder apps.

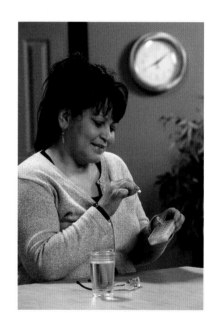

MEDS & TESTS

If you are trying to get pregnant (or are pregnant or breastfeeding), ask your doctor what medications are safe for you to take.

The Right Medications

There are many different diabetes medications. They each have different effects on your body and possible side effects as well. Some medicines lower your fasting blood sugar and others lower blood before meals. Other medications lower your blood sugar after meals. Others not only lower your blood sugar but also protect your heart from the effects of diabetes. The ultimate goals are to improve health and longevity and to improve your quality of life.

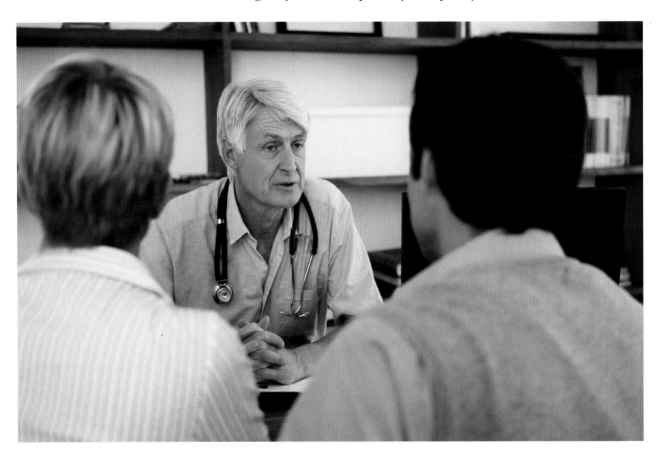

 DOCTOR'S ADVICE

Ongoing diabetes care is important.

Your diabetes care should be patient-centered. This means it's an approach that's just right for you. Your medical provider will evaluate your situation and help match you with the best medication or combination of medications. You will see the effects of medications and note any side effects. Then you and your doctor can adjust the treatment plan together. Also, since diabetes is a progressive disease, what works at one time may not continue to work. As your diabetes changes, your treatment plan will change too.

Seven Groups of Diabetes Medications

These seven groups of diabetes medications include pills and medication that you inject. Insulin is also injected but is discussed separately later in this chapter.

The drug or insulin's brand name is capitalized.

A "no-name" or cheaper version of the same drug is sometimes available. Ask your doctor or pharmacist about this.

Look for the page that describes your medication. Benefits and common side effects are listed for each medicine. Each drug helps different parts of your body: the liver, pancreas, intestine, bladder or the cells. This is why your doctor might prescribe several different ones to work in different ways.

Some companies combine drugs from two or more groups into a single tablet; for example, a combination of group 1 and group 3 or group 1 and group 5.

Drugwatch.com is a website with information on drug side effects.

If the drug you are prescribed is not listed here, ask your pharmacist which group it fits into.

Group 1: Liver sugar blocker pill / metformin
It reduces the release of sugar from your liver.

Group 2: Pancreas insulin booster pills / secretagogues
These help your pancreas make more insulin.

Group 3: Intestine insulin booster pills / DPP-4s
These stimulate your intestinal hormones that, in turn, help your pancreas make more insulin.

Group 4: Intestine insulin booster injections / GLP1s
These injections work like the Group 3 pills but are more potent. There is now also a pill version available.

Group 5: Bladder sugar mover pills / SGLT2s
These take excess sugar from your blood and move it to your bladder, then you pee the sugar out.

Group 6: Intestine sugar blocker pills / alpha glucosidase
These slow the absorption of carbohydrate into your blood.

Group 7: Cell insulin helper pills / TZDs
These help insulin move sugar out of your blood and into your cells.

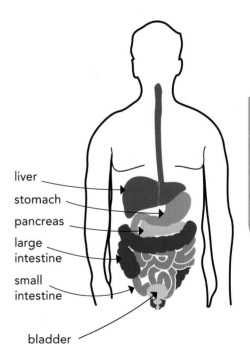

liver
stomach
pancreas
large intestine
small intestine
bladder

MEDS & TESTS

Group 1: Liver sugar blocker pill / metformin

Metformin reduces the release of sugar from your liver.

This is usually the first diabetes pill prescribed. It comes in two forms:

- metformin (Glucophage)
- metformin extended-release (Glumetza)

How a liver sugar blocker pill works

Your body stores extra sugar in your liver. When you have diabetes, sugar leaks out of your liver. This pill helps stop or reduce this leakage.

There is new research that metformin may help people with diabetes in part by helping good gut bacteria grow. These bacteria help with immunity, appetite and digestion.

When to take metformin

There are two types of metformin: regular and extended release. It is best to split the regular dose so that you take one or two pills with breakfast and one or two pills with dinner. You can take the entire dose of extended-release metformin with the evening meal if you prefer.

Metformin is often most effective when taken at the maximum dose. Don't be concerned if your doctor increases the amount to reach the maximum dose.

Benefits

- It helps bring down a high fasting blood sugar (morning blood sugar before eating).
- If you are overweight, this is a good choice, as it doesn't cause unwanted weight gain; you may even lose a bit of weight.
- It doesn't cause low blood sugar.
- It may help improve cholesterol level.

Most common side effects

- Stomach upset and diarrhea. This can be lessened by starting on a low dose and gradually going up to the full dose over a few weeks.
- Reduced vitamin B_{12} levels can result with long-term use.
- **PREGNANCY RISK:** If you are a premenopausal woman, be aware that this pill could make you more fertile.

Not recommended if:

- You have liver disease, advanced kidney disease or heart failure.
- You drink a lot of alcohol.

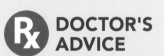

DOCTOR'S ADVICE

If you are having trouble with stomach upset or diarrhea, ask your doctor for a prescription for the extended-release metformin. It works just as well as the regular metformin but may have fewer side effects.

Group 2: Pancreas insulin booster pills / insulin secretagogues

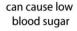

can cause low
blood sugar

Insulin secretagogues help your pancreas make more insulin.

They come in these forms:

- glyburide or glibenclamide (Diabeta)
- gliclazide (Diamicron)
- glimepiride (Amaryl)

These kinds are sulfa free:

- repaglinide (GlucoNorm or Prandin)
- nateglinide (Starlix)

How a pancreas insulin booster pill works

This medication stimulates your pancreas to make more insulin.

When to take insulin secretagogues

- Take glyburide half an hour before breakfast and your evening meal.
- Gliclazide and glimepiride are "one-a-day" versions of this drug. You take them just before or with the first meal of the day.
- Take repaglinide and nateglinide with each meal.

Benefits

- If your blood sugar is high two hours after eating, these pills can help.

Most common side effects

- Low blood sugar, especially with gyburide. This is even more likely if you are elderly.
- Weight gain, especially with glyburide: To prevent this, be careful what you eat and keep active when you start on this pill. Also, have your doctor decrease the dose if you have a lot of low blood sugars.
- Take with caution if you have liver or kidney disease.

Rx DOCTOR'S ADVICE

These pills have been around a long time, so they tend to be inexpensive. The biggest risk of using them is low blood sugar, so the dose should be carefully adjusted by your doctor. And don't skip meals when taking these pills, as this can make you even more likely to have a low blood sugar. While these pills do bring down blood sugar, they don't have the benefits of some of the newer medications, such as weight loss and protecting your heart.

MEDS & TESTS

311

expensive

Most common side effects
Side effects of DPP-4s are usually minimal.

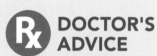 **DOCTOR'S ADVICE**

DPP-4s are not the strongest medications for lowering blood sugar. They work really well in people with mild or early diabetes when their blood sugar is not too high. Also, they work better in combination with metformin than by themselves. If you take one of these medications and metformin, ask your provider for a prescription for the combination pill.

 # Group 3: Intestine insulin booster pills / DPP-4 inhibitors

DPP-4 inhibitors help increase intestinal hormones that lower blood sugar.

They are taken on their own or combined with metformin.

DPP-4s on their own
- sitagliptin (Januvia)
- saxagliptin (Onglyza)
- linagliptin (Trajenta, Tradjenta)
- alogliptin (Nesina)
- vildagliptin (Galvus)

DPP-4s combined with metformin
- Janumet
- Kombiglyze
- Jentadueto
- Kazano
- Galvus Met

How intestine insulin booster pills work

In your body you have intestinal hormones called incretins, which help with metabolism. The most important incretin is called GLP-1. This hormone tells your pancreas to make more insulin when needed. In people with diabetes, GLP-1 doesn't work as well. The DPP-4s boost the level of GLP-1 hormone in your body.

GLP-1 tells the pancreas to release insulin only when the blood sugar is high. So, unlike other pancreas insulin boosters, they don't cause low blood sugar.

When to take DPP-4 inhibitors
- DPP-4s on their own can be taken once a day with or without food.
- When combined with metformin, the dose is usually split. You take one pill with breakfast and another with dinner.

Group 4: Intestine insulin booster injections / GLP-1s

protects the heart | helps with weight loss | expensive

GLP-1s mimic the effects of the intestinal hormone known as GLP-1.

They are available in daily or weekly doses.

Daily GLP-1s
- exenatide (Byetta)
- liraglutide (Victoza)
- semaglutide (Rybelsus) as a pill form

Weekly GLP-1s
- exenatide (Bydureon)
- dulaglutide (Trulicity)
- semaglutide (Ozempic)

How an intestine insulin booster injection works

These medications boost the levels of GLP-1 intestinal hormone produced by the human body. The high levels that can be given by injection make these medications powerful at lowering blood sugar. They have other favorable effects, such as causing weight loss and reducing the risk of heart attacks and strokes.

When to take GLP-1s
- Take Byetta twice daily with breakfast and dinner.
- Take Victoza once daily with or without food. The time doesn't matter.
- The once-weekly versions are taken once every seven days. The time of day it's taken doesn't matter.

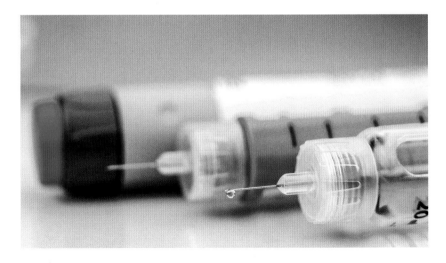

Most common side effects
You may experience some nausea with the GLP-1s. Usually the symptoms last a few days or weeks and then get better. Starting on a low dose at first can help. For some people, the nausea never goes away. They should switch to another type of medicine.

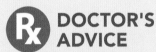 **DOCTOR'S ADVICE**

You should discuss taking a GLP-1 medication with your doctor if you have a history of or a high risk for heart disease. This could be a good choice for you! The once weekly versions are very effective and mean you only need to give one injection a week.

MEDS & TESTS

313

protects the heart

helps with weight loss

expensive

Most common side effect

- Yeast or urinary tract infections can occur.

Although rarely, men could get a serious genital infection. These infections can be treated. If they keep happening, your medical provider might suggest a different medication.

 DOCTOR'S ADVICE

SGLT2s have benefits beyond lowering blood sugar. They reduce the risk of heart attacks and strokes. They may help people with heart failure. And, they slow down kidney damage in people with kidney disease.

S Group 5: Bladder sugar mover pills / SGLT2 inhibitors

These take excess sugar from your blood and transport it to your urine. Then you pee out the extra sugar.

There are four common varities.

- canagliflozin (Invokana)
- dapagliflozin (Forxiga)
- empagliflozin (Jardiance)
- ertugliflozin (Steglatro)

How a bladder sugar mover pill works

Normally, the kidneys filter all the sugar from the blood and then transport it back to the blood. These medications reduce this transport by blocking a protein in the kidney called SGLT2. The extra sugar then leaves the body in the urine. Since sugar has calories, people often lose weight with these medications. It is important to drink plenty of fluid when taking an SGLT2 medication, as the pill makes you pee more.

When to take SGLT2 inhibitors

- All these medications are taken once a day with or without food.

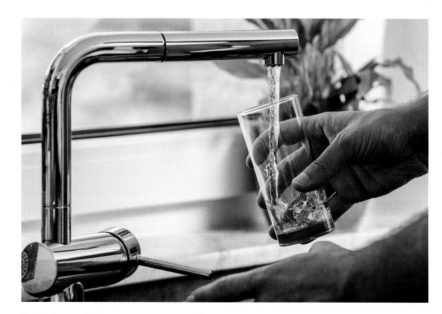

Drink lots of water when taking SGLT2s.

Group 6: Intestine sugar blocker pills / alpha-glucosidase inhibitors

These slow carbohydrate absorption from the intestines.

There are two kinds.

- acarbose (Glucobay, Prandase or Precose)
- miglitol (Glycet)

How an intestine sugar blocker pill works

Arcabose and miglitol slow the absorption of carbohydrates from the stomach and intestines. These inhibitors reduce blood sugar spikes after a meal or a large snack. Then your pancreas won't be so overworked.

When to take alpha-glucosidase inhibitors

- Take acarbose (or miglitol) with your first bite of food at each meal that contains carbohydrates.

Benefits

- It helps decrease blood sugar two hours after you have eaten.
- It does not cause weight gain or low blood sugar when taken on its own.

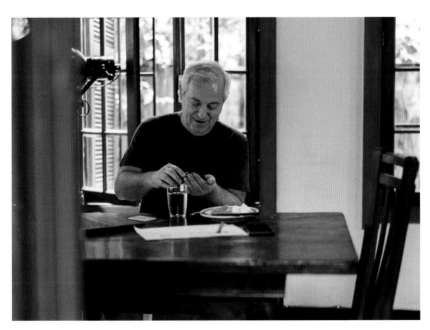

Take alpha-glucosidase pills with your first bite of food at your meal.

Most common side effects

- Acarbose and miglitol can cause stomach upset.
- Your doctor may not prescribe these if you have liver disease or intestinal disease.
- You may feel the need to pass gas more than usual.

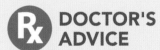 **DOCTOR'S ADVICE**

These pills are very safe. They don't increase low blood sugar episodes and they may help you lose some weight. But people who take these pills often get abdominal discomfort (stomach pain) and gas. If you don't have these side effects or the effects are manageable, alpha-glucosidase inhibitors may be a good choice for you.

MEDS & TESTS

315

Group 7: Cell insulin helper pills / TZDs or glitazones

This helps insulin work better at the cell level.

There is only one kind.

- pioglitazone (Actos)

How a cell insulin helper pill works

Most people with type 2 diabetes have a condition called insulin resistance. Even though the body usually has plenty of insulin, it isn't taken up well by the cells of the body. These cells include muscle cells and liver cells.

Pioglitazone reduces insulin resistance. It may take up to six weeks for you to notice an improvement in your blood sugar after starting to take this medication. It may take up to three months to get the full benefit.

When to take TZDs

- Take pioglitazone once a day with or without food.

R̲x̲ DOCTOR'S ADVICE

The one medication prescribed in this category is called pioglitazone (or Actos). It is one of the most effective pills for diabetes. However, you shouldn't use it if you tend to retain too much fluid or if you have congestive heart failure.

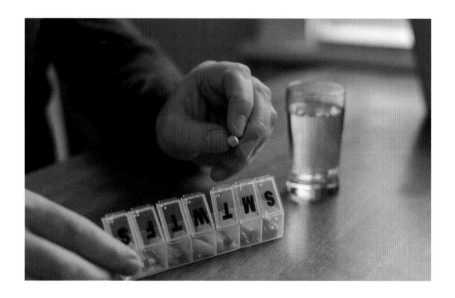

Most common side effects

- Fluid retention: If you tend to retain fluid or have congestive heart failure (fluid builds up in your heart and lungs), this is not a good choice. Fluid retention may be greater in people who take pioglitazone in combination with insulin.
- Heart failure: The risk of heart failure is greater in people who take pioglitazone in combination with insulin.
- Weight gain
- Osteoporosis: There is an increased risk of fracture, especially in women.
- **PREGNANCY RISK:** If you are a pre-menopausal woman with irregular periods, pioglitazone could make you more fertile.

Other Pills Your Doctor May Prescribe

Reduce your risk for blood clots

Doctors recommend low-dose aspirin for adults with diabetes who have had a stroke or heart attack. This is to reduce the risk of another stroke or heart attack. If you have not had a stroke or heart attack, the risk of internal bleeding (such as bleeding in the stomach) may outweigh any benefit from the aspirin, and it is not routinely recommended. Talk to your doctor about what is best for you.

Cholesterol pills

If you are at risk for heart problems, your doctor may prescribe a cholesterol-lowering pill from a group of drugs called statins. Statins help lower the LDL (lousy) cholesterol. These have names that end in "statin" such as atorvastatin (Lipitor), rosuvastatin (Crestor), simvistatin (Zocor) and pravastatin (Pravachol). These drugs have great benefit for people who have had a heart attack. Although most people do okay when they take statins, if you experience any unusual bone or muscle pain after starting on this pill, report it to your doctor right away.

Another type of cholesterol medication is TriCor, a fibrate. This is not as effective as statins, but can lower triglycerides (blood fats) while boosting the HDL (healthy) cholesterol.

Blood pressure pills

For diabetes, the two types of blood pressure pills most recommended are ACE inhibitors and angiotensin 11 receptor blockers (ARBs). ACE inhibitors have names that end in "pril" such as captopril, enalapril, fosinopril, lisinopril or framipril. ARBs have names that end in "sartan" such as candesartan, losartan, irbesartan or valsartan. These two groups lower blood pressure as well as protect your kidneys.

Sometimes, to manage your blood pressure, your doctor may give you several types of blood pressure pills, including ones that are neither ACE nor ARBs. For example, the doctor might also prescribe water pills, or diuretics.

Weight loss pills

Weight loss prescription medications were discussed in the weight loss section of the book on page 63. Most of these pills are expensive and need to be taken for life.

If aspirin gives you stomach problems, a doctor can prescribe another pill instead.

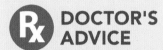

DOCTOR'S ADVICE

Pregnancy warning: During pregnancy or breastfeeding, it's good to stop taking statins, ACE inhibitors and ARBs. Your doctor can stop these and may prescribe alternatives.

Talk to your doctor or pharmacist about all your medications. Ask about side effects, how much to take and when to take it.

MEDS & TESTS

317

Q & A with DR. SHOMALI: about your diabetes medications

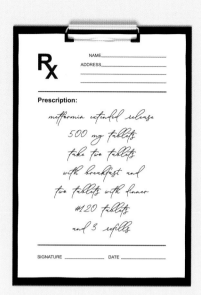

MARIA: There are so many diabetes medications. Some of the side effects sound scary. How will my doctor select the best medications for me?

DR. SHOMALI: That's a great question, Maria. We physicians are constantly learning about advances in diabetes care in order to match our patients with the treatments that will help them the most. There is no "one size fits all" solution. Here are a few of my thoughts.

1. **Lifestyle changes:** Keep in mind that diabetes medications will not work as well if you are not trying to make healthy food choices. It is also important to stay active as much as possible.

2. **Start with metformin:** Metformin has been used in Canada since 1972 and in the United States since 1994. We physicians are very comfortable and experienced at prescribing it. It is also generic now, which makes it inexpensive. It doesn't cause weight gain or low blood sugar reactions. There are some studies that show it can also reduce the risk of certain cancers common in people with diabetes. For these reasons, metformin is a good first choice of medication.

3. **Don't delay in adding a second medication:** Since diabetes is a progressive disease, using only metformin for many years is unlikely. If the A1C hasn't been less than 7%, it's a good idea to add a second medication to metformin. This can help improve blood sugar, but also helps prevent later diabetes complications. You can prevent or reduce complications such as eye disease, kidney damage and nerve damage by keeping your blood sugar in target. All diabetes medications help with this. However, the complications that hurt people the most are heart attacks and strokes, and GLP-1s and SGLT2 inhibitors reduce these. In addition, GLP-1s and SGLT2s help people lose weight and don't cause low blood sugar. I recommend adding one of these to metformin. I use the other diabetes medications as later options or if there are side effect or cost issues.

4. **Insulin:** Many patients are afraid of insulin because it's an injection, or they think insulin means that their diabetes has become more serious. I think of insulin as just another medication to help manage a patient's blood sugar. Insulin is easier to use than ever. After showing patients how to take insulin, I often see the expression on their face: "I can do that!"

Insulin

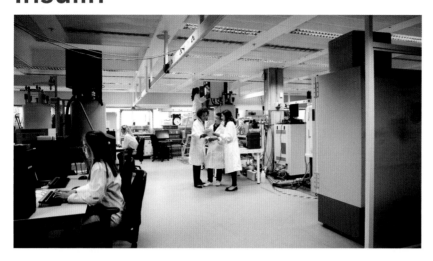

An Early Start Helps

We are learning so much than ever before from ongoing diabetes research in labs around the world. We now know that having high blood sugar for many years permanently damages the insulin-making cells in your pancreas. And we've learned that taking insulin can bring down blood sugar and protect these cells from damage. This knowledge and long-term test results have helped doctors understand why it is often the right choice to start insulin at the time of diabetes diagnosis.

Your doctor and nurse will help

The biggest concern for new insulin users is giving yourself a needle every day. There will be help and training for you from the diabetes nurse. And, it's good to know that researchers have developed really tiny needles that you hardly feel, and new ways of taking insulin (see page 321).

Your doctor will start you on a lower dose of insulin. Then in the days and weeks after you start insulin, the doctor or nurse will look at your blood sugar numbers and make adjustments to your dose of insulin. They will advise you to gradually increase the amount of insulin you take until your blood sugar improves.

Researchers have developed many types of insulin to help control and reduce high blood sugar. Some insulin doses are adjustable, especially if your meal times are unpredictable. Or, if you have a standard daily routine, your insulin dose will be the same amount each day. As your blood sugar comes down and you've made some lifestyle changes, insulin can often be reduced. Or a different type of insulin or diabetes medication may be prescribed. It is an ever-changing process.

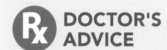

DOCTOR'S ADVICE

Starting insulin early does not mean that your diabetes is bad. Rather, it's the best way to control and bring down your blood sugar, so you will feel better sooner.

MEDS & TESTS

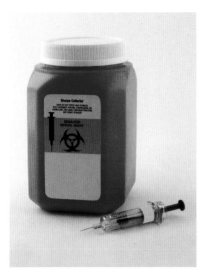

Dispose of lancets safely.

Storing insulin

If you only have a month's supply, insulin can be stored in a cupboard and kept at room temperature. Insulin can only be kept at room temperature for a month, so extra supplies will need to be stored in your fridge.

Disposing of insulin needles and lancets

You can purchase a "sharps container" from a drug store. At the time of purchase, ask where you can dispose of it once it's full. Ask if you can bring in your own container for proper disposal. You can create your own container from a hard plastic bleach bottle or similar style plastic container.

Side Effects of Insulin

Low blood sugar and **weight gain** are the two main side effects of taking insulin.

How to prevent or reduce low blood sugar

Low blood sugar happens because insulin takes sugar out of the blood and it can sometimes take too much out. This depends on many variables, such as your age, weight and activity level. When you first start on insulin and have many lows in a day or in a week, your doctor can do one of the following:

- Adjust the type of insulin or time of day you take it.
- Reduce the dose.

Your health care team will also talk to you about your food and exercise and how that affects low blood sugar.

There is more information about low blood sugar episodes on pages 329–336.

How to prevent or reduce weight gain

Weight gain happens because insulin takes sugar out of the blood and that sugar is stored as fat in your body. Weight gain while taking insulin can be prevented or reduced by the following:

- Reduce your blood sugar gradually during the first weeks or months after you start taking insulin. This can be done if insulin is started at a low dose and increased slowly. Doctors use the expression "Start low, go slow."
- Cut back on your food portions and salt, and walk every day. With these changes, you will need a lower dose of insulin. A lower dose of insulin means less weight gain.

℞ DOCTOR'S ADVICE

Always consult with your doctor if you have side effects from taking insulin. Your doctor may try a different type of insulin or combine the insulin with other diabetes medication. You may also need more help to make some lifestyle changes, and he may refer you to a dietitian, nurse or exercise specialist.

Different Ways to Take Insulin

Vial and syringe

- You pull the recommended dose out of a vial with a syringe, and inject it.
- You have to be able to see the lines on the syringe to measure the correct amount of insulin.
- Depending on how much body fat you have, you may be taught to pinch the skin and inject at an angle.

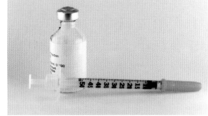

Spend time with the diabetes educator or nurse so that you learn to inject correctly with the syringe or insulin pen.

Insulin pen

- Most pen devices are disposable and prefilled with insulin.
- A reusable pen is refilled with an insulin cartridge.
- The correct dose is dialed using a knob on the insulin pen.

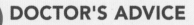

- The insulin is then injected through the skin using a tiny needle at the end of the pen.
- It's recommended to use a new pen needle for each injection.
- Most people inject at a 90-degree angle.

℞ DOCTOR'S ADVICE

Injecting with an insulin pen is more convenient than using vial and syringe. It may be more accurate, especially for people who have trouble using their hands, have poor vision or cannot read the numbers on an insulin syringe. Depending on your insurance plan and budget, using vials and syringes can be less expensive. Each method has advantages.

Rotate your injection sites

Rotate your injection sites, so you don't get a hard fatty lump under your skin. This is called lipohypertrophy. A lump doesn't look nice and could get infected. When you use the same site over and over, the insulin is not absorbed as well. Your blood sugar can go up.

Here is a picture to show you different areas of your body where you can inject.

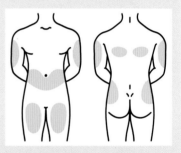

Each time you inject, keep at least one finger width away from where you last injected.

MEDS & TESTS

Inhaled insulin

Insulin can be absorbed very quickly through the lungs. Afrezza is an inhaled insulin product available in the United States and coming to Canada. You take it using a very simple inhaler that you can keep in your pocket. If you have a serious lung condition, you should not use inhaled insulin. Your doctor will perform a quick breathing test before and after you start Afrezza. Afrezza lowers blood sugar faster than any other insulin. Also, there are no needles to dispose of after use. The main side effect of Afrezza is a cough.

Insulin patch

An insulin patch is a relatively flat container of insulin that attaches to the skin. There are little or no electronics on the patch. Insulin is continuously delivered into the body through a tiny needle into the skin. An exact amount, called a bolus, can be given by pushing a button directly on the patch. Patches are less expensive than pumps and are much simpler to use. In the United States, the V-Go System is a patch that is filled with insulin and applied once a day. Other insulin patches are making their way to the United States, Europe and Canada.

Insulin pump

With these computerized devices, people no longer need to use insulin pens or syringes to inject insulin.

Insulin pump brands include the Medtronic Minimed System, Omnipod Insulin Management System, Tandem t:slim and the YpsoPump.

If you need multiple daily injections of insulin, a doctor may talk to you about an insulin pump. This device stores insulin. A small tube attached to the skin delivers the insulin. You change the insertion site every three days. Your health care team teaches you how to program your pump. Insulin automatically goes into your body. When you are about to eat or when your blood sugar is high, you program the pump to give you extra insulin, called a bolus.

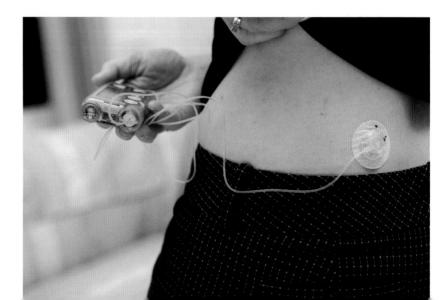

Insulin Release in the Body

Insulin release in the body in people without diabetes

In people who don't have diabetes, their pancreas makes insulin 24 hours a day. The insulin released at night and in between meals tells the body not to release the extra sugar that is stored in the liver and other areas. When they eat a meal, a matching amount of insulin is quickly released. This drives the sugar that is absorbed from food out of the blood and into the body's cells.

The normal release of insulin by the pancreas

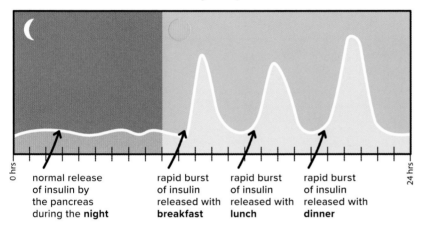

| normal release of insulin by the pancreas during the **night** | rapid burst of insulin released with **breakfast** | rapid burst of insulin released with **lunch** | rapid burst of insulin released with **dinner** |

0 hrs — 24 hrs

Insulin release in people with diabetes

In people with diabetes, insulin release doesn't occur properly, both with meals and in between meals. Some have high blood sugar in the morning or at night. Others have high blood sugar after meals. Different prescribed insulins help manage these situations.

Four Types of Insulin

Basal insulin (two types)

These insulins are also called background insulins. They are long-acting (up to 24 hours) or intermediate-acting (up to 18 hours). They work in the background while you are sleeping or awake. They help reduce the sugar the liver makes at night, so you don't wake up with high blood sugar.

Mealtime insulin (two types)

These insulins are short-acting (up to 6 hours) and rapid-acting (up to 3 to 5 hours). They act quickly and then the effect wears off. These insulins are designed to mimic how the normal pancreas releases insulin with meals.

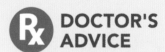

DOCTOR'S ADVICE

People with diabetes are often confused when their blood sugar is good at bedtime but high the next morning. They know they haven't eaten anything during the night. The high morning blood sugar is because the liver releases sugar at night and their body does not release insulin to compensate. Sometimes it is called the dawn phenomenon.

MEDS & TESTS

If you are pregnant

Your doctor may recommend a long-acting insulin during your pregnancy. This often helps you have steady blood sugar levels and reduces low blood sugar episodes.

Type 1: Basal insulin (long-acting)

There are four varieties:

- detemir (Levemir)
- glargine (Lantus, Basaglar)
- glargine U-300 (Toujeo)
- degludec (Tresiba)

These insulins start working in about 2 hours. They have a slow and steady effect after injected. The effect lasts approximately 24 hours. Usually, these insulins are injected once a day. They can be taken in the morning or at bedtime.

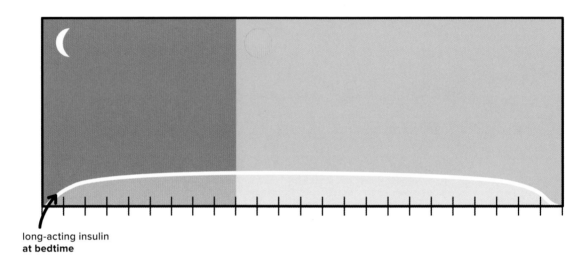

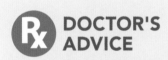

long-acting insulin
at bedtime

Rx DOCTOR'S ADVICE

Glargine and degludec insulins also come in a combination product that includes a GLP-1 medication. With each injection, you get both medications. The brand names are Soliqua and Xultophy.

Advantages

- One injection per day may be all that you need.
- They can be combined with non-insulin medications.
- Compared to intermediate-acting insulin (see next page), there is a lower chance of causing low blood sugar and weight gain.
- Toujeo and Tresiba are more concentrated than other insulins, so each injection is a smaller volume.

Disadvantages

- Low blood sugar and weight gain are still possible.
- These insulins are more expensive than intermediate insulins.
- These insulins cannot lower the excessive rise in blood sugar after eating.

Type 2: Basal insulin (intermediate-acting)

• NPH (Humulin N or Novolin N)

These insulins start working in about 1 to 3 hours. They have a peak effect 5 to 8 hours after injected. The effect lasts up to 18 hours. These insulins are injected once or twice a day. It's normal for these insulins to have a cloudy appearance.

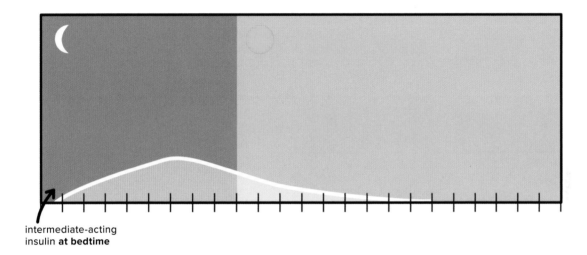

intermediate-acting
insulin **at bedtime**

Advantages
• These are much less expensive than the long-acting insulins, especially if you get the vial and syringe form.
• They can be combined with non-insulin medications.

Disadvantages
• A bedtime dose can cause a low blood sugar in the middle of the night because of the peak effect. A morning dose can cause low blood sugar later in the day, especially if you don't eat many carbs at lunch.
• The peak effect doesn't happen at the same time every day.
• These insulins can't lower the excessive rise in blood sugar after eating.

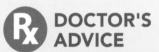

DOCTOR'S ADVICE

Intermediate insulin has been around for many years. For this reason, it is a lot less expensive than newer insulins such as long-acting insulin. If this is what you can afford, it is good to know that it is still an effective type of insulin. The rule that your doctor will use to increase your dose of intermediate insulin will be "Start low, go slow." This will decrease low blood sugar episodes.

MEDS & TESTS

325

Type 3: Mealtime insulin (short-acting)

- Regular (Humulin R, Novolin ge Toronto, Novolin R)

In the example here, you take one injection of a short-acting insulin with each of three meals and inject an intermediate-acting insulin at bedtime.

These insulins start working in about 1 hour. They have a peak effect 2 to 3 hours after you inject them. The effect lasts up to 6 hours. These insulins may be injected once, twice or three times a day.

These insulins should be injected about 30 minutes before eating, so they can start working when the food is being absorbed.

Intermediate and Short Insulins

intermediate-acting insulin at **bedtime**

short-acting insulin half an hour before **breakfast**

short-acting insulin half an hour before **lunch**

short-acting insulin half an hour before **dinner**

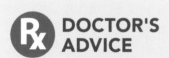

DOCTOR'S ADVICE

Short-acting insulin is cheaper than rapid-acting insulin. It is often combined with a diabetes pill such as metformin to get better blood sugar levels. It can be bought as a convenient premixed insulin with intermediate-acting insulin and short-acting insulin in the same vial, which is typically taken twice a day.

Advantages
- Compared to rapid-acting insulins (see next page), it's much less expensive, especially if you get the vial and syringe form.

Disadvantages
- You have to inject the dose before eating, often before knowing how much you will eat.
- Low blood sugar can occur as a result of the difficulty in timing with the meal.
- You need to have fairly regular meals and remember to take your insulin before each meal.

Type 4: Mealtime insulin (rapid-acting)

- aspart (NovoRapid, Novolog)
- faster insulin aspart (Fiasp)
- glulisine (Apidra)
- lispro (Humalog, Admelog)
- insulin human inhalation powder (Afrezza)

These insulins start working quickly in about 10 to 15 minutes. They have a peak effect 1 to 2 hours after you inject them. The effect lasts 3 to 5 hours. Fiasp works a bit faster than the other injectables. Afrezza works the fastest. These insulins may be injected (or inhaled, in the case of Afrezza) just before eating or even just after you finish the last bite of food.

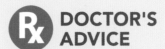

DOCTOR'S ADVICE

Consult with a dietitian or diabetes educator about how to count carbohydrates. You'll learn to match the amount of rapid-acting insulin with your food and exercise.

Long and Rapid Insulins

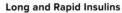

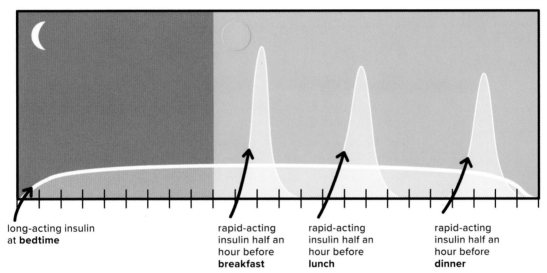

long-acting insulin at **bedtime**

rapid-acting insulin half an hour before **breakfast**

rapid-acting insulin half an hour before **lunch**

rapid-acting insulin half an hour before **dinner**

Advantages

- If your schedule changes from day to day, these insulins give you the most flexibility.
- These insulins work well if you are unsure how much you will eat.
- Since you can dose it with meals, there may be fewer lows and less weight gain.

Disadvantages

- These insulins are more expensive than the short-acting insulins.

In the example here, you get one injection of a rapid-acting insulin for each of three meals and inject a long-acting insulin at bedtime. Notice that it best recreates the pattern of insulin secretion by the normal pancreas shown on page 323.

MEDS & TESTS

327

The disadvantage of using a premixed insulin is lack of flexibility. You cannot take more of the rapid-acting or less of the intermediate-acting in a premixed combination.

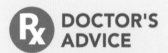

DOCTOR'S ADVICE

When you are starting insulin, your doctor may leave you on some or all of your other diabetes medicines. Most of them work well with insulin.

Your diabetes nurse can help you learn how to make adjustments to your insulin doses based on your blood sugar readings, food choices and exercise.

Premixed Insulin

- Humulin Mix25
- Humulin Mix50
- Humulin 30/70
- Novolin ge 30/70,
- Novolin 70/30
- Novolin ge 40/60, Novolin
- Novolin ge 50/50, Novolin
- NovoMix 30,
- Novolog Mix 70/30

These insulins contain a fixed amount of two different insulins. When you inject one of them, you are getting two insulins with one injection. This is more convenient than taking two injections. People who use premixed insulins generally don't make daily adjustments. It's a simpler insulin regimen.

Insulin Regimens

Your doctor and diabetes educator can find the best treatment plan for you.

One injection

If you are taking non-insulin medications and your A1C and fasting blood sugar readings are still consistently high, one injection of a long-acting insulin may work very well for you. You will start on a low dose. The dose is gradually increased, based on your fasting blood sugar readings. Once your fasting blood sugars are in target, your healthy diet, exercise and other medications may be more effective.

Two injections

If your A1C is still high with one injection of a long-acting insulin, one option is for your physician to add an injection of a rapid-acting insulin with your main meal. Alternatively, you can stop the long-acting insulin and go to two injections a day of premixed insulin. Your diabetes care team can help you figure out what works best.

Three to four injections

For the most blood sugar control, your physician may consider a long-acting insulin once a day and a rapid-acting insulin with each of your main meals during the day. This regimen is sometimes called basal-bolus insulin therapy.

Low Blood Sugar

Low blood sugar is when your level is under 70 mg/dL (4.0 mmol/L). You feel dizzy and weak and you need to eat something with sugar in it.

Who Can Get Low Blood Sugar?

Insulin or diabetes pills can build up in your blood. This can cause your blood sugar to lower. If your blood sugar is usually close to normal, you are more likely to get low blood sugar.

Insulin: Long-acting insulin (for example, detemir or glargine) is the least likely to cause a low blood sugar. The other types of insulin all have a peak action time when the insulin is the strongest. When insulin peaks, blood sugar will be at its lowest.

Diabetes pills: See page 309 for the diabetes medications that you are taking. Check in this book if there is a red low blood sugar arrow, or the words "can cause low blood sugar" appear in the description of your medication. If they don't appear in the description, your medication does not cause low blood sugar. However in rare circumstances, these other ones could cause a drop in sugar, for example, if you did a lot more than your usual exercise.

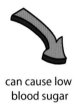

can cause low blood sugar

False low blood sugar

I am not on insulin or diabetes pills, but I sometimes feel like I am having low blood sugar. Why is this?

You may have had a large swing in your blood sugar level. For example, if your blood sugar was high and then, in a short period of time, dropped down into the normal range, that shift can cause you to feel "low." But this is not low blood sugar; you just feel some of the same symptoms.

To help the false low blood sugar symptoms go away, sit down and rest for 5 to 10 minutes. Have a drink of water. If it is time for your usual meal or snack, go ahead. Otherwise, chew sugar-free gum, or have a small sugar-free candy.

If you have a blood glucose meter, you can check your blood sugar. This will tell you if you are low and need to take sugar.

Low blood sugar terms
The medical name for low blood sugar is hypoglycemia. You can also call it a low or a reaction or a low blood sugar episode.

It takes time to adjust to normal blood sugar
When your blood sugar has been high for a while, it can take a month or two before you get used to normal blood sugar. Eventually, these false low blood sugar feelings will go away.

MEDS & TESTS

What Causes Low Blood Sugar?

1. Eating less carbohydrates than usual

2. Doing more exercise than usual

3. Taking too much medication:

- You accidentally took too much insulin or an extra diabetes pill.
- Herbs or other drugs are contributing to a low.
- Your insulin or diabetes pill prescription is too strong for you. This could be because you have lost some weight or have kidney disease.

4. Drinking alcohol without adjusting your food and medications properly

Illness

When you are ill, your blood sugar usually goes up, but sometimes it can go low. A low is more likely if you are vomiting and have diarrhea.

Think about what may cause a low blood sugar. Here are some examples:

- "My meeting went on longer than planned. My lunch was delayed an hour."
- "It was such a nice evening that I walked longer than usual."
- "I get more lows when I'm gardening, especially if I forget to cut back on my insulin."
- "My wife and I had sex when we went to bed. Later at night I woke up with a low!"
- "I was visiting with friends and we had a few too many drinks."
- "I was shopping at the mall and lost track of the time."
- "I didn't remember if I had taken my insulin, so I took another shot. I think I took it twice."

Hypoglycemia unawareness

Hypoglycemia unawareness means you won't have any symptoms of low blood sugar until you are under 55 mg/dL (3 mmol/L), or not at all. If you don't know you are low, you don't know to treat it quickly. This can be dangerous.

Why don't I realize I am low?

You may have a tolerance to low blood sugar if you have had frequent lows. Also, if you have diabetes nerve damage, this can affect the release of certain hormones. These hormones often stimulate sweating, trembling and other symptoms of low blood sugar.

Certain medications hide signs of low blood sugar. For example, a blood pressure pill called propranolol, a beta-blocker, does this. If you have hypoglycemic unawareness, ask your pharmacist if your other medications will affect your blood sugar.

What can be done about it?

Checking your blood sugar regularly is very important. Your doctor may suggest that you aim for a blood sugar that is a bit higher than the usual goal for a while. This decreases your risk of having a low.

You might benefit from continuous glocose monitoring (CGM) that can beep or alarm when you are low. See page 342–343 to read more about CGM.

Symptoms of Low Blood Sugar

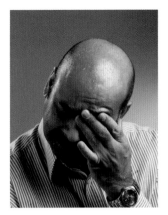

Sweating; feeling dizzy
or light-headed

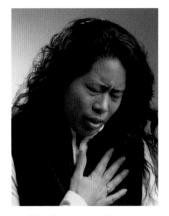

Weakness and heart
palpitations

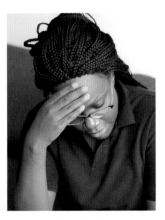

Headache

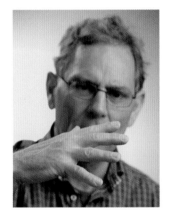

Shaking hands or legs;
feeling unsteady on your feet

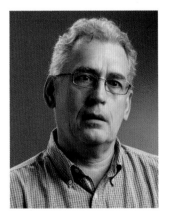

Pale skin, blue lips; feeling
a tingling around your lips

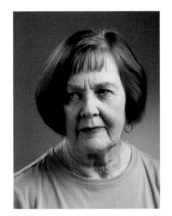

Suddenly confused or irritated,
or acting as if you are drunk

Other symptoms could include extreme hunger, tiredness,
nausea, feeling anxious, blurred vision or difficulty speaking.

MEDS & TESTS

Four Steps to Treat a Low Blood Sugar

Step 1. Check your blood sugar.

If you are under 70 mg/dL (4.0 mmol/L) go to Step 2. If your hands are shaking badly or your symptoms are severe, go straight to Step 2 without checking.

Step 2. Eat or drink sugar.

Take 15 grams of sugar to raise your blood sugar quickly. See photograph of easy choices on the next page. Pure sugars that aren't mixed with fat or protein work best. For example, sugar works best on its own and not in a chocolate bar. Glucose tablets are the fastest.

Special Note: Diabetes pills, acarbose (Prandase, Glucobay or Precose) or miglitol (Glycet) slow the absorption of some sugars. If you take these pills, glucose tablets are the recommended treatment. If you don't have glucose tablets, take 1 tbsp (15 mL) honey or 1 cup (250 mL) skim milk.

Step 3. Rest and wait 15 minutes.

Try not to panic. Sit or lie down. Give the sugar time to work. If after 15 minutes, you still have symptoms of low blood sugar, then recheck. If your blood sugar is still low, repeat Step 2 and Step 3 until blood sugar improves. Call a friend or seek medical help if your blood sugar doesn't come up.

Step 4. If you won't be eating a meal for an hour or more, have a snack.

This is so your blood sugar won't drop again. Your snack should include some protein or fat as well as carbohydrate. For example, eat a few crackers with cheese or peanut butter or 10 almonds.

If your blood sugar is under 55 mg/dL (3.0 mmol/L), take 20 to 30 grams of carbohydrate.

Do not try to treat low blood sugar with:
- sugar-free soft drink
- sugar-free candy
- low-calorie sweetener

These foods will not correct a low blood sugar.

Follow the 15/15 rule
This means take 15 grams of sugar and wait 15 minutes.

 CAUTION
If you pass out, someone needs to call 911 or an ambulance

It is unusual for a person with type 2 diabetes to pass out with low blood sugar. However, you are more at risk if you:
- Are elderly and in poor health
- Drink excess alcohol
- Have had significant change to your medication, your exercise or what you eat

To treat low blood sugar, choose one of these 15 gram carbohydrate choices:

1. **3 to 5 glucose tablets (15 g total); sold in pharmacies. This is your best choice!**

2. ½ cup to 2/3 cup (125 mL to 150 mL) unsweetened juice or regular soft drink

3. 20 g fruit roll-up

4. 3 sugar packages (1 tsp/5 mL each) stirred into a glass of water, or 5 sugar cubes (3 g each)

5. 1 tbsp (15 mL) honey

6. 6 Life Savers

7. 6 jelly beans

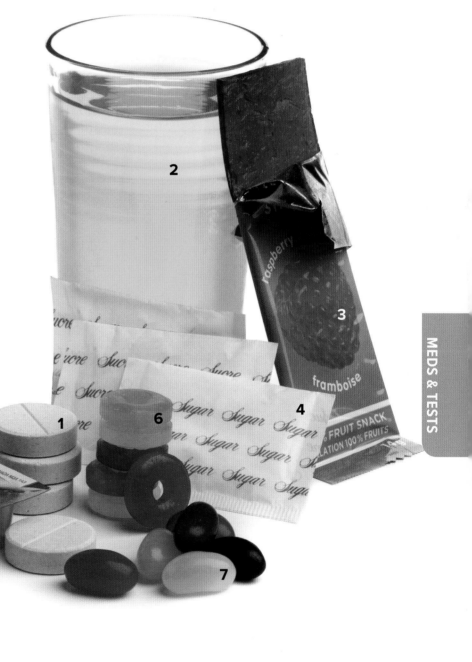

MEDS & TESTS

333

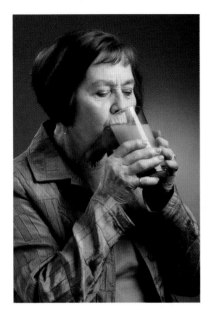

Look at how much juice she is drinking! She is drinking too much juice to treat her low. This causes her blood sugar to shoot up too high.

If you don't want to snack in the evening, ask your doctor for advice. Ask: "Can I change the kind or amount of insulin or pills I take? Can I adjust the time that I take them?"

Overtreating lows

When you have a low, you may feel panicky and ravenously hungry. As a result, you may eat a lot more than the recommended 15 grams of sugar. Perhaps you drank a large glass of juice, then ate several pieces of toast with honey. The result is like a roller coaster. You drop low, overtreat and end up with a high blood sugar. One suggestion that works for some people is not to treat with food, but only to use glucose tablets. The tablets are absorbed into your system the fastest, so you feel better sooner.

Prevent Low Blood Sugar

Each time your blood sugar goes low, your brain and organs are short of sugar. The lower your sugar, the more serious it is.

Eat meals and snacks at regular times

- Have a small snack if your meal will be delayed.
- If your meal is higher in fiber and has a lower glycemic index, you may need to delay taking rapid insulin.
- If you are taking rapid insulin, your meal time can be more flexible. Check your blood sugar before taking your rapid insulin. Take the right amount of insulin to match the type and amount of carbohydrates you'll eat.
- If you often forget to eat snacks, you might be better off taking rapid-acting insulin instead of short-acting insulin.

Include snacks as needed to prevent a low at night

Many find it helpful to eat a snack at night that includes a slowly absorbed carbohydrate with a protein and fat. For example, one or two whole-grain crackers with a small piece of cheese. The sugar then releases into your bloodstream gradually during the night. The snack portion size you choose will depend on blood sugar readings and your evening activity.

Adjust for alcohol

If you drink alcohol, have only one or two drinks. Eat extra food, or mix your drink with juice or a soft drink. You may need to decrease or omit your insulin or diabetes medication.

Rx DOCTOR'S ADVICE

Talk to your doctor or diabetes educator right away about your lows if:

- You have lows nearly every day, especially lows that drop under 55 mg/dL (3 mmol/L).
- A low blood sugar episode causes you to lose consciousness, even for a short time.

Make a record of your low blood sugar episodes and other blood numbers, and take this information to your appointment. Try to take notes about what you did before the episode. What time did you take insulin or other meds? Were you active? Did you skip a meal?

Adjust for exercise

- If you have taken your pills or insulin and then you exercise more than expected, you may need to eat extra food. For example, eat an extra slice of bread or one piece of fruit or ¾ cup (175 mL) of yogurt for each half hour of moderate exercise. High-intensity exercise requires more food.
- For planned high-intensity exercise, you can reduce your insulin or pills, or adjust the time you take them. If you are trying to lose weight, this is a better choice.
- Don't exercise at the time that your insulin peaks.
- Don't exercise soon after injecting into a muscle that you will be using to exercise. An exercising muscle absorbs insulin quickly.

Adjust for sick days

- When you are ill, your blood sugar usually goes up, but sometimes it can go low, especially if you are vomiting or have diarrhea. It is important to check your blood sugar at least every four hours when ill.

Adjust insulin or diabetes medications as needed

- Work with your doctor or diabetes educator to learn how to safely adjust your insulin. They may suggest you adjust the times when you take insulin or medication to reduce your lows.
- As you lose weight, you will generally need less insulin and fewer diabetes pills.

Check your blood sugar

If you get frequent low blood sugar episodes, check your blood sugar regularly at these times:

- Before and after exercise. Check during exercise, if your exercise is intense. Your blood sugar can drop up to 24 hours after an extended exercise session.
- Before going to bed
- When drinking alcohol
- When you are ill

MEDS & TESTS

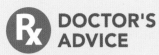

DOCTOR'S ADVICE

If you live alone

If you are elderly or in poor health, low blood sugar can cause you to feel disoriented. Your doctor may need to switch to a medication that is less likely to cause you to go low.

If you wear a "life line" device, keep it by your bedside when you sleep. Then you can press it in an emergency to get help.

You may appear drunk when you are low

If you wear a diabetes necklace or bracelet, people passing by are more likely to help you.

Low Blood Sugar Safety Guidelines

Always have some kind of sugar with you Put it in your pocket or purse, in your car in the visor or glove compartment, and by your TV chair and bed. Always have sugar with you when you are walking or exercising.

Wear a diabetes identification bracelet or necklace

Carry a card in your wallet that says you have diabetes and lists your medications. Ask your diabetes educator to give you information about a diabetes bracelet. You can also ask your diabetes educator for a wallet card.

Tell others you could have a low and how to treat it

Talk to your family, friends, work associates, gym buddies or a walking partner.

Use caution when drinking alcohol

Alcohol plus insulin can cause seriously low blood sugar. This is a particular concern when you live alone. If you have been drinking heavily and then take your insulin, someone needs to check on you every two to four hours overnight to make sure your blood sugar doesn't drop dangerously low.

Driving safety

- Check your blood sugar before you drive. Make sure it is not too low or too high. Do additional checks as recommended by your doctor or diabetes educator.
- If you are having a low, pull over, stop the vehicle and treat yourself immediately. Before driving, check to ensure your blood sugar is 90 mg/dL (5 mmol/L) or more. Eat a small protein and carbohydrate snack if a meal is more than an hour away. Check your blood sugar one hour later.
- Talk to your doctor about whether it is safe for you to drive if you have had a severe low where you lost consciousness even for a short time. Also talk with your doctor if you have hypoglycemia unawareness (see page 330) and you don't realize you have a low blood sugar.
- Don't drink alcohol before or during driving. This also applies to marijuana and street drugs, as well as prescription and over-the-counter medications that cause drowsiness.

Be safe! Check your blood sugar.

Checking Your Blood Sugar at Home

Do I Need to Check My Blood Sugar at Home?

If your doctor says yes, ask how often you should check. If you are on insulin or medications that can cause you to have a low blood sugar, your doctor will likely tell you to check your blood sugar for safety reasons. Otherwise, checking may be optional for you.

Read the benefits (pages 340–344) and the disadvantages (page 345) of checking your blood sugar.

Checking your blood is only a tool. On its own, it does not improve your blood sugar. It only tells you what your blood sugar is.

To improve your numbers, you need to change medication, adjust what you eat or become more physically active. If you go to the expense and bother of checking your blood sugar, please do something with the results to make it worthwhile.

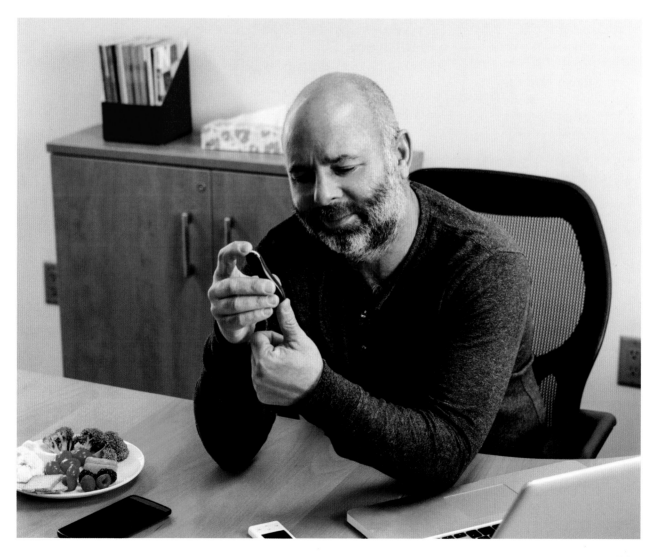

MEDS & TESTS

Benefits of Checking Your Blood Sugar

Along with A1C results, regular blood sugar or blood glucose monitoring can provide you and your doctor with valuable information. These results can show you what time of the day your blood sugar is high and when it is low. You'll learn what works with your lifestyle choices and medications and what's not working.

You can't always know by "how you feel" whether or not your blood sugar is high or low. When you check your blood sugar, you get an answer. Then you know and you can do something about it.

Manage highs

If your blood sugar is high, you can go for a walk or get on an exercise bike for 10 minutes. Another option is to cut out a snack or eat less at your next meal. If you measure your blood sugar before eating and two hours after, you can learn which types of meals tend to make your blood sugar stay high. If you take rapid insulin, you could take extra insulin to help bring down your high blood sugar.

Blood sugar results tell you if the doctor should increase your dose or change the timing or type of medication.

Manage lows

If you check and see your blood sugar is low, you can treat it yourself with sugar and prevent it from dropping lower. If you have hypoglycemic unawareness (see page 330), checking is essential. If you have had a low, rechecking can let you know when your blood sugar comes back up into a safe range.

It helps motivate you

Many people find that if they check their blood sugar regularly, it keeps them on track. Also, because they discover that certain foods make their blood sugars too high, they will cut back on eating too much of these foods.

Blood sugar checks helps you deal safely with changes such as:

- Eating or exercising more or less
- Traveling, for example, through time zones
- Drinking alcohol
- Illness, when blood sugar can go very high or low

Different monitoring devices

The next six pages cover the tools you need to check your blood sugar. These include blood glucose monitors (also called meters) and continuous glucose monitors (CGM). The blood glucose monitors give you one reading at a time, whereas CGM give you continual blood sugar readings.

There are diabetes apps available that can help you to understand and interpret the information from these monitors.

Blood Sugar Targets

An occasional high because of a large meal is less of a concern than if your numbers are consistently above these targets. If your numbers are consistently high, what can you do to bring your levels down? Do you need to see your doctor about additional medication?

Your doctor may suggest blood sugar targets for you that are a bit higher or lower than these.

You've been checking your blood sugar and have recorded the numbers. Here are some targets for healthy blood sugar levels.

Fasting blood sugar (FBG) or before meals:
under 130 mg/dL (7 mmol/L)

Two hours after eating:
under 180 mg/dL (10 mmol/L)

To avoid a low:
Always stay above 70 mg/dL (4 mmol/L)

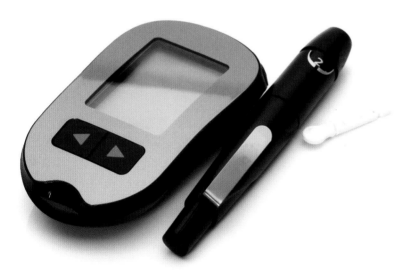

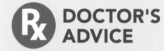 **DOCTOR'S ADVICE**

Write down your results
Although your meter may store a large number of results, it is also helpful to write them down.

This helps you own the results
If you already record what you eat or your exercise, then put your blood sugar results in the same notebook. Now you can see trends and patterns. This helps identify what you are doing right as well as your highs and lows and where you can make changes.

MEDS & TESTS

Learning to use your monitor

- Ask the pharmacy staff where you bought the monitor to show you how to use it.
- Seek assistance from a nurse or diabetes educator.
- Read the instruction manual or call the toll-free number from the manufacturer.
- Find some online resources and videos.

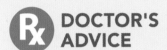

DOCTOR'S ADVICE

You may need to check more often when:

- You are ill.
- You are pregnant or planning a pregnancy.
- You have started a new medication.
- You have an infection.
- You have been having a lot of lows.
- You are going to a medical appointment. A test just before you go means you will be bringing up-to-date information to your health care provider.

Blood Glucose Monitors

These monitors, or meters, are compact and easy to carry. While they're easy to use, instructions are always helpful when you are getting started. Basically, you prick the side of your finger with a lancing device and then put a drop of blood on a test strip. Insert the strip into the meter.

Alternate site testing

Some monitors allow testing on the arm. Some people find it hard to get a drop of blood from there. Others find it less painful than testing on the fingers.

How Often Should I Check?

Discuss this with your doctor or diabetes educator. Some people check a few times per week. Others check numerous times a day. More checking gives a better picture of how well you are managing your diabetes. Here are some general guidelines.

If you are not taking insulin or diabetes medications, these are possible times to check:

- After fasting, first thing in the morning before you have eaten
- Two hours after eating a meal. Your blood sugar peaks at one hour; by two hours after a meal, it should be coming down
- Before and after exercise
- Any time you aren't feeling well

If you are at risk of low blood sugar, here are some additional times to check:

- Before meals. This is critical if you are taking meal time insulin.
- Before going to bed, check to determine whether or not you need a snack or to adjust your evening dose of insulin.
- Any time you think your blood sugar may be low
- Before driving
- After drinking alcohol
- After prolonged exercise

Understanding Blood Sugar Trends

A trend is a similar blood sugar reading at the same time of day for several days in a row. Here are some examples of trends. Understanding these trends is the key to improving your blood sugar.

Margie wakes up in the morning with good numbers. But she is usually high after her evening dinner. She should occasionally check before dinner to see how much dinner raised her blood sugar. If so, she can reduce the amount of carbs she eats at dinner or go for a brisk walk for half an hour after dinner.

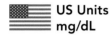 **US Units mg/dL**

Day	Before breakfast	After dinner
Day 1	102	315
Day 2	118	247

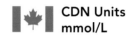 **CDN Units mmol/L**

Day	Before breakfast	After dinner
Day 1	5.7	17.5
Day 2	6.6	13.7

Claude's doctor prescribed him a basal insulin. His readings are high most of the time. The fasting sugar is usually the highest. Claude can't fix that on his own. His doctor should increase the dose of his basal insulin.

All Before Meal Readings

Day	Breakfast	Lunch	Dinner	Bedtime
Day 1	174	158	175	169
Day 2	162	189	122	144

All Before Meal Readings

Day	Breakfast	Lunch	Dinner	Bedtime
Day 1	9.7	8.8	9.7	9.4
Day 2	9.0	10.5	6.8	8.0

Martina uses both basal and mealtime insulin. On Day 1, she was low before lunch but went up really high after dinner. This was due to overcorrection of a low. The next day, Martina was actually high before lunch. Given such variability, her carb intake at breakfast and mealtime insulin dosing needs to be reviewed.

All Before Meal Readings

Day	Breakfast	Lunch	Dinner	Bedtime
Day 1	113	59	299	187
Day 2	109	276	–	151

All Before Meal Readings

Day	Breakfast	Lunch	Dinner	Bedtime
Day 1	6.3	3.3	16.6	10.4
Day 2	6.0	15.3	–	8.4

MEDS & TESTS

Embrace technology when the time is right for you. Don't feel you need to switch from a meter to CGM unless it is helpful.

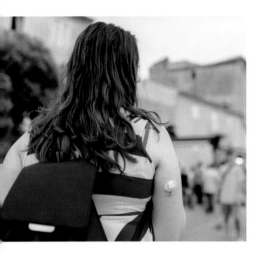

Like all new technologies, CGM is expensive and will take time to be covered under health insurance plans.

Who should use CGM?

CGM is most helpful for people who:

- Inject mealtime insulin
- Are prone to hypoglycemia
- Have hypoglycemic unawareness
- Check three or more times each day
- Are motivated to understand how insulin, food and exercise affects their blood sugar

Continuous Glucose Monitors

A continuous glucose monitor (CGM) has two separate parts.

1. **A small transmitter device plus sensor.** The transmitter device attaches to the skin, usually on the abdomen or upper arm. This device has a tiny sensor filament that goes under the skin. The sensor samples the sugar in the fluid that's just under your skin every 5 to 15 minutes. This device can stay on your arm for about two weeks, then needs to be replaced.

2. **A handheld scanner or reader.** You use this to scan the transmitter on your arm to pick up the sugar readings in the fluid. The scanner converts the information to blood sugar values. The blood sugar values are displayed on the the scanner or sent to your cell phone.

A person wearing a CGM could scan a few times a day, or many times a day. Once they scan, all the blood sugar information since you last scanned goes to the scanner. They now can know their blood sugar numbers on a continuous basis, day or night, without pricking a finger.

CGM brands include Abbott's FreeStyle Libre, Dexcom's G5 and G6, and the Medtronic system. The Medtronic CGM is used with a Medtronic insulin pump and is not covered here. Eversense brand is a new type of CGM with a sensor that is implanted just under the skin by a doctor. It can be placed and removed by minor surgery in the doctor's office. In the United States, it is approved for use for three months; it is not yet approved in Canada.

FreeStyle Libre

When you use this device, you swipe the patch with the reader or a smartphone to instantly receive information on your blood sugar. You can even swipe through clothing. When you wake up and swipe, you receive the nighttime data for up to 8 hours. This data can be used to help you make decisions on what to eat, if you need to exercise and so on.

Dexcom system

The sensor has a transmitter on it that sends useful data to a reader or smartphone. Since the device sends data continuously, alarms can be set up. These alarms warn you if your blood sugar is rising too high or dropping too quickly.

Reports can be sent by phone to a family member or health care provider.

Understanding CGM Data

The main screen of a typical CGM device displays the following information.

Current glucose reading: CGM actually measures the level of sugar (glucose) in your fluid under your skin, but the scanner converts it to a blood sugar reading.

Trend arrow: This shows which direction your blood sugar is moving and how fast it is moving. You can think of this as predicting the future. Is your sugar rising, falling or holding steady? You can learn a lot from this.

Glucose history: This shows a graph of all your readings since you last scanned. The CGM attached to your arm collects readings automatically every 5 to 15 minutes.

Target range: Your target range is shaded to make it easy to see at a glance how many of your readings are in a good range, or too high or too low. Your CGM can also determine "Time in range," the amount of time you are within your target range. "Time in hypoglycemia" is the time you have had a below-normal blood sugar level.

Notes you add: You can record your food and exercise, tied to the time. For example, you can note the carbohydrates that you ate at a meal, the exercise you did, how much insulin you took and other information. When readings are too high or too low, you can go back to this information and troubleshoot with your health care provider to look for solutions. You can also look at what you did right on days when your blood sugar is nicely in range.

How are you doing?

Time in range:
This measures the percentage of the sugar readings that are between 70 and 180 mg/dL (4 and 10 mmol/L). Most experts recommend aiming for a time in range of over 70%.

Time in hypoglycemia:
This measures the percent of the sugar readings that are below 70 mg/dL (4 mmol/L). Most experts would like the time that you are in this low range to be less than 3% of the time.

Your doctor will tell you if higher or lower range values may be better for you.

In this example, the current blood sugar is 90 mg/dL (5.0 mmol/L) and falling. The user should eat or drink some rapid-acting carbs to avoid a low blood sugar episode. If the trend arrow were level or pointing up, no immediate action is needed.

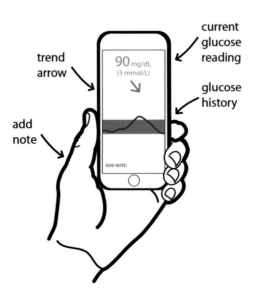

trend arrow

add note

current glucose reading

glucose history

90 mg/dL
(5 mmol/L)

ADD NOTE:

The artifical pancreas

Engineers and researchers have built devices which use the CGM data to directly control an insulin pump. These devices automatically control one's diabetes with little effort on the part of the patient. Early versions of these devices are becoming available now. They are most helpful for people with type 1 diabetes.

MEDS & TESTS

There are thousands of general health apps for smartphones and tablets available today. There are also many apps for people with diabetes. You may decide to learn and use this technology. Diabetes apps make it easy for you to track and visualize your data and share information with your doctor or diabetes educator.

Check which app works with your meter.

Diabetes Apps

Here are three examples of well-made products:

One Touch Reveal is based on the One Touch Verio Flex blood sugar meter. The meter connects to your phone via Bluetooth. It serves as an electronic log book. You can track your blood sugar data, medications and food. You can generate reports and email them to your doctor or a family member. Users receive alerts when the app detects blood sugar patterns.

Glooko makes a device that can download nearly every brand of blood glucose monitor, continuous glucose monitors, and some insulin pumps. The summarized data always looks the same to your doctor, making it easier to understand your diabetes information. You can download the app and track all the same data to better understand your diabetes.

BlueStar Diabetes is a comprehensive diabetes coaching app. It takes all of your glucose, carbs, medications, activity, weight, blood pressure and sleep data and uses an artificial intelligence system to coach you into better diabetes management. Research studies show that if you use BlueStar, your A1C will come down significantly.

 ROBERT'S STORY: Using a diabetes app and CGM

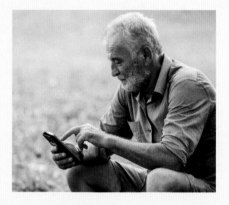

For many years, my diabetes was a moving target for me. Initially, I figured I'd learn what I could, try to watch what I eat, and beat the disease. At least until a creeping complacency set in, along with the complications of a growing and active family and intense work schedule. Fingerstick testing slipped, food was less planned, and the A1C numbers started to rise.

My doctor suggested I try using a diabetes app on my phone, called BlueStar, to track my fingerstick results, medication doses, exercise and food intake. The app helps me learn, gives me daily and weekly reports and coaches me to set weekly goals. Using the app improved my numbers. But when life got hectic again, I didn't always use it to its full potential.

A few months later, I went back to my doctor because I was having both high and low blood sugars. He told me that CGM could be used with the app, and I decided to try it. With Dexcom CGM, I now see my blood sugar readings on my phone and it even integrates with the diabetes app. The phone alerts me when my blood sugar is going low or high. This helps motivate me to eat less or to exercise more. I use the food database to learn about foods and portions. I've also learned that exercise really does work to bring down blood sugar after a meal!

Reasons Not to Check Your Blood Sugar at Home

It makes you feel stressed

You might feel upset when you see high blood sugar numbers. If you don't do something positive about it, then worrying about it can actually make your blood sugar worse. You may be unsure what the numbers mean. This can cause anxiety. Stress hormones cause blood sugar to go up. In this way, home checking could actually make your blood sugar worse. High blood sugar numbers make some people so upset that they turn to food to comfort themselves and end up eating more!

It takes time

If you check your blood sugar three times a day, that might take 15 minutes of your time (5 minutes each time). It might be more beneficial if you walked around for 5 minutes three times a day instead. That would total 15 extra minutes of exercise.

It takes learning and record keeping

You'll need to learn how to use a blood sugar monitor, but you also have to learn what to do with the numbers. If you check your blood sugar at the same time every day and find similar results, then you aren't learning anything new. If when you check, your sugar is high, but you don't change how you eat or exercise, then you need to ask yourself, "How is this helping me?" Blood sugar checks and action need to go together.

Expensive

The cost of using several test strips a day or CGM adds up.

Uncomfortable

Although lancet devices are small, testing can hurt if you have sensitive fingertips. You may not want to have a CGM attached to your body all the time.

You know yourself best as a person. It's not helpful if blood sugar checking at home makes you preoccupied with the numbers. You know how you respond to stress and what motivates you.

If you feel checking your sugars doesn't help you, then rely instead on the A1C test. Also, periodically have your fasting or random blood sugar taken at a lab.

Not everyone needs to check their blood sugar at home or use technology like smartphone apps to track their numbers. Research shows that home blood checking is only helpful when you understand and use the blood sugar numbers to make changes to your lifestyle or medication.

If you decide to not check your blood sugar at home, remember, it's still important to have the three-month A1C diabetes test taken at a lab.

MEDS & TESTS

345

Checking Blood Pressure at Home

Blood pressure (BP) is made up of two numbers, called systolic BP and diastolic BP. The systolic BP is written on top and is always higher than the diastolic BP. The American Diabetes Association recommends that your blood pressure be less than 140/90. In some cases, depending on your risk of heart disease, they recommend less than 130/80. Diabetes Canada recommends that your blood pressure be less than 130/80. If your systolic blood pressure is greater than 180 or if the diastolic BP is greater than 120, get immediate medical attention.

It is very important to check your blood pressure at home. Studies show that this often gives you more important information than blood pressure checks at the doctor's office. At the doctor's office, blood pressure may be falsely high due to what is called white coat syndrome. This means you may feel anxious at the doctor's; this can make your blood pressure go up.

High blood pressure multiplies the risk that you might get diabetes complications. For this reason, controlling blood pressure is VERY IMPORTANT.

Take the record of your results to your appointment with your doctor. This can help your doctor know how to change your blood pressure medication. Blood pressure pills often make a big improvement. See page 317 for information about blood pressure pills.

Make sure you have the right cuff size for your arm. Relax for five minutes in a quiet place. Avoid smoking or caffeinated drinks for 30 minutes beforehand. Now you are ready to take your blood pressure. Place the cuff on your bare upper arm, push a button and it will pump up by itself. It's run by batteries. It will give you a reading. If you get a high or too low reading, sit quietly for ten minutes, then recheck.

Get detailed instructions on how to use the machine at a pharmacy, from a diabetes educator, a doctor or online.

Good times to check your blood pressure

Check first thing in the morning and before going to bed. Write the results down and share them with your doctor.

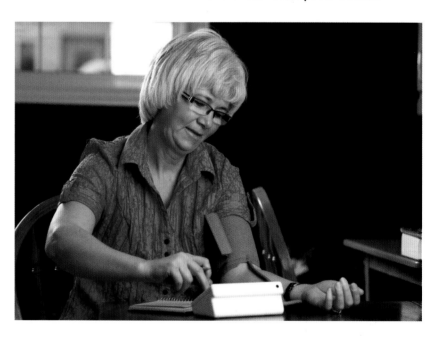

If your blood pressures readings at home are high, think about what you can do differently to help improve them. These things can help: go for a daily walk; eat some fruit and vegetables every day; cut back on your salt, alcohol and smoking; and learn better ways to relax.

Step 6: Stay Upbeat

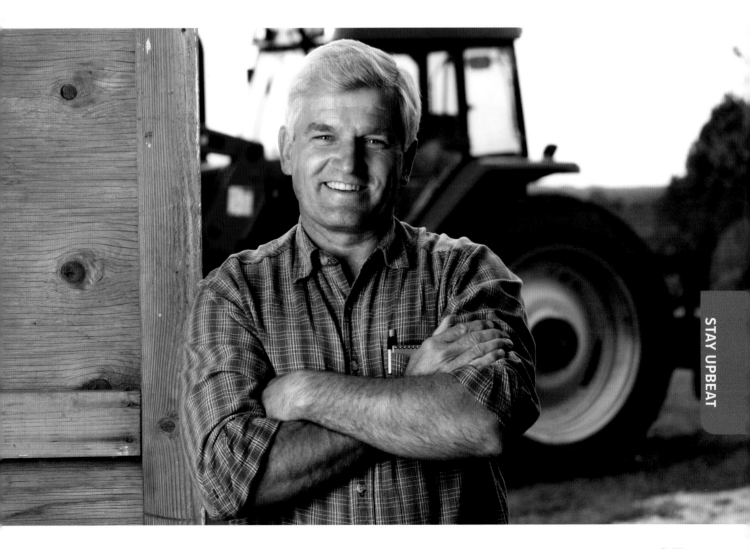

STAY UPBEAT

Coping with Stress

Learn about how stress, depression and sleeping problems affect diabetes on pages 52–53.

Stress helps you set expectations and goals for yourself.

Keep your mind healthy to keep your body healthy, too!

Stress is a normal and inevitable part of everyone's life. We put stress on ourselves because of our own expectations, or others around us can cause us stress. Stress is part of human relationships and life's realities of paying bills, work, and looking after yourself and others.

A certain amount of stress is a good thing. It helps you get up in the morning. It motivates you and moves you to get things done. It helps you live up to your potential. Stress makes life challenging and interesting.

Stress is a bad thing when it overwhelms you, and you don't know how to handle it. Then it can have a serious impact on your diabetes, blood pressure and health. Please don't ignore stress. If you have too much stress, take steps to lower it.

How Much Stress Do You Have?

How would you rate your level of stress now?

Very low, low, medium or high? Think about it for a while for yourself. At different times of your life, your level of stress changes.

Very low

This might be rare, as we all have some stress in our life. Or perhaps a person doesn't recognize their own stress.

Low

A small percentage of people with diabetes say that they have a low level of stress. This usually means they have a lot of support around them. It may also mean that they have a medium level of stress but they know how to manage it in a healthy way. With careful management and support, they can reduce stress to low levels.

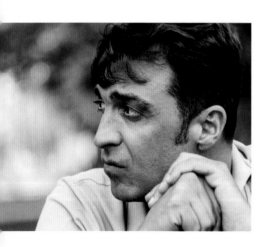

Medium

This is a common amount of stress on diagnosis. When diagnosed, you may have felt this stress. It usually isn't just the diabetes causing stress. It's also your stage of life that is most common at the time of diagnosis. Lots of things can cause stress, no matter where you are in life. You may be a middle-aged bachelor or a mother of teenagers. You could be working at the peak of your career or be a grandparent. You may be dealing with a large work load or financial debt. Do you have multiple health conditions or suffer from chronic pain? You may have family members or friends who weigh you down with their demands or complaints. Are you caring for an elderly parent or getting older yourself? Perhaps you feel frustrated with the unfair changes of aging. Although you can't make it go away, there are steps you can take to manage your stress.

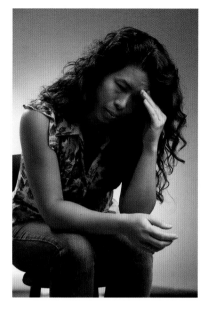

Feeling stressed

High

Your own life circumstances can push you up to high stress levels. Have you recently gone through a divorce, lost your job or the death of your spouse? This creates change that can overwhelm you. Perhaps personality conflicts in your workplace or at home have escalated. Verbal, physical or sexual abuse creates high-level stress. Your diabetes diagnosis or dealing with diabetes complications can then increase your stress further. This stress then raises your blood sugar. You probably know the source of your stress. Your stress level can improve as you learn to cope with the diabetes or as crises resolve. Bringing your stress down from this dangerous level is critical. Please read the rest of this section for tips on managing stress.

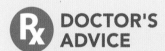

DOCTOR'S ADVICE

We can't always control the causes of stress. **We need to change how we respond to stress.**

Stress and Diabetes

Changes in your body with medium-high stress

Your body makes stress hormones when stress levels are at a medium to high level or escalate upward. These hormones circulate in your blood and affect your body in different ways. Stress hormones increase your blood sugar and blood pressure, reduce immunity, increase inflammation inside your blood vessels, and cause nerve overstimulation. You may feel unwell, have an upset stomach, sleep poorly, and feel agitated and unhappy. Over time, high stress levels increase your risk for diabetes complications, including a heart attack or stroke.

STAY UPBEAT

349

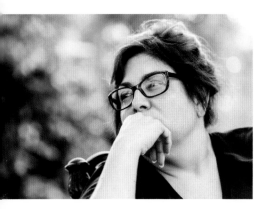

When stress becomes unmanageable

Seek help to handle stress in a healthy way before it leads to a serious health problem. Stress leads some people to addictions, including abusing food, alcohol and drugs. Addictions over the long term can devastate you and your family. If you think you need help, please ask for it.

Seek professional help if needed

Talk to your doctor or diabetes team. You may need a referral to an addictions counselor, mental health worker, social worker, psychologist or psychiatrist (medical doctor specializing in mental health). You may require medication for a short period of time to help you cope or to help you sleep better. If you are experiencing abuse, you may need shelter in a safe home.

If you experienced trauma as a child, this is real and hurtful. It was not okay and it still affects you as an adult. You are courageous. If there is ever a time you feel you need support and a listening ear, talk to a trusted friend or professional.

Tips to Help Manage Stress
Slow down
Are you feeling down, sad, angry, on the edge?

These are normal feelings when things get overwhelming. Try slowing down a bit. Get back to basics. Remind yourself that you can only do what you can do, and no more.

Stress can motivate you, but it can also cause burnout. Think about how slowing down would help. Once you've identified the main source of your stress, see if it can be reduced. If your job causes stress, can you change things? Work fewer hours, delegate some work, or change work space to reduce personality conflict? Staying in a bad situation that causes you to get sick is not worth the risk.

Take one day at time, one step at a time.
Set small, reachable goals.

Ask your doctor, health worker or friend, "What do I need to do right away?" Make a plan for other changes that can happen later, when you are ready.

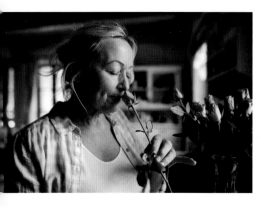

Take time to "smell the roses." Do you enjoy the aroma of a fresh pot of coffee? Some people love the smell of freshly dried clothes or the smell after a rain shower. Aromas can put you in a different mood right away.

Think in healthy ways

Some ways of thinking are like diseases.

Do you have a lot of negative thoughts?

Negative thoughts build up, one on top of another and are like poison. If you say, "I will never be able to control my diabetes" you feel discouraged, and so you may eat more and less. Try to replace this with a positive thought. For example, "I can start making one small change every few days to make my blood sugar better." Now you have changed your outlook. You work toward a positive mood and give yourself motivation to move forward. Focus on the positive changes you have made and good things in your life. This is what is most important.

Do you sometimes overthink things?

Was the situation really as serious as you thought it was? Could you solve that issue? Did your friend really think that bad thing about you that you imagine they did? We are not all good communicators. Sometimes our relationship issues stem from misunderstandings. We think we know how another person thinks and feels, or feels about us, but do we really? Words are often misunderstood, or silences taken in the wrong way. Sometimes our emotions bring us stress when that was not the intention of the other person. Don't save correspondence or reminders if it causes you stress or pain. Sometimes, as hard as it is, the best way is to let the past alone. Old grudges and arguments are very difficult to give up. If they are increasing your stress, ask yourself if you can let go of them so they don't burden you.

The world is sometimes simpler than we imagine. You may feel less stressed if you don't overthink things. Instead, step back occasionally and breathe. Things will get better.

Talk it out

It's good to share our troubles and our pain. If we don't talk, all these troubles stay inside us. They build up and we start getting sick.

There are times when what we need most is to be quiet and alone. That's okay too.

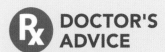

DOCTOR'S ADVICE

Thoughts are powerful
When you replace negative thoughts with positive thoughts, you start seeing good results. Tell yourself something positive — and give others compliments.

Journaling
It can help to write down how you feel. This is especially true when you are trying to find out how your emotions affect your habits. It can also be a good way to vent your emotions privately. However, this doesn't mean you need to keep what you wrote. Sometimes it's best to erase or delete what you've written because when we are upset, we don't always see things clearly.

Sadness is a part of life. It's fair to say that the good times are better when we've also gone through hard times.

STAY UPBEAT

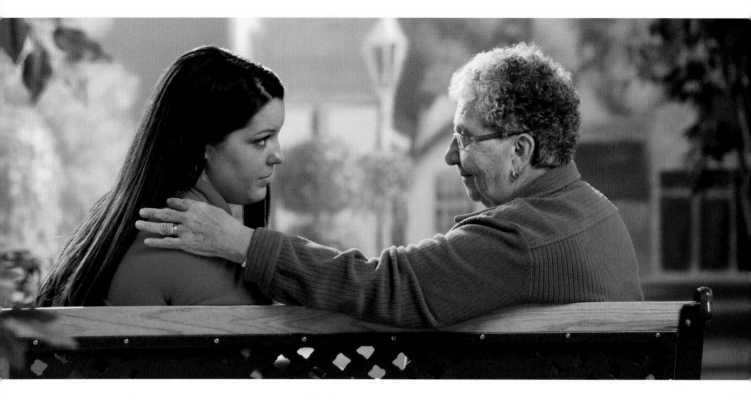

It's okay to express your emotions

Don't pretend you're happy when you're not. Sometimes we cry, and crying is good. It's a way to relieve stress and feel better afterward. Finding someone to talk to in confidence and who you trust to become emotional with may be difficult. Seek out a spiritual leader, a counsellor, a doctor or diabetes worker. Talking and having someone hear your stories without judgment is an important part of your mental health. It opens the way to healing.

Keep learning

Being bored or idle can lead to frustration. Just because we're not going to school does not mean we should stop learning or keep busy to prevent idleness.

For some, learning is best in a group situation. Attend classes at your community resource centre, library or college. If you prefer learning alone, there are many ways to bring new information into your life. Most libraries have subscriptions to a variety of magazines to borrow or read on site. Books, radio programs and podcasts are great sources of ideas and information.

To keep busy indoors, enjoy your arts and crafts, puzzles, card games, sewing, movies and writing. Outdoors in your garden or a community garden can be rewarding. Enjoy feeding birds, going to museums, art galleries and attending musical shows.

Volunteering can give back

Volunteering is a wonderful way to give back to your community and share your special skills and qualities. Participating in such social situations, you'll learn to see your worries in comparison to those of others. There are always people who have life situations worse than our own.

Have fun

Smiling helps you feel good. Sometimes it's hard to smile, but it does work!

Keep in touch with things that make you happy — friends and family, pets, keepsakes, music, plants, sports, hobbies or movies. Simple and familiar things and routines are comforting. Get out of the house for social outings. Enjoy a cup of tea, an occasional beer or glass of wine with friends or family. Laugh and have fun. Start planning a vacation now!

Laughter is a wonderful medicine

What could be funny about having diabetes? About having to follow a meal plan and take pills or insulin? Well, nothing really! That's exactly why we need some humor and laughter to help cope with challenges and stress.

Laughter balances our lives. It helps us realize that some problems are not the big events they seem to be at the time. It helps us accept our limitations. Then we can get on with taking care of ourselves.

Amazingly, laughter helps improve our resistance to disease and infection. It encourages healing. When we laugh, we breathe deeper. Then the oxygen-enriched blood and "happy hormones" (endorphins) flow through our body. Laughter helps us live longer and happier lives.

Keep good things close to you. Focus on short, happy moments. Tuck these moments away, folded like a napkin. Take it out when you need a good thought. Write down happy things or look at photographs that you love. Happy memories are the ones to keep.

Have fun — do things you enjoy!

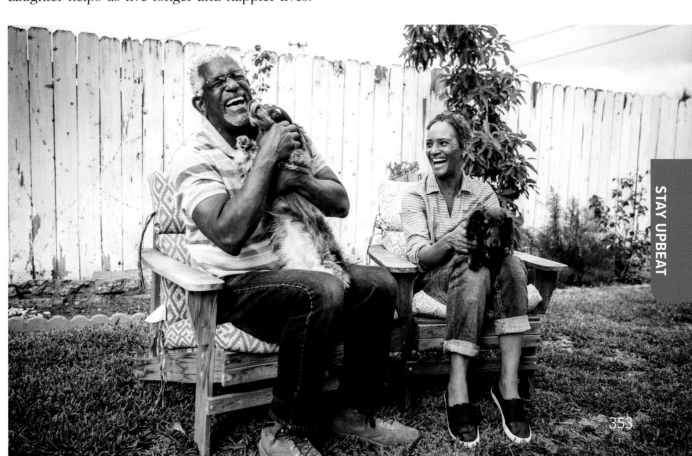

STAY UPBEAT

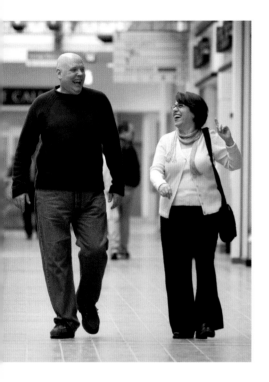

A good hearty laugh can also:

- Lower blood pressure and protect your heart
- Improve your brain functioning
- Help you relax and feel good
- Help take away anger
- Connect you to others

For the most part, small everyday moments make up our lives — not great occasions or successes. Enjoy those moments.

Bring laughter into your life

Kids have a wonderful way of laughing and giggling, even in the face of adversity. We don't have to always be grown up. Sometimes we feel good when we act like kids again. Let's learn from the children in our lives, and play and laugh along. If you have grandkids or young kids around, it can be healing to play in the sand or make things out of play dough.

Who helps you laugh? Spend more time with those people. Some of us laughed more when we were young. You may want to try to reconnect with your friends from when you were young. If you can't connect with old friends, do activities where you might meet new friends.

What makes you laugh? Go ahead and enjoy a favorite radio or TV show, a movie, a book or comic strip, an email joke, or that old family story. If it makes you laugh, it's good and you need it. Better yet, share it with someone else who has the same sense of humor as you, and the laughter will be even better. Laughter is contagious.

Believe in something

Our beliefs give us hope. Hope renews itself, like flowers in the spring after every long hard winter.

The most important thing is for you to believe in yourself. Be proud of who you are and where you have come from. Don't measure success by the position you have in life, but by the obstacles you overcame to get to where you are today. You may have had some big obstacles to overcome. Good for you.

Attending services regularly at a place of worship is like scheduled stress reduction. You become part of a network of support with others in your community and around the world. It's also a chance to relinquish your everyday worries to a higher power, if even for a short time. Prayer and meditation provide an opportunity for quiet reflection. When you sing hymns and chants you may feel an emotional connection, but you also breathe deeply and that relieves tension. Hearing familiar songs can calm you.

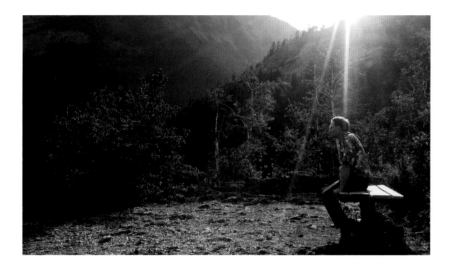

Outdoors is where you feel the wind on your face, hear the leaves and the birds, see the clouds and the evening stars. Time alone outdoors is time to reflect, rethink and restart.

Find your healing path

Being in nature can be a spiritual and healing experience. Many of us live in cities where wilderness is out of our reach. Modern life draws us away from the outdoors as we spend more hours in front of screens. Yet, deep inside us, we need to connect with nature.

Cities have parks and nature paths. Find them and use them. Take a daytrip to a national, state or provincial park; make time for a picnic or a walk in the forest. Closer to home, many people enjoy gardening in their backyard as a way to be outdoors.

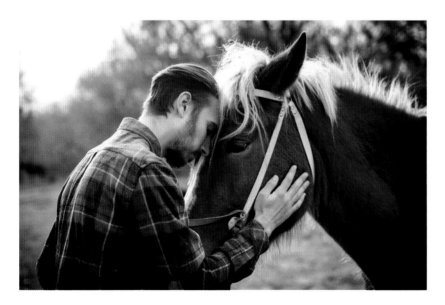

Pets can be steadfast companions, reduce boredom, have calming effects, and they provide unconditional love. Owners have silly playful times together and quiet cuddling times with their pet, all of which can prove to be healing. In return, pets need to be properly fed, groomed and cared for, and walked regularly.

STAY UPBEAT

Animals can help us with emotional healing

Ask your doctor about a referral to animal assisted therapy (ATT). There is significant research about people who experience anxiety or depression, who have successfully overcome their mental health issues from interacting with animals.

Reducing clutter in your home can help you lose weight. Here's why:

- Clutter causes stress and a feeling of failure. This can lead to overeating.
- If your fridge, freezer, counters and cupboards are cluttered with high-calorie food, you'll be tempted.
- When your dining area is clean and tidy, you'll enjoy eating at home more.

Seasonal affective disorder, or SAD, is a kind of "winter blues." It's more common in people who live in northern latitudes or are shift workers. A lack of light may be part of what causes these blues. Spending a half an hour a day near a specially designed fluorescent lamp that acts like daylight helps some people. For more information, ask your doctor or your local mental health association.

Make your home your nest

Keep your home tidy, comfortable and safe. A vase of flowers can pick up your mood for days. Easy renovations can cheer you up. Try different pillows on your couch or hang up a new picture. A fresh coat of paint on your walls can make quite a difference. Consider calming wall colors of pastel or paler colors (try a pale sage green or light sky blue) complemented with shades of white or ivory. Soothing scents in your home, such as cinnamon, orange or lavender, help relax you.

Feed your brain good food

Your brain controls your mood. It needs nutrients to work properly. Adequate magnesium, B vitamins especially niacin, vitamin B_6 and folic acid, and omega-3 fats, help improve mood and reduce stress. Foods that have tryptophan, a type of protein, also help boost your mood and help you sleep better. Milk is rich in tryptophan. Other good sources are yogurt, cheese, eggs, bananas and peanuts. To get the nutrients you need, eat a colorful variety of healthy foods in the right amounts for you. Eat regular meals and eat slowly. Share meals with family and friends. Enjoy the occasional indulgence. If your weight causes you stress, think about getting rid of your scale. As long as you monitor your weight with your doctor, you don't need to weigh yourself every day.

Exercise and sunlight

Keep active at home or work. Walk away from stress. Walk, bike or do other exercise. All bodies can be fit and strong. When you exercise, you pump out "happy hormones." These relax you and bring down your blood sugar and blood pressure. This reduces inflammation in your body.

An extra bonus of walking outside is that you get exposed to light. Sunlight, even through a window, helps stimulate your senses and lift your spirits. The vitamin D from outdoor sunlight may also help lift your mood.

ALICE'S STORY: Walking lifts my spirits

When I started walking, I could only walk for 5 minutes. Then I went to 10, then 15, then 20. Then I was really happy with 30 minutes. And I found that it helped me in many ways. It didn't just help me physically but I feel it helped me emotionally too. I was in a better frame of mind. Whatever came up, I was able to handle it better. As we age, we have children and grandchildren and there's always something going on. I found walking helped me to be more positive.

Look your best

Enjoy a relaxing shower or short bath daily. Keep your nails and hair well groomed. Wandering around your home in your pajamas or sweat pants is comfortable, yet dressing up is one way of making you feel better about yourself.

> Your smile is the most important thing you can wear.

A few clothing tips

- Clothes that are too oversized or too tight may simply not be comfortable. Tugging and pulling and readjusting clothes is distracting for yourself and others. Sort your closets and drawers and keep only the clothes that fit you well.
- It's not just the shoes that must fit properly. Have a special athletic or walking outfit. They say red is a powerful motivating color. When you put on that outfit, you are already feeling good about starting your walk or exercise.
- When you go out, wear your "happy sweater" or clothing item, such as jewelry or a belt, that has brought compliments in the past. When people notice you and compliment you, you will automatically feel good.
- Whatever you wear, good posture is essential. Keep your shoulders back and relaxed. Keep your head up, look forward and smile.

Music

Research into music therapy shows it increases social skills in children and reduces dementia in the elderly. Music can help you too. Reduce your stress and play your familiar tunes and sing along. Enjoy music videos. Sing along with family to the musical score in children's movies. Music often compels us to sing, dance or tap our feet, and that's a great thing. Music also provides the opposite, relaxation and pleasure by stimulating the brain to release the hormone dopamine, the pleasure chemical.

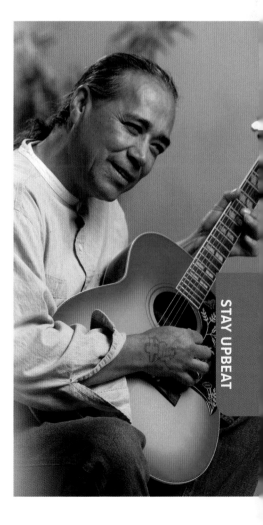

STAY UPBEAT

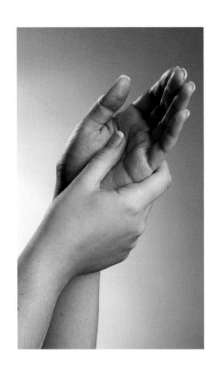

Touch

Appropriate and invited touch comes in many forms. Touch has the power to relax and improve health. Shaking hands, holding hands, hugs and kisses, cuddling, hand manicures, foot or back massages, a "wash and cut" at the hairdresser, brushing a child's hair, holding a baby or child, or dancing with a partner can all be good touches. Petting a dog or cat is a wonderful opportunity for touch. Pets need our attention as much as we need theirs.

On your own, have a relaxing bath or shower and feel the touch of the warm water. When you feel stressed, your circulation decreases. This can make your hands feel cold. Massage and warm your hands by working in hand cream. Start at your wrist and work down to each individual finger.

When sex is enjoyable, you release "happy hormones," whether you are with a partner or flying solo.

Get seven to eight hours of sleep

As discussed on page 53, lack of sleep or too much sleep can make stress worse, as well as increase your weight and your blood sugar. You may function on more or less sleep, but if you're stressed, it's good to get seven to eight hours of sleep. Sometimes, making one small change can make a difference. Try one of these tips.

Have a regular bedtime routine
- Try to go to bed and get up in the morning at a regular time.
- Have a "before bed" routine; for example, brush and floss your teeth, then have a shower or short bath.
- If you have a phone, tablet, TV or computer in your bedroom, turn them all off 15 minutes before bedtime. Your mind and eyes need a chance to settle down. If you read just before turning off the lights, settle for something light rather than something that will keep you awake. Try to save arguments with family members for other times, so your body can relax.

Avoid or limit caffeine, nicotine and alcohol at least three hours before bedtime. Also limit drinking fluids one to two hours before going to sleep, to reduce getting up at night.

If your bedmate snores…

If this disrupts your sleep, think about options to resolve it. Consider earplugs or a fan to provide white noise. Can you sleep in a different room? Can your partner change something that will reduce his or her snoring such as treating allergies or sleeping on his or her side? Snoring can be a symptom of sleep apnea. Talk to a doctor to learn more.

Exercise during the day or earlier in the evening will tire you out so you sleep better at night.

Avoid or limit large bedtime snacks. If feeling hungry prevents you from falling asleep or wakes you up, you may need to have a small evening snack. A glass of milk or a small banana is a good choice, as the tryptophan helps you sleep. Large, heavy snacks will disrupt your sleep.

Limit long daytime naps if possible.

A comfortable mattress helps. If your back is sore, see page 228 for information about using pillows and changing sleeping positions.

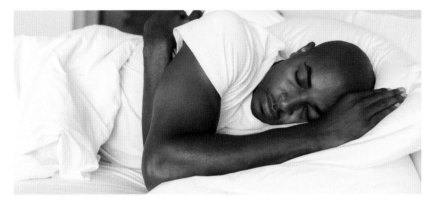

Keep your room temperature cool, about 65°F (18°C), if possible. If your feet are cold, wear warm loose socks.

A dark and quiet room makes a big difference.

Other ways to relax

Are you feeling stressed? Try one of these ideas to relax. The first one takes less than a minute, the second one a couple of minutes. The third ones take 10 or 15 minutes.

If you have one minute, do some deep breathing.

Deep breathe during the day whenever you are feeling stressed. Just stop and take a couple of deep breaths. It only takes a minute, but it gives you an immediate oxygen boost and helps relax you.

If you have up to three minutes, try these short exercises.

Doing a few short exercises can relieve tension building up in your muscles. For example, try shoulder shrugs, ankle rotations or stretches. If the tension is in your neck, drop your neck to your chest, hold for 10 seconds, then slowly move it from side to side.

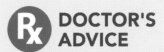

DOCTOR'S ADVICE

Talk to your doctor if insomnia continues. You may benefit from seeing a counselor to work out what's on your mind. Consider going to a sleep clinic if you think you might have sleep apnea. Sometimes taking a sleeping pill for a short time helps get you through a stressful time.

If you spend only 1% of your day focusing on relaxing, that's just 10 minutes. Yet, it can make a significant improvement in your blood sugar and blood pressure.

STAY UPBEAT

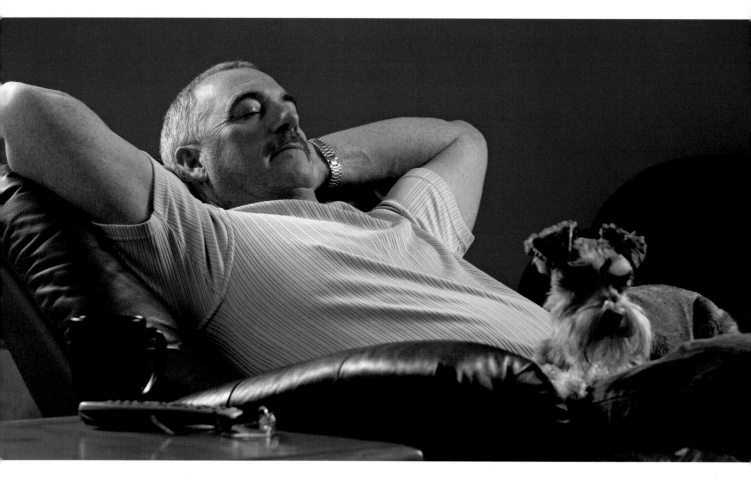

If you have 10 minutes, try focused relaxation.

For complete relaxation, find a quiet place with lights dimmed. Then:

1. Sit in a comfortable chair or lie down.

2. Breathe deeply and slowly with your eyes closed.

3. Concentrate on slowly relaxing all the muscles in your arms and legs. Try to not think about anything else, just focus on your muscles relaxing.

4. Then focus on relaxing your stomach, bottom, back, face and neck. Keep relaxing until you feel no pressure on your muscles. You will feel like you have softly sunk into your chair or bed.

5. Continue breathing deeply.

If you have 15 minutes or more, try yoga, Pilates or tai-chi.

These types of exercises all include some relaxing movements or poses. These slow, controlled exercises focus your attention away from outside distractions. They require different levels of fitness and flexibility. If you have never tried them, talk to an instructor at a local fitness club about whether it might be a good exercise for you. If so, consider giving it a try.

Coping with Depression

Depression is different from stress. Depression can be like a black cloud that hangs over your head. One day, for a reason, or sometimes for no reason, that black cloud drops down. You feel its pressure. It affects everything you want to do. It makes it difficult to get out of bed, to talk to family or friends and to do your work. It takes away joy, and it takes you away from people who love you. If you think you might be depressed, please talk to your doctor or a mental health professional. Also, consider taking the depression test below.

A Short Test for Depression

Over the last two weeks, how often have you been bothered by any of the following problems? (Circle your answer then add up your circled answers.)	Not at all	Several days	More than half the days	Nearly every day
Little interest or pleasure in doing things.	0	1	2	3
Feeling down, depressed, or hopeless.	0	1	2	3
Trouble falling or staying asleep, or sleeping too much.	0	1	2	3
Feeling tired or having little energy.	0	1	2	3
Poor appetite or overeating.	0	1	2	3
Feeling bad about yourself — or that you are a failure or have let yourself or your family down.	0	1	2	3
Trouble concentrating on things, such as reading the newspaper or watching television.	0	1	2	3
Moving or speaking so slowly that other people could have noticed? Or the opposite — being so fidgety or restless that you have been moving around a lot more than usual.	0	1	2	3
Thoughts that you would be better off dead or of hurting yourself in some way.	0	1	2	3
If your score was 5 or more, go to the next page and read _When to Seek Help_.	0	+_____	+_____	+_____
				TOTAL SCORE: _____

These questions are from the PHQ-9 Patient Health Questionnaire. It was developed by Drs. Robert L. Spitzer, Janet B.W. Williams, Kurt Kroenke and colleagues, with an educational grant from Pfizer Inc. To access the original questionnaire, which is designed for use by health professionals, go to www.pfizer.com. It includes ways to determine if depression is mild or severe.

STAY UPBEAT

361

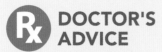

DOCTOR'S ADVICE

Some, but not all, anti-depression medications can contribute to weight gain. This may make your diabetes worse. Talk to you doctor about your options.

Depression and Diabetes

When you are depressed you feel lethargic and uninterested in making healthy choices. Coping with diabetes is challenging, and this can contribute to depression. Treating the depression is an important first step. Once your depression improves, you feel better. If you feel better, it's easier for you to manage your diabetes.

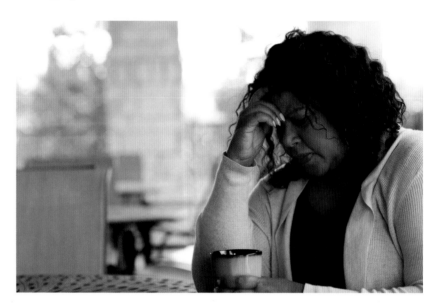

When to Seek Help

You *may* be depressed if you scored 5 or more on the test on the previous page. Talk to your doctor or a mental health professional so they can assess you further. This is particularly important if your score was high or you have feelings of depression that don't go away. If you have thoughts of hurting yourself or someone else, please seek medical care. If needed, call an emergency help phone line.

Some people have success in managing their depression through exercise and by making changes to help manage stress. A health counselor can support you in making some of these changes. Other people benefit from also taking anti-depressant pills or other medications. Your doctor may prescribe meds for a short time, or you may need them for longer.

Step 7: Manage at Other Life Stages

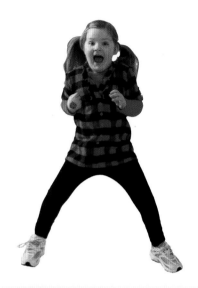

Preschoolers to Teenagers

For every five youth in North America diagnosed with diabetes, one of these will be diagnosed with type 2 diabetes. The other four will be diagnosed with type 1 diabetes. A lot more children and youth now get type 2 diabetes because they do less exercise and weigh more than ever before. Oversized foods and drinks are sold everywhere. Many kids get driven to school rather than walk or bike. Kids play outside less. Lives are filled with technology and screens. This can all seem overwhelming. Yet, even one change, like eating more meals at home with your family, makes a difference.

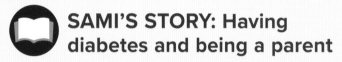

SAMI'S STORY: Having diabetes and being a parent

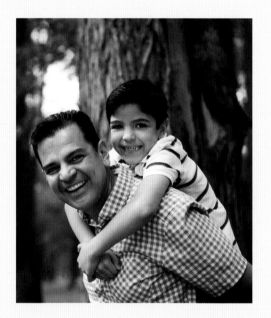

I am 45 and I was told I had type 2 diabetes when my son was just three. I was pretty heavy at the time. My mother, my mother's mother and my uncle all have diabetes, so I guess it wasn't really a surprise. But it was a surprise. I couldn't believe it because I was so young, and they got diabetes when they were a lot older. That first month I was pretty upset, but when I looked at my son, I knew I wanted to live a long time and see him grow up. So, I promised myself that I would do whatever I could to get healthy.

I asked my wife how we could start eating healthier at home. First thing she said was no more soda pop in the house. Then we talked about limiting the screen time for all of us. We wanted to give him an active, busy childhood just like what we had when we were kids. We spent more time in the yard playing with balls, taking him on walks and bike rides and playing more games in the house. My wife joined a preschool play group and met new neighbors that way. Now my son is nine and involved in more organized team sports and eats healthy food because we were committed to a better life for him. Of course, this also meant my wife and I ate better, I lost weight and I am proud to say my diabetes is well managed.

If you're an adult who has struggled with overeating and being inactive, it's important to seek help as part of your wellness. This can be an important step to help you care for your children. Children have an amazing capacity to love and be resilient but they need the help of a supportive and healthy caregiver.

Tips to Prevent Type 2 Diabetes in Young Children

To begin, consider trying just one or two of the following suggestions.

- **Offer water regularly.** Limit juice, soft drinks and all other sweetened drinks. Limit juice to 4 to 6 oz (125–175 mL) per day, especially for toddlers and young children.

- **Provide healthy snacks.** These snacks between meals lessen hunger pangs. They provide energy for a child's muscles and brain. When you limit high-calorie, junk food snacks, children will be hungry when they sit down at the table to eat a healthy meal.

- **Provide balanced meals at regular times.** This encourages good eating habits. Children love routine. They like to know what is going to happen and when. It's good to learn early to wait until the next meal or snack.

- **Allow for occasional treats.** Your shelves and refrigerator should hold mostly healthy foods. Offer occasional treats, in reasonable portions. Kids love chocolates, cake, ice cream and candies as much as adults do. As long as they recognize that these are not everyday foods, they can go ahead and enjoy them.

- **Cook with children.** Children can learn cooking skills at three or four years old. Show them the meal pictures in this book. Let them "help" you put together a meal. Start with easy meals, such as cereal with fruit (page 156), a wrap (page 164) or Hot Chicken Salad (page 176). By the time they are teenagers, they should be able to prepare most of the meals found in this book. This will give them the knowledge and confidence to cook and try new recipes and healthy foods.

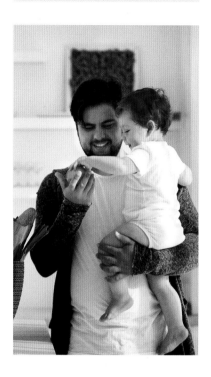

At home and school, make water the number one beverage choice.

Set a good example – eat healthy foods yourself!

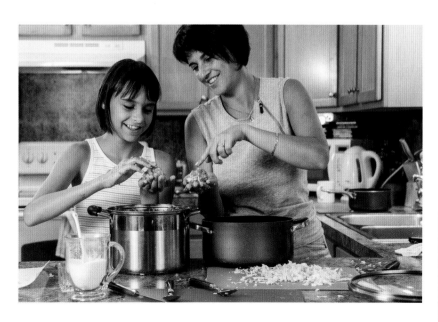

Use hand portions as a guide. See the Food Guide on pages 55–57. A toddler needs only portions that fit in their small hands on most days. At times they will have growth spurts and be hungry and will need more. As your child grows older, their hands get bigger, and so will their appetite.

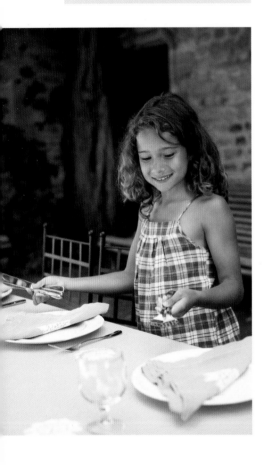

- **Make time to eat together.** Eating together helps families talk and develop a support network for life. Studies show that children who eat dinner often with their families:
  - Are less likely to smoke, drink or use drugs
  - Earn higher grades at school
  - Eat healthier foods

- **Don't force food.** Allow and promote new foods in small amounts. Don't demand that they eat all the food or that they clean their plates. We all have likes and dislikes, and kids have sensitive taste buds! For some kids, certain foods don't taste good. Children's appetites also vary from day to day. Sometimes they need more, and sometimes less.

- **Keep conversation light.** Turn off electronics and screens. Serve meals in a calm and casual way. Let everyone talk about their day.

- **Encourage good table manners.** Kids can help set the table and clear the dishes. Teach them to sit up properly at the table. Eat slowly and put the knife and fork down between some bites. It's not good manners to say "I hate that" or "I don't like that." Teach them to say "No, thank you" instead. Give your children praise and attention when they make positive remarks like "This is really good." Model saying thank-you to the person who cooked during and at the end of the meal.

- **Teach children to respect food.** Offer small portions of food. Let your toddler or child feed themselves. If your child doesn't want to eat some or all of the food, remove it from the table when the meal is over. Praise them for what they ate. Don't comment on the food they didn't eat. Don't get in the habit of always offering your child alternative foods to what you are serving the rest of the family.

- **Deal with fussy eating early.** Otherwise it can become a habit. Offer your toddler regular meals and snacks at regular times. When toddlers — and people of all ages — are hungry, they get miserable! If you've offered your toddler a variety of choices and your child still fusses and complains, try to change the conversation away from food and distract your child. If the fussing becomes a tantrum, remove your child from the table. Give them a toy or activity. This takes their focus away from the food so your table doesn't become a food battleground. Your children won't starve because they've missed a food group or even if they don't want to eat and miss a meal here and there.

When you are on a routine of regular meals and snacks, the next food is always in just a few hours' time, at least during the day. Be consistent. You will find your child will start enjoying their meals and leaving little on their plate.

- **Encourage outdoor play, summer and winter.** When active, children have a better appetite when it's time to eat. This can reduce picky eating.

- **Keep kids active and limit screen time.** Kids with less screen time have fewer behavioral problems and more time to be active. Some electronics such as a Wii device can keep kids active indoors, and some TV or tablet activities can be educational. Generally though, less is better for good health. From an early age, restrict kids' use of electronic devices, phones, computer and television. Make use of parental control apps for phones and tablets. Less screen time then opens time for kids to play. Play includes structured time where you play with your child and unstructured time where the child plays on their own or with other children. Visit a playground regularly. Hang a swing in a backyard tree. Once outdoors, most kids are moving and burning calories.

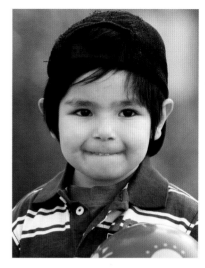

The American Academy of Pediatrics recommends limiting screen time to less than an hour for children two to five, and less for under two.

Are there safe options for your kids to walk to school or partway to school?

What about safe ways for them to walk to see friends and do activities? When we drive our children places, they forget to hop on a bike or walk to get to where they are going. They may come to expect to catch a ride everywhere. Are there older siblings, 12 or older, who can assume the responsibility of walking with those that are younger?

- **Put toddlers and young children to bed at a regular time.** Sleep is important for appetite control. Inadequate sleep is associated with becoming overweight and getting diabetes. One of the biggest benefits of getting your children into a regular sleep pattern is that it gives you, the caregiver, a break every night. Then you can be fresh to look after your kids the next morning. Try to be consistent. If young children learn that bedtime is 7 or 8 o'clock, they adapt to this. If they are active earlier in the evening or day, this will tire them out. For the last half hour before bedtime, create a healthy routine that works for you. It's a good idea to get rid of distractions. Turn off all technology. Give them a bath, brush their teeth, and read a bedtime story.

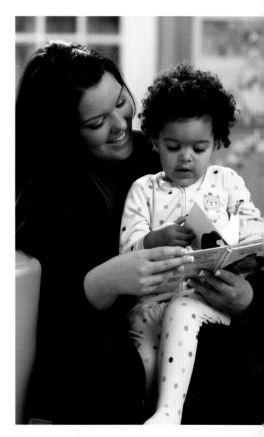

The best gift you can give your child or teenager is your time. Listen and keep talking.

Teenagers with Type 2 Diabetes

JESSA'S STORY: I'm 13 and the only kid with type 2 diabetes

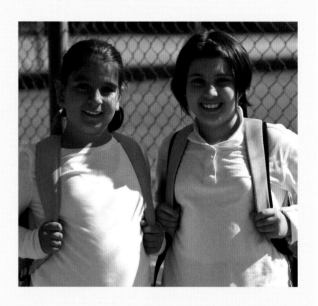

My name is Jessa and I'm 13. A year ago my mom took me to the doctor 'cause I was telling her I was always so thirsty. After a bunch of yucky tests, the doctor told us I had type 2 diabetes. My mom started crying in the doctor's office. OMG just because I was thirsty.

Anyway, me and my sister Jennie, she's 16, we live with my mom during the week and see my dad as much as he can find time. When I was seven, they separated and I was really sad but also glad we didn't have to listen to them fighting all the time. I think my dad felt bad for us girls and he bought me a PS4. First game I played I loved it. I spent hours and hours playing all the games I could get. Mom bought me my favorite foods so I'd be happy. I love pineapple juice, iced tea and every kind of chips. It got that the only time I'd leave the house was when we went to McDonalds. I hated all stuff to do with exercise; I hated walking the stupid dog. And just 'cause my dad loves soccer, doesn't mean I want to kick the ball with him. Anyway I was getting pretty fat and that's another reason I didn't want to go out much.

When the doctor said I had diabetes he also said I'd have to have injections. That scared me but my sister helped me. My mom said that Nana had diabetes and it wasn't my fault. But then she was mad and telling me to do this and stop doing that, and asking me for my blood sugar numbers all the time. And she stopped buying my favorite foods and it was horrible, like it was my fault.

When I had to go see the nurse, I couldn't believe how nice she was. She listened to me when I told her how sad I was and how when I played video games I could forget all that stuff about my mom and dad. I told her my BFF likes gaming just like me, and that's her with the short hair in the picture. So that's when the nurse said that the two of us should try doing different things together. We'd started going to the ball park to watch her older brother 'cause he was the pitcher. And now, we do more stuff than video games and I've even lost 10 pounds.

PARENTS

Don't focus on the diabetes. Focus on what your child is doing and how they are feeling. Rather than ask them over and over about their blood sugar numbers, ask them how they feel and talk about what steps they can take to manage right now.

Limit soft drinks, juices and other sugared drinks

Did you know that soft drinks, ice tea, juice, sports drinks and energy drinks can make you gain weight? (See pages 87–89 for more info). It's okay to have sweet drinks now and then, but drinking them every day is not good for your waistline. When you have diabetes, these drinks are really bad for your blood sugar.

Be in the driver's seat

It's hard to avoid all the unhealthy choices around you. Friends might be smoking or vaping near you. Wherever you go, there are temptations like fast food, chips and soda pop. Take this one step at a time. The first change is to take your medications. Then make one more positive change. In a week or so, ask yourself if you feel ready to make another change. Consider these:

- Go to medical appointments. Just showing up is important.
- Drink more water instead of soda pop, juice or sweet coffees.
- Start walking or using a treadmill.
- Check your blood sugar at least once a day.
- Think carefully about the problems that go with smoking, drinking and drugs. Do you want those problems?
- Seek help. You don't have to deal with diabetes all by yourself. Talk to your family, a doctor, nurse, school counsellor or someone you trust who has helped you before.
- Be realistic and be the best you can be. With each new change, you can start feeling better. This will give you new strength. Often when one person makes a change, this can influence others to make healthy changes too.

If you need to talk to a counsellor

There is free online or phone support for teens. Search online free telephone counselling hotline, and in Canada search Kids Help Phone.

Teaspoons of sugar from 16-oz (500 mL) servings:

- **Zero teaspoons:** Water
- **7 to 9 teaspoons (28–36 g of carbs):** Sports drinks, including Gatorade, Thirst Quencher or PowerAde
- **11 to 15 teaspoons (44–60 g of carbs):** Energy drinks, soda pop, unsweetened orange juice or apple juice; chocolate milk; Slushees or Slurpees, or iced sweetened coffees
- **24 teaspoons (96 g of carbs)** Gatorade Energy Drink

Sports drinks are for endurance athletes. They have sugar, sodium and potassium added to replace those from excessive sweating. Check with your coach, diabetes professional or doctor to see if it is ever safe for you to drink one of these after a workout.

Energy drinks often have even more sugar than sports drinks, plus they are also high in caffeine. That is why they raise your blood sugar and are fattening. Energy drinks can also cause you to become dehydrated.

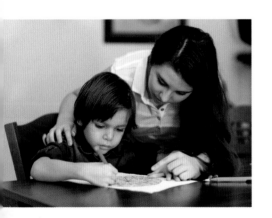

Reduce screen time to fight diabetes

How much screen time do you have each day? Keep a record for one day.

The more time you spend in front of a screen, the less time you have for moving around and being active. Health experts recommend that as a youth, you should get at least 90 minutes (1½ hours) of exercise each day to prevent diabetes and to move to wellness.

Set a goal. Cut out one hour of tablet, television, phone or computer time on most days.

Here are 10 things you could do with this hour:

1 Get active outdoors. Go for a walk with family or friends.

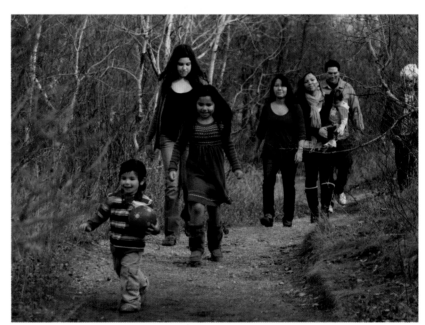

2 Take up an active hobby or activity. You'll be moving around more than sitting looking at a screen. Try nature or landscape photography using your cell phone. Help a parent or neighbor with carpentry. Join a community-based group, garden club or a teen training program such as Caring4Youth.

3 **Spend time with grandparents.** They may have diabetes, too. You may be able to learn from them. Hike in to your favorite fishing hole. Fishing forces you to slow down, forget your worries for a while and relax.

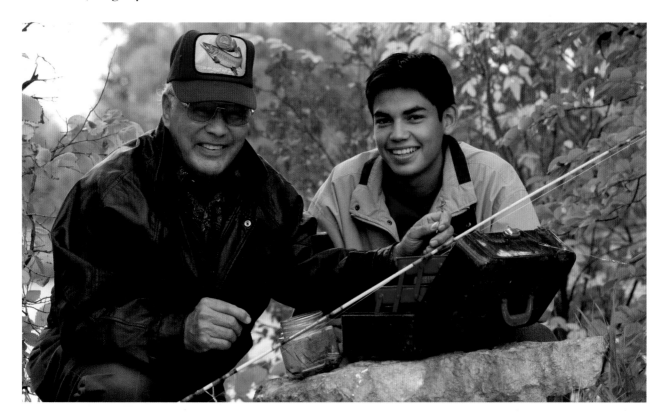

4 **Learn to cook.** Does grandma, grandpa, mom, dad, uncle or auntie like to cook? Cook together with the healthy recipes in this book. Learning to cook and eat well will help you grow strong. This is an important step to looking after your diabetes.

5 **Walk outdoors or on a treadmill or elliptical.** It's hard work but it pays off. Test your blood sugar before and half an hour after exercise — and see it go down.

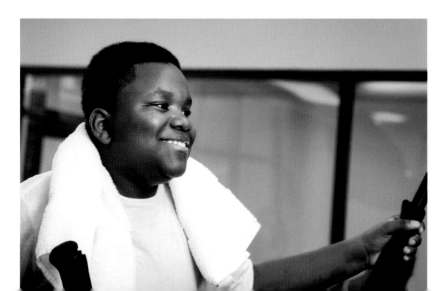

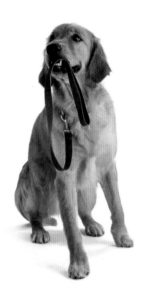

6 Earn some money and stay active with an after-school job. If you love animals, become a paid after-school and weekend dog walker for a neighbor's dog. Help out around the house or cut the lawn or deliver flyers. Babysit your neighbors' kids and play with them indoors or take them to a park to play outdoors. If you are an older teen, do you have a parttime job? Working isn't always easy but it can offer you new experiences. It keeps you from sitting on the couch.

7 Set up an area for street hockey with movable nets. Stock up on hockey sticks and soft pucks or tennis balls. Other things to do: shoot some hoops, kick a soccer ball around, or go swim or play with flutter boards in a leisure pool. Are you interested in a team sport like soccer?

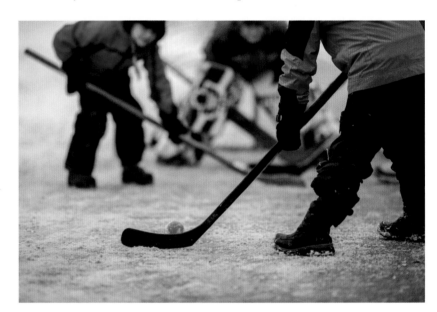

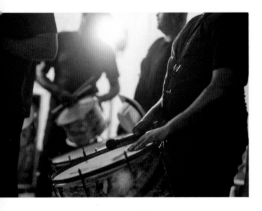

8 If you are musical or like to dance, join a marching band, drumming group or step team. Step team is a form of percussion dance where you use your body to make sounds and rhythms. Be inspired by stories on youtube about different forms of dance, search "school step team" or "teens dancing to beat obesity." You may want to first try these dances at home while following along with a video.

9 Go for a bike ride with your brother, sister or friend. Or ride a stationary bike or recumbent bike at home or in a gym.

PARENTS

Take walks or go biking with your kids. Throw a frisbee or football. Or take them skating or bowling. If you go on vacation, can you do active things like kayaking, horseback riding or hiking? You are your kids' role model! And your kids may inspire you too.

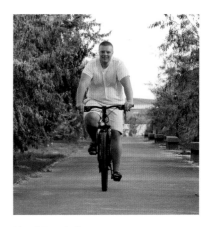

Hey! Don't forget to put on a bike helmet.

10 Stay in school to keep active. Think about it: you walk to go to classes, you walk up and down hallways and you may also walk to school.

PARENTS

Encourage your kids to develop interests and hobbies. Help them get involved in activities around the home and outside the home. Value their schoolwork so they stay in school.

Physically active kids do better in school and are less likely to smoke and take drugs.

The good news is that even small changes can make a big difference.

Try one of these changes in the first month. Check your blood sugar, and monitor what a difference eating better and exercising can make to your sugar levels. You will feel proud when your A1C level starts coming down, and you stop gaining weight.

LIFE STAGES

can cause low
blood sugar

Low blood sugar risks

Your blood sugar can go low (see pages 329–336) if you are taking insulin or a pill such as glyburide (see page 311). Low blood sugar is especially dangerous if you are driving or drinking. Alcohol can cause you to have a seriously low blood sugar. Consuming alcohol, marijuana and street drugs can impair your judgment and can mask low blood sugar.

When you have diabetes and are on medications, it's safest to not drink. If you are going to drink, then talk to your parent or doctor about this. Your doctor will likely advise you to skip your insulin or pills before and during the drinking. **Be safe, not sorry.**

> ⚠️ **CAUTION**
> **Low blood sugar and being drunk can look the same.**
>
> If your friends are also drinking, they won't realize you have low blood sugar. They won't be able to give you the sugar you need.
>
> Blood sugar can be low for up to 24 hours after you drink alcohol.
>
> For more information on alcohol, see pages 134–137.

> 👤 **PARENTS**
> If you find your child is drunk or high on drugs and you think they might have taken their insulin, you need to monitor them, including while they are sleeping. You may need to wake them every two hours to make sure their blood sugar isn't going seriously low. If needed, call a toll-free health phone line or emergency department for advice.

Dehydration risk

Beware of mixing energy drinks with alcohol and medications. High blood sugar plus drinking energy drinks, which are high in caffeine, in combination with alcohol can cause dehydration. This is more likely to happen if you are exerting yourself, maybe dancing or playing a sport. See page 138 for signs of dehydration.

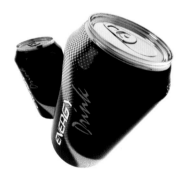

> ⚠️ **CAUTION**
> **Energy drinks**
>
> Energy drinks don't always list caffeine sources, such as from herbs like yerba matte. Just one 16-oz (500 mL) can of energy drink usually has 11 to 15 teaspoons of sugar (44–60 g of carb) plus as much caffeine as 5 cups (1.25 L) of coffee.

Medications and insulin

Doctors often recommend insulin for young people with type 2 diabetes. When blood sugar improves, the doctor will usually stop the insulin. While you are taking diabetes pills or insulin, it is still important to always eat well and to exercise to control your weight.

Are you sexually active? Birth control and STI prevention

Using the pill and a condom is a lot easier than getting a sexually transmitted infection (STI) for life or having a baby in your teenage years.

Ask questions and get the help you need. Search online "birth control hotline" or "STI hotline." Then you can call and talk to someone, without anyone else knowing.

When you learn more and you feel confident, it is easier to follow up with your school nurse, counsellor, parents or doctor.

As a teenage girl with diabetes, your birth control options are the same as for a girl without diabetes, including:

- Abstinence
- Condoms or the diaphram or cervical cap combined with spermicidal gel or foam
- Low-dose hormone contraceptives (such as the pill, patch or vaginal ring)
- The IUD (intrauterine device) inserted by your doctor.

For more information on birth control, see page 389.

If you have had unprotected sex and are worried you might have got pregnant, attend the walk-in clinic right away. You may want to ask about emergency birth control ("the morning after pill"). If you have an unwanted pregnancy, don't delay; talk to the people you trust about your options.

The best type of pregnancy is a planned pregnancy!

Read the *Type 2 Diabetes Pregnancy and Gestational Diabetes* section on pages 377–389.

Don't get an STI!
All sexually active teens, girls and boys, should know about safer sex and use birth control. Read the section on Cautions about STIs and how high blood sugar worsens your risk on page 390.

Girls with diabetes are also more likely to get a vaginal or urinary tract infection with sex. See pages 46–47 and 287–290 to learn more about ways to reduce your risk.

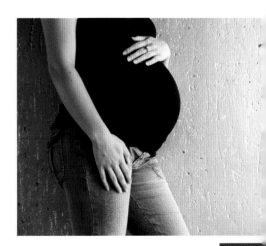

You can succeed with diabetes

Having diabetes isn't easy. It may help to realize that all your friends have challenges too. If you make small, gradual changes, it's easier to cope. This helps you feel better day by day. The things you need to do to be healthy are the same for everybody. Set goals. Eat well, be active and stay in school.

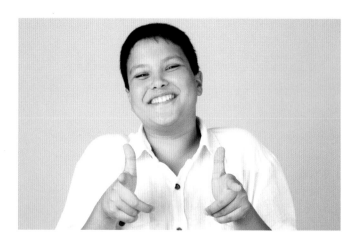

PARENTS

Your child has grown into a teenager and is experiencing all the normal struggles of teenage pressures and demands. Managing diabetes is one more extra burden on your teenager. This is a time when children don't want to be different; they want to fit in and be like their friends. They may not eat healthy foods, they may give up exercising, they may start vaping and they may challenge your rules and limits.

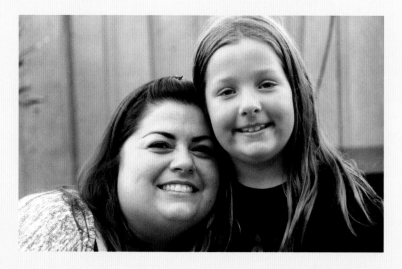

However, as tough as it is, your rules are essential to provide healthy limits for your child. They are learning to make their own decisions, yet still need your guidance and support. Managing diabetes and being a teenager can have workable solutions.

If rules are being seriously ignored and you have concerns for the health and safety of your teen, consult with a diabetes educator or nurse. They can help you with new ideas and suggestions on how to approach and speak to your child. A school social worker or counsellor are also good contacts, since they're trained to deal with teenagers' emotions and mental health issues.

Rules are like the guardrails along the edges of a bridge. They help keep kids loved and safe.

Type 2 Diabetes Pregnancy and Gestational Diabetes

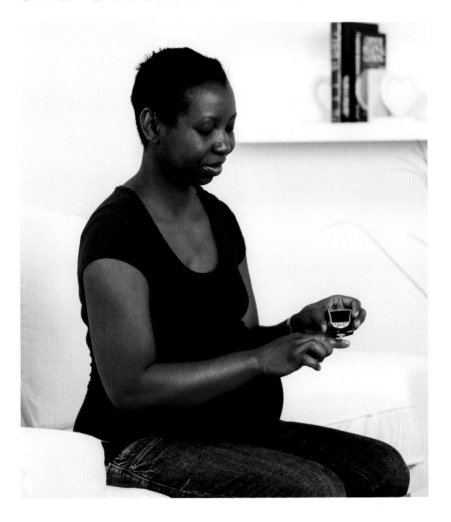

Women without diabetes are screened at 24 to 28 weeks pregnant to see if they have gestational diabetes. Gestational diabetes means you develop diabetes during your pregnancy (see page 15).

Whether you have gestational diabetes or are pregnant with type 2 diabetes, your doctor or obstetrician may order various tests. For example, you may have one or several ultrasounds. An ultrasound is sound waves that take a "picture" of your fetus. Looking at this picture, your doctor can estimate the size of your fetus. This information is useful in determining if you need to start on insulin.

Avoid Problems

You can have a healthy pregnancy, a healthy baby and a healthy you! Read on to learn more.

See your diabetes team regularly and ask about prenatal classes.

℞ DOCTOR'S ADVICE

If your family has a history of diabetes, your fetus may carry a gene for type 2 diabetes. Research shows this diabetes gene can actually be switched off if the mother has a healthy pregnancy. This means that during your pregnancy you gain a healthy amount of weight (see page 380) and maintain good blood sugar levels during your pregnancy.

LIFE STAGES

Once you have your baby, gestational diabetes normally goes away. However, you are at risk of getting it again with your next pregnancy. You and your baby also run the risk of developing type 2 diabetes later in life. You can reduce these risks. Follow the steps in this section.

Problems that May Occur

If your blood sugar is consistently high and you gain too much weight during your pregnancy:

- Your blood pressure could go up during your pregnancy. This extra stress can also affect your kidneys, eyes and heart.
- Your fetus could grow too large. It is harder to deliver a large baby. You may need a Caesarean section, or C-section.
- If your baby isn't healthy, you may need to deliver early. Then your baby is more likely to have breathing problems or jaundice.
- You are more at risk of having a miscarriage in your third trimester if your blood sugars have been high throughout your pregnancy. You can lower this risk with good blood sugar levels.

If your blood sugar was too high during pregnancy, then after birth, your baby may have these problems:

Breathing problems

When a baby is large or premature, his or her lungs may not have developed fully. Your baby is likely to need oxygen and, in some cases, may need resuscitation.

Jaundice

Jaundice is yellowed eyes and skin. It occurs when the baby's normal body chemical called bilirubin builds up. Normally, the liver removes excess bilirubin from the blood. Jaundice means the liver isn't fully developed and can't work properly. Putting the baby under special lights helps treat the jaundice.

Low blood sugar

Breast milk is ideal to bring up your baby's low blood sugar. This is why mothers should be supported to start breastfeeding as soon as possible after baby is born.

If your blood sugar was high in late pregnancy, your growing baby gets some of this extra sugar and, in response, its pancreas makes extra insulin. Then after birth, your baby's pancreas continues to make extra insulin and this causes your baby's blood sugar to be low when first born. A newborn with low blood sugar will be jittery and crying. Comfort your baby with skin-to-skin contact (see page 387). This closeness along with early breastfeeding helps to bring up your baby's low blood sugar.

Seven Steps to Having a Healthy Baby

1. Keep Active

Exercise will help you:

- Prevent too much weight gain during your pregnancy.
- Use insulin more effectively and improve your blood sugar.
- Prevent back pain and constipation.
- Get in good shape for your labor and delivery.

Walking, using an exercise bike or doing low-impact aerobics are good exercises when you are pregnant. Swimming is also very relaxing, especially in the last trimester. Aim for a daily hour of walking. Split this into a few walks, especially after meals. Use common sense. Avoid sports or exercises that increase the chance of jolts or falling.

When shouldn't you exercise?

Your doctor will tell you if you need to reduce your exercise or be on bed rest. Common reasons for bed rest include high-risk pregnancies, persistent vaginal bleeding or if your doctor thinks you may go into labor too early.

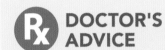

DOCTOR'S ADVICE

If your blood sugar is higher in the morning, this is an especially good time to go for a walk.

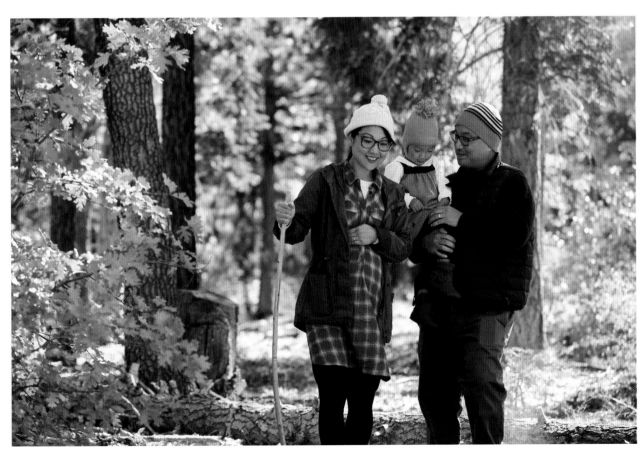

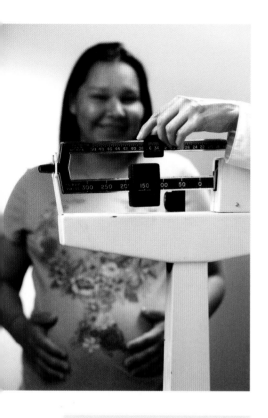

2. Gain a Healthy Weight

You can't eat whatever you want just because you are pregnant! Keep your portions under control. Aim for a slow, gradual weight gain during your pregnancy. The amount of weight you should gain depends on your weight just before you got pregnant.

Healthy weight during pregnancy	
Overweight by more than 30 lbs/14 kg (BMI* of 30 or more): Gain 11 to 20 lbs (5–9 kg). Your doctor may recommend you gain even less than this.	**Overweight up to 30 lbs/14 kg (BMI of 25–29.9):** Gain 15 to 25 lbs (7–11 kg).
Normal weight (BMI of 18.5–24.9): Gain 25 to 35 lbs (11–16 kg)	
Underweight (BMI of under 18.5), a teenager or expecting multiples: Doctors recommend a larger weight gain than suggested for women with normal weight.	

Weigh yourself once a week or at your doctor appointments. Adjust your food portions and exercise as needed. It's a good idea to spread your food out throughout the day by including three meals and three snacks. The size of your snacks and whether you choose the small or large meals (see page 151) will depend on your appetite and weight gain.

*BMI, or body mass index, is a calculation based on your weight and height. BMI calculators are online.

The faster you gain weight and the more you gain during pregnancy, the larger your baby will grow. During the first three months you only need to gain a couple of pounds (1 kg) in total. After that, your weight should gradually go up, and you should gain most of your weight in the last trimester (months 6 to 9). If you are overweight, your average weight gain should be about half a pound (0.25 kg) a week averaged over the last two trimesters.

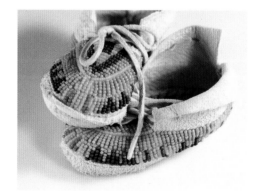

3. Make Wise Health and Nutrition Choices

- **Use the small or large meal plans in this book** as a guide. Your portions will depend on your weight gain. You may need a bit more protein and less carbs at meals or snacks to manage your blood sugar.

- **Choose foods rich in iron, folic acid, vitamin C, calcium and vitamin D.** See good food options on pages 132–133. Fish are excellent sources of omega-3 fats, which are healthy for a growing baby. Choose fish that are lower in mercury such as salmon, trout or sardines.

- **Take a prenatal multivitamin and mineral pill every day** during your pregnancy. If planning a pregnancy, start taking this three months before you get pregnant. Continue the supplement when breastfeeding.

- **Eat high-fiber foods, drink water and walk every day** to lessen or avoid constipation.

- **Limit caffeine:** Avoid or limit caffeine to no more than 200 mg a day. This would equal a 12-oz (355 mL) cup of coffee. A cup (250 mL) of tea or can of cola each have about 45 mg.

- **Avoid cyclamate or saccharin sweeteners.**

If you are nauseous or vomiting, try some of the meal suggestions on page 148. It may help to eat a few soda crackers, kept at your bedside, before you get up in the morning.

Caffeine: Researchers don't know for sure if high amounts of caffeine cause miscarriage. You may choose to reduce caffeine or skip it during pregnancy.

⚠️ **CAUTION**
Don't smoke, drink alcohol or take any unknown drugs or street drugs when you are pregnant. These go directly to your baby. There is no safe limit.

Talk to an addiction counselor if needed. They can discuss harm reduction if quitting is not possible.

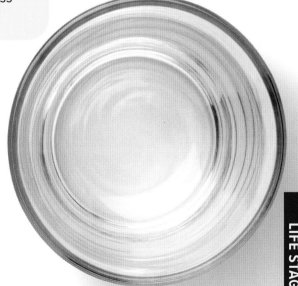

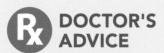

DOCTOR'S ADVICE

Try not to overeat. The doctor can keep the insulin dose lower. Aim for the recommended weight gain (see page 380) or as advised by your doctor.

Talk to your doctor about all your medications before you get pregnant or as soon as you know you're pregnant.

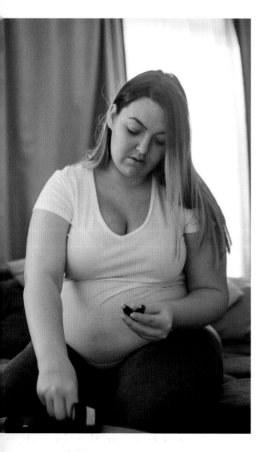

4. Take Insulin If Needed

If you are not on insulin, your doctor may prescribe some during your pregnancy, especially in the third trimester. This is when blood sugar usually goes up the most. *Insulin is safe for your baby.* Taking insulin allows you to manage your blood sugar and still eat enough for proper weight gain. The doctor usually stops the insulin when you go into labor. If you have type 2 diabetes and took insulin before you got pregnant, you may need less, or none, while breastfeeding.

During pregnancy, doctors commonly prescribe:

- An evening dose of intermediate-acting or long-acting insulin
- If needed, short or rapid insulin during the day
- If you are vomiting, rapid insulin is often the best choice. You can take it when you feel you will be able to hold down the meal.

Other medications. Your doctor may tell you to stop some medications when you are pregnant or breastfeeding. This can include some diabetes pills, blood pressure or cholesterol pills. In some cases, alternative pills or treatments may be suggested. For example, low-dose aspirin may be recommended to reduce your risk of preeclampsia (high blood pressure).

5. Check Your Blood Sugar

Your doctor will likely ask you to check your blood sugar during your pregnancy, especially if you are taking insulin. He or she may recommend checking both one hour and two hours after a meal. If you're taking rapid insulin, you'll also need to test before meals.

To help protect your growing baby, doctors recommend that your blood sugar levels be a bit lower than at other times. See usual targets below. These may be increased if you're having low blood sugars.

Recommended blood sugar levels during pregnancy	
Before meals	less than 95 mg/dL (5.3 mmol/L)
One hour after a meal	less than 140 mg/dL (7.8 mmol/L)
Two hours after a meal	less than 120 mg/dL (6.7 mmol/L)

Your doctor may recommend you take insulin if your blood sugar stays above these levels.

To avoid a low, stay above 70 mg/dL (4 mmol/L).

6. See Your Doctor Regularly

During pregnancy

Your doctor will check your blood pressure, and order lab and urine tests. She will check the growth and health of your fetus.

After your baby is born

If you have gestational diabetes, have your doctor check your blood sugar about two to six months after your baby is born. Then have it checked annually or as recommended by your doctor. This is to see if you have any early signs of type 2 diabetes.

It's also a good idea to get your iron levels and thyroid checked after your baby is born. This is especially important if you feel tired or sad or have a hard time losing weight.

Feeling down? Do you need help or support?

Pregnancy and the birth of a baby brings many changes to women's bodies and lives. Some women feel upset or stressed during pregnancy or after their baby is born.

A doula (see page 386) can be a great support to you and your baby in the early days and weeks to help you through some difficult times. If you don't have a doula, call a friend or family and ask them to come by and be with you. If needed, your doctor can refer you to a counsellor specializing in postpartum depression.

Appointments during pregnancy

Take care of your whole self. Here are appointments you should keep besides your doctor and diabetes educators.

Optometrist

When you have diabetes, pregnancy can affect your eyes. See your optometrist before your third month of pregnancy.

Dentist or hygienist

The hormonal changes during pregnancy can lead to more plaque and gum disease. See your dentist during your pregnancy.

LIFE STAGES

383

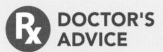

DOCTOR'S ADVICE

Breastfeeding gives many other lifetime health benefits to both mother and child.

Benefits to mother:

- Reduces risks for breast and ovarian cancer
- Reduces risks for high blood pressure and heart disease

Benefits to child:

- Healthy brain growth
- Protects against ear and lung infections (asthma)
- Protects gums and teeth
- Protects stomach and bowel (less diarrhea)
- Helps prevent food allergies and eczema
- Protects against childhood cancers

Human milk is always available at the right temperature. It saves money. And it has no packaging, so is good for the environment!

7. Breastfeed to Protect Against Diabetes

Breastfeeding benefits women with type 2 diabetes. They often see a lowering of their blood sugar and may need less diabetes medication while breastfeeding. Breastfeeding helps some mothers lose the extra pounds put on during pregnancy, which if kept off, has long-term benefits to their blood sugar levels.

Breastfeeding reduces the risk of developing type 2 diabetes:

- For mothers who do not have type 2 diabetes
- For mothers who had gestational diabetes
- For babies who were breastfed

Why are breastfed babies less likely to get diabetes?

Breastfed babies tend to have a slow, but steady weight gain in the first six months. It is recommended that breast milk be the baby's only food or drink for those first six months. This protects them from gaining excess body fat, which helps them keep a healthy weight in their early years.

When babies gain excess body fat (often associated with formula-fed babies) this tends to stay with them as children, and into their teenage and adult years. This excess body fat can increase the risk of getting type 2 diabetes.

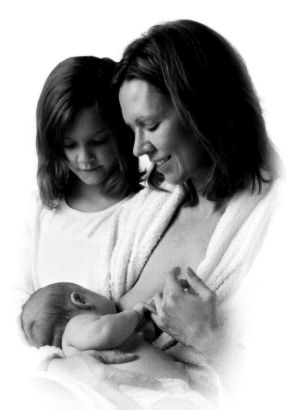

Breastfeeding supports

Think about breastfeeding in your last trimester of pregnancy

Talk to your partner and family members. Some may not be sure of the health benefits, for both you and your baby, or they may be uncomfortable with the idea of breastfeeding. Look for easy-to-understand information and share it with them so they can know the benefits. Search online for this recommended free resource, "My Breastfeeding Guide — Best Start," available in many languages.

Your last trimester is a good time to attend a prenatal class and learn more about a healthy pregnancy, labor and breastfeeding. These nurses may be available by phone for questions you have between classes. Also think about whether you want a midwife or doula (see below).

Talk to a family member or friend who has successfully breastfed. Ask them about their experience. Could they support you in the hospital or in the early days? You can also attend a community breastfeeding support group while you are pregnant to make important connections. Then, after your baby is born, you'll know who to call if you need a helping hand with breastfeeding.

Labor and delivery health care team

With a hospital birth, the doctor or nurse is usually your first support directly after birth.

Your family doctor or obstetrician. Before your delivery, talk to your doctor about your wish to breastfeed as soon as possible after birth. If your doctor is at the birth, she will give directions to the ward nurses to help you with breastfeeding early. If you have a C-section, the obstetrician can consult with the surgeon and nurses about early skin-to-skin contact (see page 387).

Midwife. A midwife may work independently to deliver your baby, or work alongside your doctor. During labor, midwives are by your side to provide ongoing support. This support helps a woman better manage pain without medications.

Your doctor or public health nurse can recommend a midwife, doula or lactation consultant, or breastfeeding support group where you live.

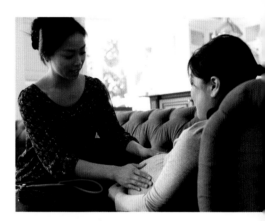

LIFE STAGES

If you have a health plan, see if the cost of a doula is covered. If not, the cost of a doula is generally a lot less than the cost to buy formula for a year.

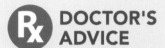

DOCTOR'S ADVICE

If a mom breastfeeds in the first hour after birth, the amount of milk she will make will significantly increase within the first month. This is why immediately after birth, mom and baby should be kept together, except for a medical emergency.

Certified doula. Doulas don't provide medical care or deliver babies but they are trained caregivers to be by your side before, during and after birth, and to help with breastfeeding following an uncomplicated birth. When you go home from hospital, a doula will help with your baby, and care for you so you are rested to breastfeed.

Lactation consultant. This is a specialized breastfeeding professional who is skilled to help all mothers breastfeed, including moms with preterm babies and moms who are having breastfeeding difficulties.

During labor and after delivery

Take minimal or no medications, if possible. Medications taken during labor go directly to your baby. Your baby may be too sleepy from the drugs to latch on after birth. When the baby becomes more alert, they sometimes are overly hungry and crying, which also can affect the first latch. A midwife, doula, nurse or doctor who supports the natural birth process can help you get through labor without medication or with less medication.

Labor medications induce labor or reduce pain during labor. Pain medicines include nitrous oxide and strong narcotics such as morphine or fentanyl. Some medicines are given via spinal or epidural.

Ahead of time, learn about the risks to breastfeeding of taking these. When pain medication is considered essential, there are alternatives that will leave your baby's body sooner and so interfere less with breastfeeding. Ask about these.

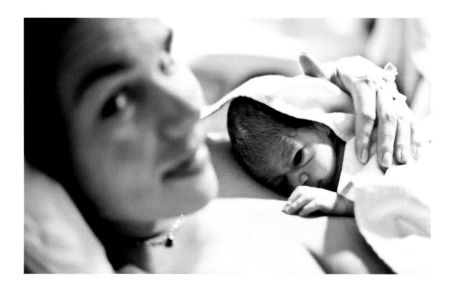

Benefits of early skin-to-skin contact. Skin-to-skin means your baby wears only a diaper and is placed upright on your bare chest. A light blanket can be draped over your baby. It's best to have uninterrupted skin-to-skin contact for at least one hour or longer after birth, including for babies born by C-section and premature babies. Skin-to-skin is so important because it regulates your baby's heart beat, body temperature and blood sugar.

Early breastfeeding helps. During the first uninterrupted hour of early skin-to-skin contact, your milk can start to flow, and your baby may be ready for their first feed. This is when your baby has a strong instinct to suck.

If you or your baby are not well, it's not always in your control to have your baby right away. Once alert, your baby should be put skin-to-skin. Your baby will want to feed, and with the help of the health team, latch-on will be more successful.

If you have a C-section, a regional anesthetic (epidural) is a good choice, if possible, as you will either be fully awake or mildly sedated. You may see your baby being born, and hold your baby skin-to-skin while the surgeon closes your wound, and be able to breastfeed sooner. With a general anesthetic, there will be some delay, but you can breastfeed once you're awake and able to hold your baby, skin-to-skin.

Keep the baby with you during your hospital stay and maintain skin-to-skin contact. Most hospitals allow your baby to stay with you, if your baby is well enough to do so. This helps you know when your baby is hungry and that it's time to try feeding. The more your baby feeds (both during the day and night) and the more skin-to-skin contact you have with your baby, the more milk you make and the more content your baby will be.

Avoid bottles, especially in early days. Sometimes doctors recommend supplemental feeding with formula or expressed breast milk. Your baby sucks differently from a bottle than from your breast. If you offer a bottle in the days and weeks before breastfeeding is well established, this may interfere with success.

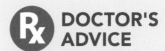

DOCTOR'S ADVICE

More hospitals are implementing practices that place the baby on the mother's chest, skin-to-skin, immediately after a C-section, while you are still in the operating room.

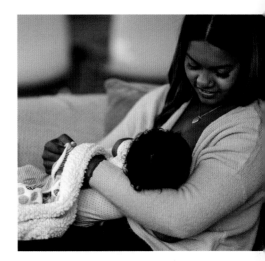

Did you know?
If your baby needs supplemental feeding, a bottle is not the only way to do this. A newborn can feed with a small spoon or cup, or through a tiny tube taped to the mother's breast. If you or your baby are ill, a feeding tube may provide intravenous nutrition.

LIFE STAGES

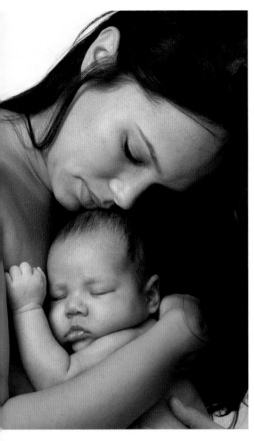

All babies need to be held skin-to-skin.

Bottle-feeding tips for parents

A mother may not have been properly supported to breastfeed, or to pump, by health providers, family and friends. A mother may have to return to work early, and breastfeeding or pumping may not be supported by the work place. Or a mother may be pumping and the baby is being fed human milk exclusively by bottle.

There are rare times when, for health reasons, a woman can't breastfeed. If a woman has had breast surgery for breast cancer or has a condition called insufficient glandular tissue, breastfeeding may be limited and require some supplemental feeding or, in some cases, not be possible. Another example is when certain adult medications can interfere with the health of her baby by passing through the breast milk. In this case, for the woman's personal health and well-being she must take her medications and bottle-feed her baby with donated human milk or formula.

Sometimes, a parent may understand the benefits of breastfeeding but has made an informed decision to bottle-feed.

Once you have decided you are going to bottle-feed your baby, still talk to your public health nurse about:
- Learning to express milk from your breasts if you're able, by hand or using a breast pump. Then your baby can be fed expressed breast milk or formula, or a combination of the two.
- The type and amount of formula you should feed your baby, and how to properly prepare it
- A healthy baby's weight gain

Bottle-feeding time
This is a time for parents and other family members to pay special attention to the baby. Skin-to-skin time is still important. Hold your baby close to your body so your baby feels secure and can see your face. Your baby feels loved when you look at him or her, and learns language when you talk and sing during the feeding. This is bonding time that also boosts your "happy hormones." These are bonding times that will last a lifetime.

⚠️ **CAUTION**
Don't feed your baby canned milk, juices, sugar water, coffee or soft drinks. This is harmful to your baby's growing body and brain.

If You Want Another Baby, Start Planning Early

Once you've had gestational diabetes, you are at risk of getting gestational diabetes again or getting type 2 diabetes after the pregnancy. With more pregnancies, your risk increases. This is because you may be at a higher weight at the beginning of your next pregnancy, and you'll be older.

You can reduce your risk of getting diabetes after your baby is born.

- Continue to eat well after birth, but eat less, so you can gradually lose weight. Try to get back to your pre-pregnancy weight or a lower weight if you are overweight.
- Continue daily walking and other exercise as soon as you recover from the birth or C-section.

Birth control

Discuss birth control with your doctor or public health nurse, and be clear about your wishes. Ask about any side effects and their effectiveness. For more information, search "birth control helpline" on the internet to find a toll-free number. You can talk to someone confidentially by phone.

As a person with diabetes, your birth control options are the same as someone without diabetes. For example, permanent birth control for a man is a vasectomy, and a woman could have her tubes tied. For temporary birth control, a man could use a condom or a woman could use a low-dose hormone pill or patch, IUD, or a diaphragm or cervical cap with spermicidal foam. For unexpected and unwanted pregnancy, discuss your options with your family and your doctor.

> **If you have type 2 diabetes and want to get pregnant:**
> It is best to have a good A1C before you conceive. The first trimester is when the fetus' organs are developing. Good blood sugar in the first trimester and throughout pregnancy reduces your baby's risk of health problems.

> ⚠️ **CAUTION**
> **For women who have reached menopause**
> Two diabetes pills, metformin and pioglitazone, can increase your fertility and you may get pregnant. Talk to your doctor about how long you need to continue birth control.

Birth control if you are breastfeeding

Birth control that contains estrogen is not usually recommended, as it can reduce your milk supply. It's also recommended that progestin-only options be delayed for the first six weeks. The lactational amenorrhea method is a natural birth control method that has high effectiveness under the following circumstances only: you are exclusively breastfeeding (no table foods and no other liquids fed to your baby), you are feeding on demand (during the day and night), your period has not returned and your baby is less than six months old. Talk to your doctor about the best birth control option for you.

To talk to a health practitioner by phone about STI precautions; search "STI hotline" and the area that you live.

For **birth control information**, see previous page.

Sexuality and Diabetes

When you have diabetes, you may notice changes in your body and have concerns about your sexual life.

Learn about sexual changes that may be caused by diabetes on pages 49–50. Read about the benefits of sex and intimacy (pages 391–392) and precautions (below). The rest of this section has seven approaches to help manage sexual changes, with lots of practical information. Most of all, know that as a person with diabetes, you can still enjoy your sexuality.

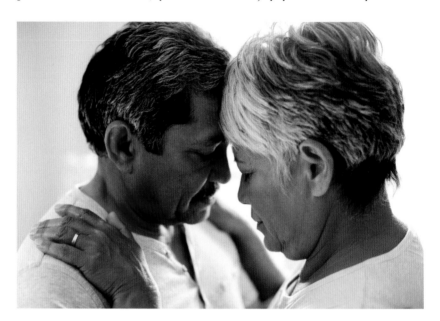

 CAUTION
Protect against Sexually Transmitted Infections

Sexually transmitted infections (STIs) include infections such as herpes from cold sores, HIV and HPV viruses and syphilis. Intimate contact can pass sexual infections between partners.

Always use a condom to protect yourself and your partner, unless you are in a long-term monogamous relationship with no STIs. If you're unsure of your partner's health, ask your partner to be tested and share the test results. Condoms used properly are very effective in stopping the spread of chlamydia and gonorrhoea, but they only partially protect from herpes, genital warts and syphilis, which can spread from infected areas not covered by the condom.

Use a water-based or silicone-based lubricant with a condom. This reduces friction, so the condom is less likely to break during sex. A lubricant also helps keep tissue smooth and reduces the chance of tiny cuts during sex. HIV and other STIs and germs can enter the body through these tiny cuts.

Anal sex has the highest risk of injury and HIV and other infections for the receiving man or woman. Delicate tissues can get cut, even when lubricants are used. If the receiving partner has diabetes neuropathy with reduced feeling, they may not know when to say stop to prevent injury. With diabetes, infections can be serious and medical treatment difficult.

Solutions for Sexual Changes and Diabetes

Lovemaking offers the following benefits:

- It expresses your love and feelings for your partner.
- It increases your circulation.
- It tightens and then relaxes muscles.
- It releases hormones that relax you.
- It can help you sleep.
- It decreases blood sugar, if your session is active or long lasting.

Some gradual sexual changes are a natural part of aging. A woman's sexual response may be slower than when she was younger. A man's penis may not get as firm as quickly as when he was younger. Sex may take longer. This is normal and shouldn't be confused with not being able to have sex. There is still room for pleasure.

Talk with your partner

Today's society bombards us with sexual images, yet sex still remains one of the hardest things to talk about. You are not alone if you find it embarrassing to talk about sex with your partner, even if you've shared a bed for five or fifty years. If you are a man who enjoyed sex in your relationship, and then began to have a slower or softer erection, you may feel uncomfortable about it. Some people decide it's just easier to stop having sex. If you are a woman with dryness or lack of desire, you may turn away from your partner and lose an important part of your relationship. These changes might lead to frustration and even resentment. Consider talking with your partner about what is important to you as individuals and as a couple.

Talk with your doctor

It's worth it to look for solutions if you or your partner struggle with sexual changes. Hopefully, after you read this section, it will be easier to start the conversation. Along with talking to each other, try talking to your doctor or another health professional — this gives them permission to bring up issues of health and sexuality. Please don't suffer in silence.

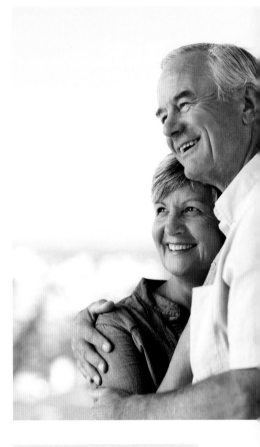

Sexual change isn't easy, but it doesn't mean giving up sexual intimacy.

Good news!
Just because you have diabetes, or are getting older, does not mean you will develop sexual changes. It helps to keep an open mind, do regular exercise, quit smoking or smoke less, and eat well.

LIFE STAGES

The past affects us

How others treated you as a child, teenager or adult affects your sexuality. If there is hurt or abuse in your past, this affects how you feel about yourself and sex. It may be difficult for you to get close to another person through sexual intimacy. You may have had an unhappy sexual relationship in the past, and struggle to be comfortable with sex with a caring person who is now part of your life. As a result, you may not choose sex to be part of your life.

What is consent?

Consent means both partners have agreed to be sexual with each other. It also means that if you want to try something new, ask if your partner also wants to try it. If one partner is silent this does not ensure consent. If you aren't sure, always ask.

Sexuality and sexual intimacy

Much of our sexuality is between our ears, rather than between our legs. Sexuality is how you feel about yourself, your body and your gender. It's the way you express yourself in how you dress, hold yourself and smile. It's the friends you have and the compliments you give each other. Talking, laughing, sharing and touching are all part of sexuality. It's about others appreciating you, for who you are. You may not have a sexual partner, but you are still sexual. This is part of all of us.

Sexual intimacy is something you share with another person. It is the knowledge that you have of how your body, and your partner's body, functions. Pleasure and fun are key — even as you get older and your body changes.

A couple's sexual life can vary like different kinds of car rides. Everyone likes a different kind of ride: fast, slow, smooth or bumpy, frequent, just occasional, or not at all. Some couples have the same or differing sexual appetites.

Some feel sex is a disappointment or chore. Perhaps it's an invigorating and important part of life, especially as you get older and have more time. Many men and women reach their peak sensuality in their forties or fifties and beyond.

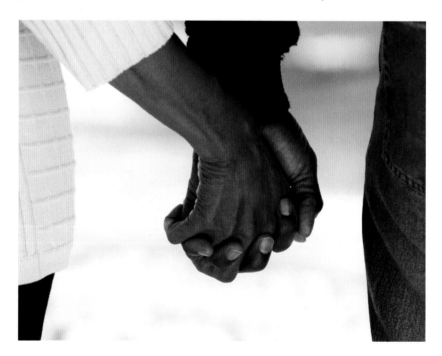

Seven Approaches to Sexual Changes

These seven approaches offer some choices and potential to make your sex life better.

1. Boost Your Circulation and Nerves

- **Improve your blood sugar.** In some cases, this actually reverses some of the damage to your blood vessels and nerves. Then vaginal sensitivity or erectile dysfunction can improve. When your blood sugar is better, you are energized and ready for sex.
- **Keep your blood pressure and blood cholesterol at a good level.** These changes improve the health of your blood vessels, and now more blood flows to the vagina or penis.
- **Try to quit smoking.** If you are a man who smokes, you are more likely to have difficulty with erections than someone who doesn't smoke. This is because smoking narrows your blood vessels. Please think of this as one more important reason to quit.
- **Eat a healthy diet.** Nutrition that is good for your diabetes and heart is also good for the nerves and blood vessels in your sexual organs.
- **Exercise regularly.** Exercise increases the flow of blood and oxygen to your sexual organs. Exercise stimulates your blood vessels to produce nitric oxide, which helps arouse sexual organs.

  When you walk regularly and keep fit, you will have more flexibility and stamina for sex. You may also need less of blood pressure or antidepressant medications. This is good, as they can have side effects (see sidebar).

  Kegel exercises for women (see page 290) and for men (see page 291) strengthen the pelvic floor muscles, which can improve blood flow to the groin. Doing these exercises may later have a role in sexual sensitivity. It may also help with a man's erection.
- **Limit or avoid alcohol.** While the first drink can relax you, the second drink or more can slow or stop a man's erection. Also, if you've drunk too much, receiving or giving consent to have sex, can become unclear.

Schedule a doctor's appointment for a complete physical

- Your doctor can rule out other causes (besides diabetes) for erection changes, vaginal dryness or decreased interest in sex.
- Your doctor may refer you to a urologist or gynecologist, or a sex therapist. You can further discuss sexual concerns with these specialists.
- Ask about going to a diabetes education center. There, you can get advice on how to improve your blood sugar, cholesterol and blood pressure.
- Medications such as some blood pressure pills and anti-depressants can lower interest in sex or affect erections. If you are on these pills, ask if there are other options.
- If you have had a recent heart attack or surgery, talk to your doctor about when it is safe for you to have sex. Generally sex is safe if you can tolerate light to moderate exercise.

2. Self-Fulfillment

Masturbation helps your body make "happy hormones," or endorphins. It can help you relieve tension and sleep better at night. It also helps keep your erectile tissue (in a man's penis or woman's clitoris) elastic and healthy. Some women and men use a lubricant or vibrator (pages 395 and 409), and find this enhances their experience.

- **Women:** Some women say that as they got older they became more comfortable with their own body. They now know what feels good, and what visual stimulation or thoughts they need to orgasm. Masturbating may be more natural.
- **Men:** Erection enhancement medications or devices used by couples, can be used by a man alone to either enhance or enable masturbation. This would include erection pills, vacuum devices, penis rings or local therapies (creams, pellets or injections) used on the penis itself to get or maintain an erection. All of this information is discussed on pages 399–405.

3. Lubricants

If you feel dry during sex or masturbation you may want to consider buying some "personal lubricant." You can buy it at any drugstore in single packets, tubes or small bottles. It can be used by men or women. If you put it on your genitals, it helps them feel slippery, so sexual activity is easier. For women who are dry during sex, using a lubricant can also help reduce the risk of a yeast infection. Apply lubricant with clean hands to prevent bacteria getting into the lubricant, or use single-packet lubricants only.

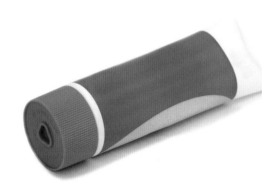

- Start with a water-based lubricant such as K-Y Jelly, Astroglide, Wet or Sliquid, or less expensive generic brands.
- If you find the water-based lubricant dries out too quickly, try a silicone-based lubricant. However, this type is difficult to wash off yourself and your sheets.
- Don't use oil-based creams or Vaseline as a lubricant! These can break a condom. They are also more difficult to wash off.
- Avoid "warming" lubricants or those with flavors or colors which can irritate your skin. Flavored lubricants may also have sugar added. This might make you more likely to get a vaginal or urinary tract infection.

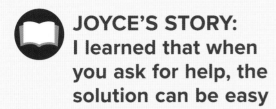

JOYCE'S STORY: I learned that when you ask for help, the solution can be easy

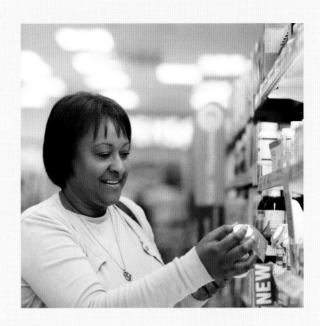

I started having dryness, and intercourse was painful. After a while I started finding reasons not to do it. I knew it was affecting my relationship with my husband and we talked about it, but I didn't know what to do about it. At my next appointment with the diabetes nurse, I decided to talk to her about this.

She asked me if I had ever tried a lubricant. I didn't really even know what this was. She explained that you could buy a little tube for under ten bucks in the pharmacy. She suggested a water-based lubricant. This may seem funny to you, but I had to ask her what do I do with it. She told me that just before intercourse, to squeeze out a blob of lubricant (about the size of the tip of my pinky finger to begin with). Then, to use my fingers to spread it over my clitoris, labia, around my vagina and even a little bit inside my vagina.

I tried it, and you have no idea what a difference this made. It removed the dryness, and sex was comfortable again. When I think back, the solution was simple, and yet it took me so long to discover it.

Vaginal moisturizers

Vaginal moisturizers are not the same thing as lubricants. This is a product used by women to keep their vagina feeling moist for several days in a row. It's a good idea to try lubricants first. Then, if you are still having pain with vaginal dryness, you could try a vaginal moisturizer. Common brands are Replens, Gyne-Moistrin, Hylafem and K-Y Liquibeads.

You use an applicator to insert the moisturizer up into your vagina. Usually you put it in every day for a week, and then two to three a week for ongoing moisturizing. Some of them can cause a harmless white discharge to later leak out of your vagina.

Vaginal estrogen creams
These are prescription only and are discussed on page 402.

LIFE STAGES

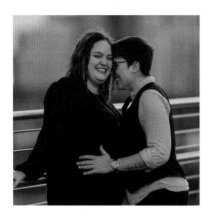

Improve your sexual relationship through good communication. Talk about what's important to you.

Sex is as individual as each of our personalities. Remember, good communication is essential to building intimacy.

4. Build Intimacy

Nurture your relationship. Celebrate each other. Eat meals together so you have time to talk. Help each other with household chores.

Every day, do something with your partner, even if it is something small. Give each other compliments. Say thank-you. Go for a walk together. Hold hands. A touch, kiss and hug are good too. Be gentle and kind. Make your partner feel good, and you will feel good too.

Plan a regular date night — and stick to it. Watch a movie or enjoy a meal, just the two of you. Read old love letters. You're never too old for romance.

In your relationship with your partner, focus on each other as individuals with unique feelings. You each have your own bodies — bodies that aren't perfect, but that can be sensual and sexy. No matter your size or shape, what makes you sexy is what is inside — your desire to give and receive.

When you nurture each other, then you will be more comfortable talking about and considering new approaches to managing sexual changes.

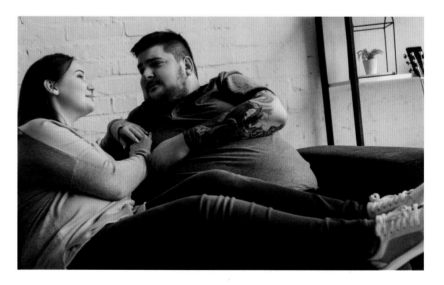

Set the mood. If you'd like tonight to be the night, then build it up a bit that day. Give your partner a call or send a romantic text to see if the interest is mutual. If you have nicknames or code words for intimacy, use those.

Prepare your room for what appeals to your sense of sight and smell. Turn down the lights or leave one on. Use a battery-operated candle or scent that your partner loves. Play music to get in the mood.

Prepare yourself. Take a shower. Put on the sexy clothes. All of us can be turned on by what we see.

Invest in foreplay. Go for lots of sensual foreplay with passionate all-body kissing and touching, to get you in the mood.

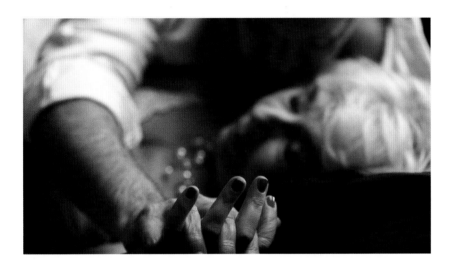

Helpful tips prior to sexual activity

- Be well rested.
- Relax. Try not to think about your worries.
- Don't drink excess alcohol.
- Don't eat a heavy meal.
- Choose a room that is comfortable, not cold or hot.
- Men, you may find erections are more likely at certain times of the day or evening. This will depend on when you take your pills, and how you and your partner feel.

5. Accommodate Your Special Needs

You may have aches and pains or you may have a disability. Small changes in your sexual pattern can enhance or bring back sex and intimacy into your life.

A short session or a long one?

Sometimes you may be up for a short session. Maybe only one of you needs relief at that moment. It's okay to make it a quickie and move on. Other times it's nice to stretch out lovemaking when you have time. Don't always leave sex until later. At bedtime, you may have no energy left.

Comfortable positions

Do you have arthritis, back pain or a disability that makes sexual activity difficult or painful? Sometimes a simple change like a pillow to support your back, or a pillow under a woman's hips, can make a difference. Discuss different positions with your partner. Just talking about this can build excitement and intimacy.

For men with a sore back, it may also help to use a hip-hinging motion rather than thrusting. With a hip hinge you push your bottom back and come in, rather than thrusting from the same position.

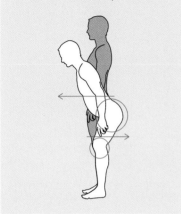

Here are some ideas for more comfortable positioning.

While these positions are for a man and a woman, you can adapt them if you are a same-sex couple.

- *If a woman's back, knees or hips hurt:* If lying on your back, place a small pillow beneath your lower back or a wedge pillow behind your knees for support. To take pressure off hips, your partner on top can put his legs outside your legs. Placing a pillow under your buttocks can be helpful if both of you are large.

- *If a man's hips or knees hurt (or he is quite large):* Try sex with your partner on top; then you don't have to support your own weight. And try the missionary position, where you are on top, but you support your weight with your elbows, not your hands.

- *If you both have sore knees:* Try standing. The woman can lean on a high bed for support (to take weight off her knees) and the man enters from behind. This position can work for some larger couples. And try lying in spoon position (man behind woman, with his chest to her back, with both of you facing the same direction); a pillow between your knees can help too.

- *Books or videos on sex* can give you sex position and lovemaking ideas. Look for resources that present sexual options for adult couples in a respectful way for both of you. Just because you see it on the internet, don't feel pressured to use anything or do anything with which you are not comfortable.

If fatigue, pain or reduced erection hardness makes intercourse too strenuous or difficult, you may want to consider other options. (See pages 406–409.)

Do you worry about a low blood sugar episode during sex? Check your blood sugar level before sex. Have glucose tablets on your bedside table.

Do you have a fear of urinary incontinence during sexual activity?

It helps to empty your bladder and shower just before sexual activity. Taking other steps long before intercourse also helps. Drink water to keep your urine clear, pee regularly, and limit coffee, tea, alcohol and smoking. This helps reduce bladder irritation, so you are less likely to have leakage. If odor is a concern, try a product like Vagisil. Constipation can contribute to incontinence, so exercise daily, eat lots of fiber and drink water. Doing Kegel exercises regularly (see page 290 and 291) is important to keep your pelvic muscles strong.

If you have a physical disability such as a spinal cord injury or are fully dependent on a wheelchair, search for "DHRN sex manual" on the internet.

6. Medications and Erection Devices

If getting or maintaining an erection is a concern, talk to your doctor. Your doctor may suggest and prescribe either medications or erection devices, or both. This section explains these and how they work. In some cases your doctor may refer you to a urologist.

Doctors most commonly recommend erection drugs, such as Viagra and other similar drugs, called phosphodiesterase type 5 inhibitors, or PDE5s. If these aren't well tolerated, there are other erection drugs. If your hormones are low, the doctor may recommend taking testosterone for men or estrogen for women. Rather than medications, your doctor might recommend a penis pump. This is a device shaped like a cylinder, which creates a vacuum to make the penis go hard.

> Medications and devices are important options, but it's important to remember that they are not a cure. You still need to take care of your health so that the erectile dysfunction doesn't get worse.

℞ DOCTOR'S ADVICE

Medications and devices have varying levels of effectiveness and safety. If one option isn't appropriate for you because of your health or other medications you are taking, your doctor will likely suggest something else. If you try a treatment and it doesn't work, your doctor can recommend another option. It's important to know how to take a medication and how much, and how to safely use an erection device. All treatments have both benefits and side effects.

Herbal products or other over-the counter products

Before Viagra and the other PDE5s were available, doctors or herbalists sometimes prescribed the herb yohimbine hydrochloride or epimedium to help with erections. Today, doctors prescribe PDE5s, as as they are much more effective.

The variety of erection herbs and drugs sold over-the-counter and on the internet may have risks. These drug advertisements and lower prices may be tempting, but beware. Some of these products have been found to have no medication, while others have a dangerous amount of medication or additives.

Please talk to your pharmacist first.

⚠ CAUTION

Beware! It can be risky to buy any medication through unsolicited emails. If you order online, only use reputable pharmacies.

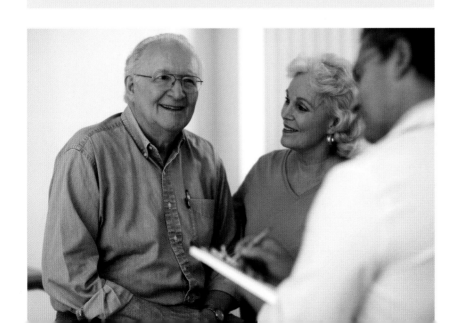

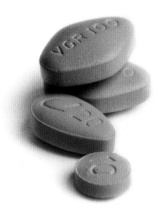

Talk to your doctor about which PDE5 to use and the correct starting dose. If one type of PDE5 does not work for you, your doctor may recommend you try one of the others.

⚠ **CAUTION**
Doctors don't prescribe Viagra or the other PDE5 inhibitors if you take nitroglycerine. They also may not recommend them if you have:

- Decreased liver or kidney function
- Very low or high blood pressure
- Recently had a heart attack or stroke, or other heart conditions
- Certain eye disorders

It's wise to learn about the risks as well as the highly advertised benefits.

Talk to your doctor.

Viagra and other PDE5 inhibitors for men

These pills help fill the penis with blood. They will not increase your sex drive, per se. To make this kind of drug work, you need to combine it with foreplay or visual stimulation, so you will feel excited and get hard.

Phosphodiesterase type 5 inhibitors, or PDE5s, include:

- sildenafil (Viagra)
- vardenafil (Levitra)
- avanafil (Stendra)
- tadalafil (Cialis)

Sildenafil, vardenafil and avanafil work for four to six hours. Tadalafil (Cialis) lasts in your system for up to 36 hours, which means you could consider having sex anytime over the next one to two days. Whichever PDE5 drug you use, wait about one hour after taking it before you have sex. Never take more than one pill in 24 hours.

If you eat a high-fat meal, it affects your body's ability to absorb short-acting PDE5s including Viagra, Levitra and Stendra. **Take it on an empty stomach.** Drink a glass of water to keep hydrated. What you eat does not affect Cialis.

Some people wonder if drinking alcohol affects how these pills work. You can drink alcohol with these pills, but drinking too much alcohol affects everyone's sexual abilities. Avoid alcohol or limit to one drink.

If you use PDE5s regularly, it can get costly. They are not covered under most drug plans. Generics (non-brand names) are often cheaper.

Although PDE5s are a great option for many men with diabetes, they may not be right for you. Talk to your doctor.

Side effects of PDE5 inhibitors

After taking one of these pills, you may get a headache, stuffy nose, flushed face, mild vision changes or indigestion. If this happens, tell your doctor. He may reduce your dosage or suggest you try a different PDE5 or try another drug or device. Although it rarely happens, if your erection lasts longer than four hours, see your doctor right away (or go to an emergency department). If you experience vision or hearing loss, which is also very rare, stop using the pills, and see a doctor right away.

Applying erection drugs on or in the penis

Alprostadil is a prescription erection drug that contains a natural compound called prostaglandin EI. This drug can boost blood flow into the penis. It can be delivered in three ways: (1) injected into the penis (ICI), (2) put into the end of the penis as a small pill (MUSE), or (3) dispensed on the head of the penis as a cream (Vitaros).

ICI penis injection

The medical name for this is intracavernosal injection or ICI. Alprostadil (prostaglandin) often works better in combination with another two drugs, papaverine and phentolamine, in a trimix (or "Triple P"). Another combination is a bimix and it doesn't have the alprostadil. You inject the drug(s) into the side of your penis. You give the injection about 10 minutes before intercourse or masturbation. It can last up to an hour. These drugs create an erection by increasing the blood flow to the penis. They work best when you are relaxed, aroused and stimulated. This isn't effective for all men with diabetes. Yet some men find ICI produces a more firm erection than PDE5 inhibitors.

MUSE penis pill

MUSE is short for "medical urethral system for erection." You gently put a tiny pellet that contains a small dose of alprostadil in the end of your penis. This is done about 10 minutes before intercourse. It stimulates an erection, but is not as effective as ICI in men with diabetes, and is expensive. However, if you don't like the idea of using an injection, this might be worth a try.

Vitaros penis cream

This is an alprostadil cream that you drip into your urethral opening and rub on the head of your penis. It is quickly absorbed and can work in five minutes. This application is a good option for men without severe erectile dysfunction.

Side effects of alprostadil

Alprostadil can cause aching in the penis for some men. If this is happens, bimix (which doesn't have alprostadil) might be an alternative. If you give yourself an ICI injection regularly, there is a small risk of scarring at the injection site. In an occasional case, your erection may stay hard and hurt. If that happens, try ejaculating or an ice pack to reduce the erection. Although it rarely happens, if your erection lasts longer than four hours, see your doctor right away (or go to an emergency department). This problem can be prevented with proper technique and dose of medication. Discuss this with your doctor ahead of time.

Work together with your partner when using an erection medication or device. Before you buy or use an erection medication or erection device, talk to your partner. If you think you might be interested in trying one of these, go together to see your doctor or urologist to learn more about them. This may help you feel more comfortable talking about it with each other.

To increase togetherness and fun, incorporate the erection medication or device into your sexual experience with your partner. For example, your partner can place the pill or vacuum pump (see page 404) on your bedside table as a seductive suggestion. As part of your sexual foreplay, your partner might do the ICI injection for you, or help you pump up your penis. This involvement can enhance sexual desire and intimacy.

Hormones for men or women

If your blood tests show a hormonal imbalance, your doctor may recommend and prescribe hormones such as testosterone or estrogen.

Taking testosterone may not improve your erection, but it usually improves your sexual desire and energy.

Testosterone: Both men and women have testosterone in their bodies, but men have a much larger amount. Men typically have a steady decrease in their testosterone levels as a natural part of aging. Men with diabetes are more likely to have low testosterone levels. Bringing the testosterone level back to a normal level can help a man have more interest in sex. This helps him ejaculate or reach orgasm easier. It may not help erections. In addition, for erections, men usually need to take PDE5 pills or use an erection device. The PDE5s work better with a normal level of testosterone. A doctor will assess your health, and may prescribe testosterone as a pill, a gel or cream, or by injection.

Like all treatments, testosterone can be associated with certain risks. It can stimulate the growth of the prostate, and it can cause an increase in red blood cells, which makes blood thicker and more likely to cause a stroke or heart attack. These risks can be reduced when health care providers monitor blood work and adjust the doses carefully.

Estrogen can increase blood sugar. Women often find they have blood sugar swings during their period. Their blood sugar usually increases before and during menstruation. When estrogen levels change during menopause, this also causes blood sugar swings.

Estrogen: Both women and men have estrogen in their bodies, but women have a much larger amount. As a woman gets older, estrogen continues to have benefits, including keeping her bones strong. Estrogen helps with natural vaginal lubrication and comfort. Estrogen decreases in women after menopause. To enhance a woman's sex drive or decrease vaginal dryness, a doctor may prescribe estrogen. This can be prescribed as a pill, a skin gel that you rub on your arm or a patch to stick on your skin. Alternately, an estrogen cream can be put around the vagina, or a tablet, cream or ring containing estrogen can be placed inside the vagina.

While estrogen has many benefits, doctors may suggest post-menopausal women avoid taking it. Estrogen may increase the risk for breast cancer, heart disease and stroke. It also increases blood sugar. However, in many cases, the benefits of taking estrogen may be greater than the risks. Fortunately, lower doses of hormones (both estrogen and testosterone) carry less risk. Low doses still have benefits.

Please discuss the pros and cons of taking hormones with your doctor.

Penis rings and vacuum pumps

When used properly, a penis ring or vacuum pump can be a good nonmedicinal option for men with varying degrees of erectile dysfunction. You can buy them without a prescription. But beware, there are many poor quality products sold online. So you don't harm your penis, buy good quality products and *always follow the manufacturer's directions.*

Penis rings

If you get an erection but can't hold it as long as you'd like, a penis ring is an inexpensive, effective option for you. It's a special rubber ring that you can stretch and place at the base of your penis once you start getting hard. Some find that a little lubrication at the base of the penis, or on the ring, eases the ring on. The ring then helps keep you firm. *Don't leave the ring on longer than 30 minutes.*

Some men with poor hand strength buy a device especially designed to help them put on the penis ring. Or they use a hard plastic pipe fitting from a hardware store called a "coupling" (that looks like a napkin ring) and comes in different sizes. It should fit over your erection but not be too big — so you can stretch the ring over it. Slip the device with the attached ring over your penis as far as it will go. Then carefully slide the ring off the pipe to the base of your penis.

> ⚠️ **CAUTION**
> If you have a bleeding condition or are on blood thinners such as Warfarin, penis rings and pumps can increase your risk of bruising.

> ⚠️ **CAUTION**
> Use common sense! Remove a penis ring that is hurting, or so tight it is causing the penis to swell or go cold.
> Never use a rubber band as a penis ring; this could cause serious harm.

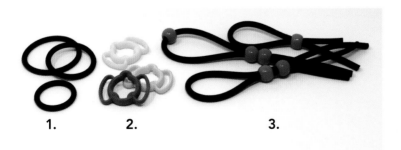

1.   2.   3.

1. **Rubber penis rings** come in different sizes. It's best to start with a larger size and move to smaller if needed. Two can be used with the smaller one closest to the base of the penis.
2. **Rubber penis rings (three sizes).** Use the "wings" to stretch the ring open so you can gently slide it over the penis to the base.
3. This ring can be adjusted for the right tension using the **toggle-hold.** One can be on the penis and the other around the scrotum. However, the single ring may work better, as the scrotum ring may make you take longer to ejaculate.

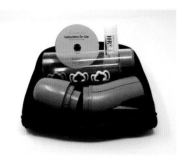

A penis vacuum pump

A vacuum pump is an option for men who are unable to get an erection. It is also an alternative for men with erectile dysfunction who don't want to take erection medications.

This uses a specially designed pump *and* a penis ring. The vacuum pump is a hard plastic tube (or cylinder). You manually pump out the air around your penis. This creates a vacuum. The ring will hold the erection. If your hand strength is poor, consider buying a pump that is battery-operated. Using the pump takes a bit of practice, but can be an effective solution with few side effects.

Hinge effect

The vacuum pump helps the small tubes in the outer part of your penis become erect, but not the inner tubes of your penis that attach to your pelvic bone (so there is no strut, or brace, for the erection). This means the erection you get with a vacuum device and held by a ring, may pivot at the base (this action is called the "hinge effect"). During sex, some men find it helpful to adjust their angle to avoid slipping out of their partner, especially for missionary position. Some heterosexual couples who use the pump find that the female-on-top position works well.

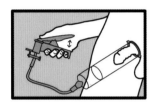

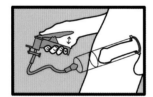

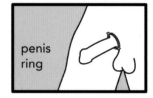

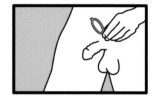

Step 1. Place sterile lubricant on the base of your penis to allow for a good seal. Then, place the plastic tube around your penis.

Step 2. Using a stop-and-go action, pump out the air around your penis using the handheld pump. This creates a vacuum and helps draw blood into your penis. An erection will usually be created within a few minutes, but could take 10 minutes.

Step 3. There is a penis ring attached to the base of the plastic tube. Once your penis enlarges, you slip the ring off the tube and over the base of your penis. This holds the erection. Then you remove the plastic tube. If you use a condom, have it ready. Put it on at this time.

Step 4. After sex, you remove the penis ring and the erection will go down. The ring should not be left on longer than 30 minutes.

(You can watch an instructional video online at youtube.com search "Osbon ErecAid.")

Where to get a pump

If you feel comfortable, ask your doctor or urologist to recommend a brand of vacuum pump or penis ring. The doctor, or doctor's nurse, can explain how to use them.

Where to buy a pump: (1) at a medical supply store, (2) at a pharmacy, by special order, or (3) at an online store such as Amazon.com, or brand-name suppliers' own online stores. A top-of-the line quality pump is about $500 from Osbon, and lower-cost acceptable versions are available from Encore or Augusta for $150 to $250. The penis rings bought on their own usually cost under $20. Some drug plans cover these costs. After a year or two, the one-time cost of a vacuum pump is for many people a cheaper option than erection medications that cost $10 or more for **each time.**

RON'S STORY: Sexual changes can be challenging — find something that works for you

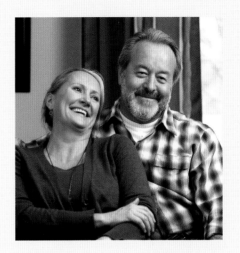

My wife and I have enjoyed a loving sex life. But about a year ago I noticed changes. I couldn't get as hard as I used to or I'd lose it quickly. I thought this was just because I was getting older. Then I was reading that diabetes could cause this, and I have had diabetes for 15 years.

We tried Viagra, but it gave me headaches. I didn't want to take any more medications. We looked into other options and decided to order a vacuum erection device (a pump).

We laughed when we got the pump, as it was kind of bigger than we expected! The instructions said that if you haven't had erections for a while, that it is important to take your time learning to use the pump. The first time I used it, I pumped slowly, and released the vacuum, and pumped slowly again, and repeated this a few times over 10 minutes. I felt a pulling, but I didn't get an erection. I felt disappointed, but then I realized that it wasn't going to work the first time. So, like the instructions said, over the next two weeks I practiced on my own. After about a week of practice, I was able to get an erection. I held the pump on and kept my erection for about a minute, then released the vacuum, and repeated it once or twice. Soon I felt comfortable to pump at the right speed and pressure to create an erection. The second week I also practiced a couple of times, putting the ring on to keep the erection. Now I can get an erection in about two to three minutes using the pump.

Then it was time to try it together! I got ready for bed, then I pumped myself erect and slipped on the ring to keep me erect. I came to bed and we started with foreplay. When we were ready, my wife went on top and we got it to work! My wife did mention that my penis felt less warm than normal, but otherwise she said I felt hard — and we had fun again.

That was about six months ago. Now that we're intimate again, I feel happier and I have a reason to be healthy and fit, so I've started walking more. I'm even thinking about quitting smoking. Now that my wife and I have tried this, we both feel more open to talk about these things. Sometimes we can have intercourse using just the penis ring, without the pump, but more often we need them both. The vacuum pump is probably not for everyone, but it's worked for us.

Penis implants surgery

Surgically placing inflatable rods into the penis would be the last resort for the treatment of advanced erectile dysfunction. This is surgery done by a specialized urologist who is a surgeon. After the surgery, a man can get an erection by squeezing a pump that the urologist implants in the scrotum. Fluid then flows from a small implanted reservoir into two silicone rods implanted in the penis. With this surgery, a man can have sex spontaneously, without planning as you need to do with the PDE5s.

For more information about this surgery, search "penis implants" online.

LIFE STAGES

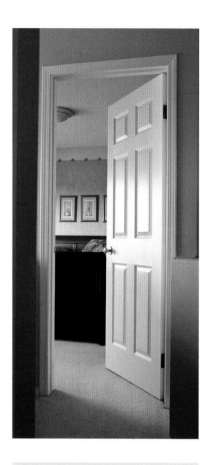

Healthy sexuality means not focusing on specific acts. Instead, focus on giving each other pleasure and having fun.

Never try to force or coerce a sexual partner. Sexual activities should be comfortable for you both.

7. Other Options

For some couples, pills or devices aren't effective or are medically unsafe or too expensive. Maybe pills or devices just aren't the right fit for them. The couple may have physical limitations to intercourse, or the male partner may be unable to have or maintain a hard erection. Therefore, you may be looking for alternatives to intercourse.

Perhaps you would consider new ways of lovemaking? It's okay if you feel embarrassed about it. Don't let this stop you from trying to make each other feel good. Your sex life doesn't have to end. In the past, your sex may have included foreplay, followed by intercourse. Now, consider having more touch and foreplay, with or without the penetration. A massage could lead to one of you masturbating (or both of you together), or one of you helping the other.

Pleasuring a woman with vaginal dryness, decreased sensation or desire

It's exciting to see your partner aroused. If you are not sure what feels arousing for your wife or partner, then ask her what she enjoys and what she'd like. Don't assume you know everything about what feels good for her. Even if you've been married for 40 years, it's never too late to ask! Remember, people change over time, and there's likely still something you don't know about your partner.

For many women, gentle lips, hands, and kind and encouraging words make you a great lover. Say words that you can think of that means she is beautiful and sexy. She needs to hear this, over and over. She needs to know you want her. She needs you to communicate with her so you know she wants to be touched in her special places.

Kiss and touch her — perhaps her neck, back, earlobes, lips, fingertips, nipples and vagina area. Keep asking her, "Where does it feel good?" Her clitoris is tiny compared to a penis, but you might be surprised to know it has all the same parts — a covering like a foreskin, a shaft and a head. Save touching her sensitive clitoris for last. Ask her to tell you if she needs lubrication, or wants less or more touch.

Women can have orgasms from direct genital stimulation without intercourse. For men who don't want to attempt penetration due to erection difficulties, it may be stimulating for you both to try something else. Ask her if she would like you to enter her slowly with your finger or a vibrator, or to give her oral sex. Bringing your partner to orgasm can be exciting for you too. Women do not have orgasms every time they have sexual intimacy with their partner, but they can still enjoy being intimate.

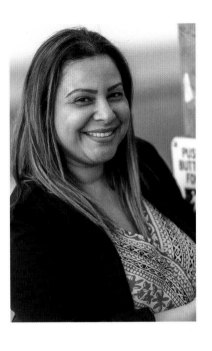

For women with a Urinary Tract Infection

When you have a urinary tract infection (a UTI), you need to take care of yourself. Hold off on sex until your infection has healed.

To prevent UTIs

Showering — together or separately — is a good way to start a lovemaking session. This helps you relax and leaves you fresh and clean. It's important that the woman's genitals are well lubricated. Without lubrication, friction causes tiny cuts and can lead to a yeast infection. Both partners need to avoid spreading germs, especially from the anus area.

If your partner has a mouth infection related to their diabetes (or other cause), then this is not the time for mouth-genital contact.

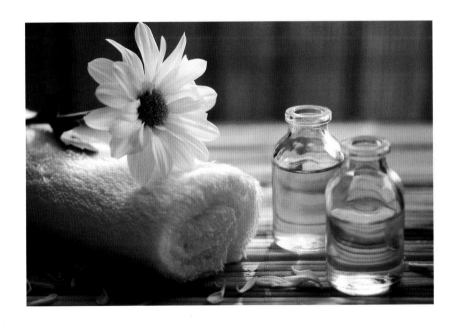

For more information on preventing UTIs, see pages 290–291. For information on sexually transmitted infections, see page 390.

Pleasuring a man with erectile dysfunction or decreased desire

When you care about your partner and relationship, and want intimacy, it's sometimes helpful to take a more active role sexually. One of the things that may turn on a man the most is seeing you excited. If you tend to let him take charge, then think about a change.

Intimate touch is a very personal thing. What is comfortable for one person may not feel comfortable and safe for you. Staying close with the one you care for is important, so help each other discover your way together.

He needs to know you want him. Ask him what feels good and to show you. Talk together about what is comfortable for you both. Trying new things in the bedroom can be intimidating, and feel awkward, but over time, it becomes more comfortable. Giving pleasure to him using your hands or with your mouth is something to consider. Oral sex is so stimulating that some men can experience an orgasm without an erection, although it may be less intense. For protection against infections, or if you aren't comfortable with this very intimate contact, a man can wear a condom.

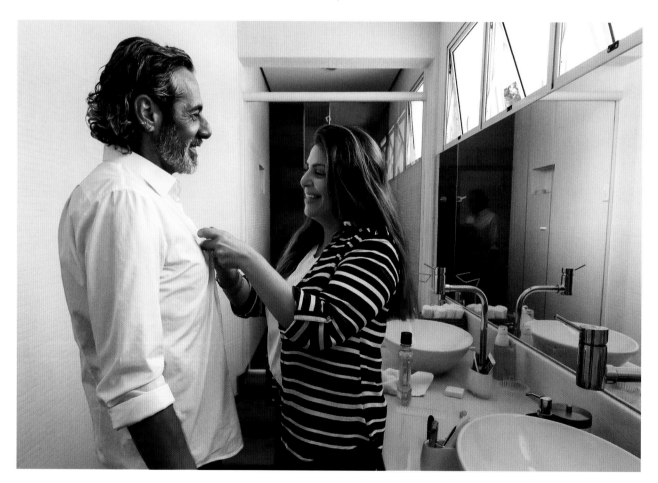

Intimacy products

Do you like to use something for fun in your bedroom — such as a tie, lingerie, romantic lighting or massage oil? Then, you are already using a type of adult toy! At some point you may be curious to experiment with other sex toys for men and women, such as a vibrator. These toys are best used with a water-based lubricant. With a little humor and adventure, one of these toys could become a part of your sexual life. These are sold at online stores like Amazon or at adult sex shops.

If this is new, you might feel uncomfortable with having or using a sex toy. These are normal concerns, but if you're facing other health challenges, these could be ways to still have fun and sexual intimacy. If your energy level is low, these can help you make love for longer. If you have a sore back or knees, these may allow for pleasure without stressing your joints. If you or your partner has full erectile dysfunction, you may be bold and consider a strap-on dildo, search "strap ons for ED." This product helps you enjoy the pleasure of natural and familiar hip movements of intercourse, without stress and worry about erections.

Always ensure sex toys such as a vibrator or dildo are are in good condition and clean before each use.

To avoid causing injury or irritating tender tissues, don't insert a sex toy too deeply. Don't use it roughly or too frequently. Use a lubricant. A woman with diabetes may have reduced feeling in her vagina due to neuropathy. Be careful to avoid injury.

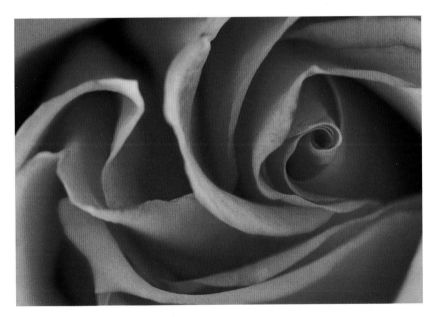

Diabetes brings some changes.

Some will be about having different sexual experiences. Some will be about learning to eat healthier. But all changes will help you take better care of your body so you'll live a happier life.

Diabetes Glossary

A1C: A blood test that measures your average blood sugar over the past three months.

ABCs: Three important diabetes blood tests: A1C, Blood pressure and blood Cholesterol.

ace inhibitors: A type of recommended blood pressure pill for people with diabetes.

albumin creatinine ratio (ACR): A urine test that measures the amount of albumin (a type of protein) in your blood; a sign of kidney damage.

alpha-glucosidase inhibitors: These pills slow carbohydrate absorption from the intestine and so can reduce blood sugar after a meal.

ARBs: Recommended blood pressure pills for people with diabetes (drug names end in "sartan," as in valsartan).

atherosclerosis: Hardening and narrowing of blood vessels.

basal insulin (background insulin): These are long or intermediate insulins that work in your body over a longer period of time.

blood sugar trends: Looking at blood sugar numbers over several days to try to understand underlying causes of high or low blood sugar readings. Some apps identify trends from your readings.

carbohydrates: Starches, natural sugar from fruits, vegetables and milk, and table sugars.

CGM: See continuous glucose monitoring.

continuous glucose monitoring (CGM): Using a computerized device that attaches to your skin, this monitor reads your blood sugar on a continuous basis and sends the information to a computer or your phone.

diabetes apps: A large variety of phone apps are available, from apps that list calories and carbohydrates to apps that can be used to analyze detailed blood sugar results from blood glucose meters or CGM.

dialysis: A machine that works like a kidney to filter and clean your blood.

dilated eye exam: A special test done by an optometrist or ophthalmologist to make your pupil get larger so the back of your eye can be examined.

DPP-4 inhibitors: A type of diabetes pills that increase intestinal hormones that lower blood sugar.

erectile dysfunction: For a man, difficulty getting hard or maintaining an erection.

gastroparesis: Nerve and blood vessel damage in your gut that causes poor digestion.

gestational diabetes: Diabetes that develops during pregnancy.

GI: See glycemic index.

GLP-1s: This diabetes medication is injected. It has a similar action to the DPP-4s, but in the injected form is more powerful at lowering blood sugar.

glitazones: See TZDs

glomerulus: Part of the kidney that helps filter and clean your blood.

glycemic index (GI): A rating of how quickly a carbohydrate food raises your blood sugar.

gum disease: A serious bacterial infection of your gums and jaw bone.

hypoglycemic unawareness: This is a condition that can occur when someone has had repeated low blood sugars over a period of time. After a while they don't have normal low blood sugar symptoms.

infection: A growth of disease-causing germs in your body or on your skin.

inflammation: Swelling and redness of your tissues.

inhaled insulin: Insulin is in an inhaler, like an asthma inhaler, and you breath the insulin in through your lungs.

insulin: A hormone made by your pancreas that moves sugar from your blood to your brain, muscles, tissues and organs.

insulin pen: A device shaped like a pen that is used to inject insulin.

insulin pump: A computerized device that stores insulin and has a small tube that is attached to the skin through which insulin goes into the body.

insulin receptor: These are areas on your body cells inside your body that allow insulin to work properly.

insulin regimen: This describes different patterns of taking insulin, for example, a different number of injections each day, and mixing basal and mealtime insulin.

insulin resistance: This means that the receptors on your body cells are blocked and cannot remove sugar from your bloodstream. It is associated with higher levels of insulin in your blood and weight gain.

insulin secretagogues: These diabetes pills stimulate your pancreas to make more insulin.

low blood sugar: When your blood sugar is under 70 mg/dL (4 mmol/L).

low-calorie sweeteners: Products that taste sweet but are not sugar. They have few calories.

macroalbuminuria: Advanced kidney damage with loss of large amounts of protein (albumin) in your urine.

mealtime insulin: These are short-acting or rapid-acting insulins that work in your body over a short period of time and help bring down blood sugar after a person eats.

metformin: The most common and often the first diabetes pills prescribed for type 2 diabetes. This pill helps to stop or reduce the release of sugar stored in the liver.

microalbuminuria: Early kidney damage with loss of small amounts of protein (albumin) in your urine.

nephron: Part of the kidney that helps filter and clean your blood.

neuropathy: Nerve damage that can cause a variety of problems such as skin pain or numbness, particularly in your feet.

non-proliferative retinopathy: Early diabetes eye damage.

pancreas: The organ in your body, behind your stomach, that makes insulin.

prediabetes: Your blood sugar levels are higher than normal but lower than what is diagnosed as true diabetes.

proliferative retinopathy: Advanced diabetes eye damage.

retinopathy: Diabetes eye damage to the back of the eye.

SGLT2 inhibitors: These diabetes pills increase the loss of sugar from the urine, which lowers blood sugar.

statins: A type of pill that helps lower cholesterol.

type 1 diabetes: This is generally diagnosed in children or teenagers. People with type 1 diabetes must take insulin, as their pancreas does not make insulin.

type 2 diabetes: This type of diabetes most often occurs in adults and is related to being overweight, physically inactive and family genetics.

TZDs: A diabetes pill that helps insulin work better.

ulcer: An open wound (sore) with severe skin breakdown.

urinary tract infection (UTI): Infection that affects the kidney, bladder or urethra (urine tube).

Index

Library and Archives Canada Cataloguing in Publication
Title: Complete diabetes guide : advice for managing type 2 diabetes / Karen Graham, RD, CDE, Registered
    Dietitian & Certified Diabetes Educator, Mansur Shomali, MD, CM, endocrinologist & diabetes expert.
Other titles: Complete diabetes guide for type 2 diabetes
Names: Graham, Karen, author. | Shomali, Mansur, author.
Description: Second edition. | Series statement: Health & wellness series | Previously published under title:
    The complete diabetes guide for type 2 diabetes. Toronto, Ontario : Robert Rose, ©2013.
Identifiers: Canadiana 20200203231 | ISBN 9780778806530 (softcover)
Subjects: LCSH: Diabetes—Popular works.
Classification: LCC RC662.18 .G73 2020 | DDC 616.4/624—dc23

Other Books in This Health & Wellness Series

Diabetes Essentials
TIPS & RECIPES TO MANAGE TYPE 2 DIABETES

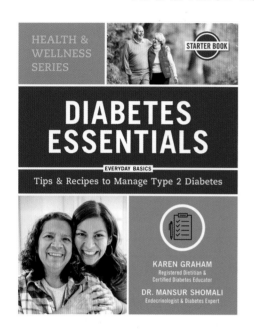

When you are first diagnosed, or even if you have had diabetes for a while, it can be overwhelming. This book is a perfect place to start. These pages give you easy things you can do right away. For example, discover 10 ways to bring down a morning high blood sugar or 10 steps to manage your stress. There are 10 easy meal plans, and 10 recipes each of soups, salads, dinners, desserts and snacks. At the end of the book, there are 10-question quizzes on topics such as weight loss, diabetes and relationships, and a diabetes health quiz.

Diabetes Essentials is the first book in the *Health & Wellness Series*.

The Diabetes Meals for Good Health Cookbook
COMPLETE MEAL PLANS & 100 RECIPES

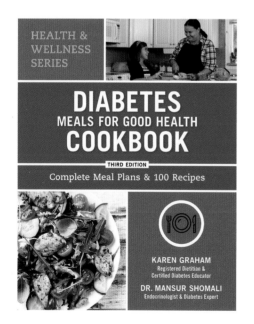

Easy-to-follow meal planning format with life-size photographs of complete meals. There are 100 delicious recipes made with everyday ingredients. This bestselling cookbook, now fully revised and updated, will help you choose a meal plan that's right for you. This third edition also includes carbohydrate counts. If you have type 1 or type 2 diabetes and are adjusting your insulin or carefully controlling portions, you can use this information to individualize your intake. Handy food charts help you learn about sensible portion sizes.

The Diabetes Meal for Good Health Cookbook is the second book in the *Health & Wellness Series*.